Secrets of
Seduction
for Women

Brenda Venus

Secrets of Seduction for Women

A DUTTON BOOK

DUTTON
Published by the Penguin Group
Penguin Books USA Inc., 375 Hudson Street,
New York, New York 10014, U.S.A.
Penguin Books Ltd, 27 Wrights Lane,
London W8 5TZ, England
Penguin Books Australia Ltd, Ringwood, Victoria, Australia
Penguin Books Canada Ltd, 10 Alcorn Avenue,
Toronto, Ontario, Canada M4V 3B2
Penguin Books (N.Z.) Ltd, 182–190 Wairau Road,
Auckland 10, New Zealand

Penguin Books Ltd, Registered Offices:
Harmondsworth, Middlesex, England

First published by Dutton, an imprint of Dutton Signet,
a division of Penguin Books USA Inc.
Distributed in Canada by McClelland & Stewart Inc.

First Printing, February, 1996
10 9 8 7 6 5 4 3 2 1

 REGISTERED TRADEMARK—MARCA REGISTRADA

LIBRARY OF CONGRESS CATALOGING-IN-PUBLICATION DATA
Venus, Brenda.
Secrets of seduction for women / Brenda Venus.
p.   cm.
ISBN 0–525–94103–7 (acid-free paper)
1. Sex instruction for women.   2. Women—Sexual behavior.
3. Sexual excitement.   4. Man-woman relationships.   I. Title.
HQ46.V45   1996
613.9'6'082—dc20   95–20548
CIP

Printed in the United States of America
Set in Sabon
Designed by Julian Hamer

To all women—

Your life is similar to a song. Not only do you compose, arrange, and play it; you sing it as well. You instinctively choose the tone and the key. And the man you love should complement your melody with his harmony. But each man will have his own special voice—no two men are the same. And when you meet your soul mate, your song will carry his name . . .

—BV

Acknowledgments

From my heart I thank:

My magnificent editor, Ed Stackler, for giving shape and perspective to the material and for being sensitive to my artistic needs. My wonderful agent, Alan Nevins, for always finding a good home for my books. My heart's blood, choreographer Yuri Smaltzoff, who keeps my life moving in a positive direction. Poet Clive Brewster, who inspired me to reach higher goals. Rocket scientist Dan Bloxsom, for donating generously of his time throughout the final stages of production. Attorney Mark Ukra, for his legal expertise and invaluable support. My personal physician, Dr. Harvey Cantor, who not only kept me physically alive but also apprised me of all the newest medical advances. Patty Formeca, who on short notice dropped everything to further and enhance my work. And Dr. John Minoli, who, in spite of being on call around the clock, always found time to contribute his invaluable insights and endearing humor.

And finally, all the warm and beautiful souls who contributed their private thoughts and expertise and lent me a shoulder.

Contents

4—Acts of Love

5—If Things Go Wrong: Troubleshooting

Introduction

Love looks not with the eyes, but with the mind,
And therefore is winged Cupid painted blind.
— SHAKESPEARE

Do you want to know what men are dying to tell you about their secrets, their innermost passions, but can't?

I have been in love with the "brotherhood of the sperm" ever since I became conscious of them at age six. I had some starry-eyed notion that they were like us, except for their large outer organ, of course. They are not. And yet . . .

Years later, after experiencing great love and even greater pain, and growing from those experiences, I wanted to understand more about men deep inside their souls—their very thoughts and dreams. So I got busy —studying, traveling, investigating, and interviewing over one thousand men of diverse age, race, and wealth from around the world.

Of course, it wasn't easy getting to the core of men's emotional sensibilities, but it was rewarding. And I will share with you this rich and hard-won knowledge of men's needs, wants, and sexual desires. To really understand your man—to understand what he wants in a woman—you have to breathe him, taste him, and get inside his blood. Therein lies the reason for this book.

At times, gathering information was like stealing their most guarded secrets; underneath their brazen veneer, many men were actually shy, socially reticent, and full of mistrust. But once comfortable and relaxed, they courageously poured forth their true feelings and insights. My heart was touched many times while hearing some very moving and intimate revelations. And, yes, I gained a new respect for the men with whom we share our planet.

Consequently, my goal is to offer you the tools to understand your man's inner thoughts and feelings, interpret his masculine behavior, peel away his protective armor and reach into his soul, thereby becoming a magnificent, loving seductress.

In the process, you will also discover a man's turn-ons and turnoffs, his likes and dislikes. I'll teach you how to cope with rejection by turning negatives into positives and . . . how to choose the *right* man while staying away from the *wrong* man.

It all begins with us females. Ever since the day Eve enticed Adam to bite the apple, *you* have been choosing the time, the place, and the man with whom you wish to interact. You have the power to say either yes or no—to accept or reject. So take an honest look at yourself and decide what you really want. Learn exactly what you can and cannot live with in a man.

Never forget: you are a woman. You are a goddess. You are in control. Make your move! If you want a good man, picture him in your mind and nurture the same qualities you wish to attract. Self-awareness, self-improvement, and self-esteem are your keys. Remember, you must first become that which you hope to find. It's not about a season, fashion, or fad. It's about *real love*!

Chapter 1

....

What Makes a Seductress

WHAT MAKES A SEDUCTRESS

Someone who does not run
toward the allure of love
walks a road where nothing lives.
                                    —RUMI

You can be a magnificent seductress. At this very moment you may already be one in someone else's eyes whether you know it or not. Do you find that hard to believe? You must have had some hope that it could be true or you wouldn't be reading this book. So take a deep breath and relax . . . your hope led you to the right place, a place where the seductive arts *can* be learned and the secrets are revealed with every page you turn.

Many women don't think of themselves as seductresses because their understanding of seductiveness is too narrow. They think of Marilyn with her gorgeous body and raw sexuality combined with her vulnerable fragility. Or they think of Cher with her terrific figure, outrageous clothes, and intrepid attitude. Then they look in the mirror and if they don't look like Marilyn or Cher (and, after all, very few of us do), they decide that they're not seductress material. What utter nonsense!

Seductresses come in all shapes, sizes, and ages. Was Marilyn a seductress? You bet! Is Cher? Absolutely! Their sexual energy and magnetism could never be mistaken or overlooked. But in a different way, Grace Kelly was also a seductress. Men sensed (correctly) that her cool exterior concealed a volcanic na-

4 • BRENDA VENUS

ture. Audrey Hepburn? Oh, yes. Her charm and vitality drew men and women to her. Ingrid Bergman? Her freshness made men long to be loved by a woman like her. No one who saw *Casablanca* had any problem believing that Humphrey Bogart and Paul Henreid both wanted her.

Garbo's air of mystery made men dream. Dietrich with her suggestion of the dominatrix made them thrill. Michelle Pfeiffer, slinking on a piano in *The Fabulous Baker Boys* or cutting a swath through old New York in *The Age of Innocence*, is a lesson in seductiveness. Meg Ryan, with her exuberance, made us glad that Tom Hanks finally found her at the end of *Sleepless in Seattle*. Lena Horne becomes more bewitching with every passing decade. And it's more than mere beauty that makes Julia Roberts light up the screen.

In fact, being a seductress has very little to do with beauty but everything to do with a confident attitude, energy, humor, charm, playfulness, genuineness, sensuality, and *knowing*. These qualities turn men on.

Most of the men I interviewed envision their dream girl as follows: she is sensitive to my needs. She is spontaneous. She loves to make love. I feel all of her focus is on me. She seems to sense when to be aggressive and when to submit. She's not afraid of her womanhood or her vulnerability. She never fails to compliment the way I please her. She's vocal about her pleasure, and she is quick to guide me in pleasing her. She's always different, never predictable, never indifferent. She suggests role playing. She's always inventive, fun, exciting, and willing to try something new. She's like Sheena of the Jungle one minute, delicate and demure the next. She doesn't mind if I watch while she turns herself on. She's not ashamed of her body even when she feels overweight. She knows exactly what turns me on and what doesn't. She talks sexy to me on the phone. She teases me in restaurants and driving home in the car. She lets me know when she wants to make love in a seductive and feminine way. If I'm tired, she doesn't pout and make me feel guilty. And when she's not in the mood, she's very gentle and sensitive to my feelings. She makes me feel like a combination of Don Juan, Casanova, and Rudolph Valentino. She knows what to do when I'm feeling down. She understands when I need silence. She makes sounds during lovemaking, and she expresses her fantasies. She's full of surprises—the kind I like. She's smart but not so much that she intimidates me, just enough to arouse thought. But *most important*, she touches my heart, and that's a mystery I can't explain.

To be a skillful seductress, you need to find out your man's likes and dislikes—what excites, hurts, tickles, or makes him uncomfortable. Just as you may want your clitoris stroked through your panties, he may want his testicles held and properly squeezed. Maybe that makes him feel terrific. Then again, maybe he hates it. You need to explore his body gently. Does he respond to a lot of pressure or a little? When stroking, does he prefer light or firm, long or short, or both? Does he want you to use both hands together or one hand on his shaft with the other hand on his scrotum? Does he like slurping sounds, hummms and ahhhs, or no sound at all? Does he like it when you talk to his penis, or does it make him feel silly? Watch his facial expressions, listen to his moans and groans, and pay close attention to the way his hands move your hands.

What does he like when he's really hot, and what does he enjoy when he's not? Do you know how to make him more aroused? Do you know how to cool him down? His mind and body are in the power of your magic hands, your magic mouth and tongue—your magic spell.

Learn to vary your rhythms and draw the utmost

pleasure from his body. Watch how he touches, strokes, and plays with himself, if he's not shy. Be sensual and passionate with both yourself and him. Give him lots of love and understanding, and don't force him to perform. It isn't the circus. He's only a man. Most men have plenty of secret desires that they may find difficult to express. Give him time and space. Be patient. Eventually, he will trust you enough to expose all of himself to you.

It's best to keep a little something in reserve for a special evening. Every day is not the Fourth of July, nor should it be. The Fourth of July is a spectacular display of fireworks exploding and floating through the night sky accompanied by the rousing music of a Sousa march. Magnificent! But every night? Some nights you might prefer the quiet beauty of moonlight reflected on the water, while listening to soft strains of a violin.

Don't give everything you've got all at once. Remember—the art of seduction is the science of restraint!

Always please yourself first and never, ever do anything that makes you feel uncomfortable. Whatever you do, do it with your whole heart, body, and soul, and you will find yourself greatly loved in return.

HOW TO BE A SEDUCTRESS

Pursuit and seduction are the essence of sexuality. It's a part of the sizzle.

—CAMILLE PAGLIA

- Genuine confidence begins with knowing your own body and mind.
- Knowledge is your ultimate love power.

- Develop good communication skills both in and out of the bedroom.
- Listen more than you speak, unless talk is related to both of you. Your conversation should always be positive and sensual.
- Be relaxed and self-assured.
- Know exactly what you're doing and why. Learn your man's mind, emotions, body, and sex organs.
- Appeal to all his senses: touch, taste, smell, sight, and sound.
- Find the right lighting for the mood you want to set.
- Create a romantic atmosphere. Arrange furniture to suit your sexual expression.
- Make him feel comfortable and relaxed in your environment. Welcome him with his favorite beverages, snacks, and music.
- Show enthusiasm when he speaks; have a twinkle in your eye. Flirt.
- Value cleanliness. Both you and your man should be able to lick, suck, probe, rub, squeeze, massage every square inch of one another without hygienic concerns or inhibitions.
- Go slow with all thoughts and actions. Be gentle and tender. Savor every moment. Tease.
- Kiss your man as though it were the first time, every time. Imagine that your lips are your nether lips and your mouth is your clitoris and his lips are the tip of his penis and his tongue is the shaft. That will be a kiss to remember!
- Learn the art of massage—of both body and mind.
- Listen to his body language and sounds. He will tell you all you need to know, even if silently.
- Do what pleases you both.

- Explore. Be adventurous. Find the things that really turn him on. If he doesn't like something you're doing, move on. If he does, stay with it.
- Don't be afraid to experiment.
- Relish every part of his body as though it were your "last supper."
- Create your own fantasies and then *live* them.

WHEN MEN WANT IT

Sex is impersonal, and may or may not be identified with love. Sex can strengthen and deepen love . . .
—HENRY MILLER, *The World of Sex*

Men are *always* ready to love and be loved, and that *sometimes* may translate into sex. For example, when men come home to relax from a hard day at work . . . they want it. After they fulfill their daily obligations and chores . . . they want it. Even while walking down the street . . . they *want it*! The bottom line: the penis is crying out for love—touch me, kiss me, suck me, fondle me, stroke me, take my gondola down your warm, wet canal—anything . . . just pay *attention* to me, woman!

And if there is no one around to fill his dance card, he just might have to take matters into his own hands. Marlon Brando said of playing Stanley Kowalski in *A Streetcar Named Desire*, "I think Stanley was like me —very physical. And I think that Stanley would have liked to put his hands in his pockets and feel himself." Marlon is putting his finger on the fact that most men are driven by a common and mischievous motivator: namely—testosterone. The sheer enthusiasm of watching his penis rise from a snooze is part of man's identity; and, in large part, it is what guides and rules a man's thinking and behavior.

A man's "glands" stand especially at attention on weekends—Friday night, Saturday morning, Saturday night, Sunday morning. Vacations are also a fabulous time for sex. It's playtime! After exercising and sweating at the gym, a man walks away feeling particularly good about himself . . . and Willie wants sex. After watching a provocative movie, reading a titillating story, or talking to his girlfriend over the phone, he wants sex. If he could, he might actually climb through the phone!

A man wants sex in different ways, too, based on his mood. Sometimes he wants wild, steamy sex; sometimes he wants gentle, soft, and romantic sex; sometimes he wants role-playing. One of the more popular fantasies revolves around aggressive, dominating women. (You play the teacher, he plays the student; you play the goddess, he plays your slave; you play the doctor, he plays the patient; you play the figure skater, he plays the fan; you play the Playmate, he plays the photographer.)

A lot of times, a man would like to do something about the yens of his penis but it's neither the right time nor the right place. That in itself can be very erotic. At such moments, he remains civil, cultivated, and controlled. But deep in his thoughts, even while reviewing statistics or going over the numbers, there are subliminal longings simmering.

Some men carry out their fantasies to such a degree that these dreams become part of their lifestyle. One such couple with whom I spoke are Margo and Sam. They are a respectable couple; they live by outward appearances. But they carry on a wild fantasy life behind closed doors. She plays mistress to his submissive tendencies and reduces him to the role of sex toy—his only purpose in life is to please her. He does the housework, cooks meals, and at her whim drops to his knees to serve her with his silver tongue and his golden organ.

On a typical evening, Sam arrives home from work clad in his proper business suit. He immediately changes into his black jumpsuit and nail-studded leather collar. Margo, meanwhile, dons her thigh-high black leather boots, straps on her corset and garter belt, and sits down to watch TV. She likes scotch and soda and little cigars, which Sam provides at the snap of her fingers. Sam then sits in the corner of the room, waiting for her orders.

On any given night, Margo lets Sam stroke himself while she masturbates. But on special nights, when she, of course, is in the mood, she directs him to explode quickly. Sometimes, she lies down, parts her legs, and orders Sam to kneel between them. If she feels Sam has been good, she lets him part her lips with his tongue. After a long while, she orders him deeper inside. After these sessions, Sam falls back and fixes Margo a nightcap.

Ladies, you don't have to work as hard as Margo to get the same results. Why don't you start by whispering your fantasies in your lover's ears between kissing and nibbling on them. He would love hearing a story (note: story!) from you of domination, or of him joining you with another woman, or any lascivious picture that pops into your pretty head. Remember: you don't care where he gets his appetite, as long as he eats at home.

CONFIDENCE

To love oneself is the beginning of a lifelong romance.
—OSCAR WILDE

Although youth's for an hour and beauty's a flower, confidence will win you the world. Confidence is an aphrodisiac. When you have it, everybody wants a taste. That is the very reason that nothing is more sexually appealing to a man than a confident woman.

Have you ever been at a party or social affair and wondered what a certain woman surrounded by a bevy of interesting and attractive men had that you didn't? Confidence! It makes up for any lack of physical endowment.

You're not born with confidence. You acquire it. It's a learned skill. Granted, some people come by it naturally, but that's uncommon. More often, arrogance, snobbery, or plain pushiness masquerade as confidence, and in time people discover the ruse. But anyone can gain confidence if the desire to learn is genuine. Be determined. Learn to love yourself by readjusting your mind-set.

It requires practice but presents pitfalls because many of you have been taught, either deliberately or unconsciously, *not* to love yourself. *Now* is the time to relearn. Whether you were raised by loving, caring parents, dysfunctional parents, or no parents, the choice is yours. Practice making the correct choices so that they become as habitual as brushing your teeth. Then you'll be on your way to making it a way of life.

I've talked to women who were raised in a storybook family and grew up with low self-esteem. On the other hand, I've talked with women who were raised by abusive, insensitive parents, yet have acquired self-respect and success because they disciplined themselves. Let's explore some ways to build, maintain, and reinforce your self-respect.

1. Set high but reachable goals.
2. Work hard and complete one goal before moving on to the next one. Finishing a task or goal,

however menial (such as waxing your floors),
produces a sense of accomplishment.
3. Appreciate and reward yourself for a job well
done.
4. Cultivate friends who appreciate you. Develop
your own support group.

Conversely, fear and lack of self-respect are very
destructive enemies. A man comes to a woman for reassurance and a shoulder on which to lean—someone
to tell him he's okay. If you appear confused and afraid,
you'll have no power to reassure him and he will probably go to a woman who feels secure and can do the
job.

If you find yourself in a tragic situation and it's
tough to face the day, read this poem. Then pick yourself up and get busy. I keep it on my refrigerator door
as a constant encouraging reminder. It helps immensely.

Don't Quit

When things go wrong as they sometimes will,
When the road you're trudging seems all uphill,
When the funds are low and the debts are high
And you want to smile, but you have to sigh,
When care is pressing you down a bit,
Rest, if you must, but don't you quit.

Success is failure turned inside out—
The silver tint of the clouds of doubt,
And you never can tell how close you are,
It may be near when it seems so far;
So stick to the fight when you're hardest hit—
It's when things seem worst that you must not quit.
—Unknown

Remember: a winner never quits, and a quitter never wins.

The first step on your road to success is having a *positive attitude*. Your attitude toward life, yourself, and men in general, can lead to success or failure. Everyone has imperfections and bad days, but you can be a compelling person as long as you don't make a big deal out of your shortcomings. And please, ladies, when you're on a date with a man, don't tell him about your cellulite and excess weight. He does not care. What he does care about is that you're comfortable with yourself, flaws and all. A little cellulite, a few extra pounds, and a tiny bump on your nose are not the end of the world.

A man asks a woman for a date because he obviously likes what he sees. Mark, a thirty-eight-year-old tennis pro said, "I hate going out with a drop-dead beautiful woman who poses, acts uncomfortable with herself, and always looks around the room. I'd rather date a confident woman with a good sense of humor. If she likes herself, I know I'm in for a good time."

Know exactly what you want and go after it with all your might. Be specific. Visualize your goal as though you already have it. That means you can imagine what you want and *will* it to happen. The power of the mind is very potent indeed. Take your time and see every detail in your head—imaginatively feel it, smell it, touch it. But be realistic. Don't visualize yourself married to the desirable John Kennedy, Jr., or some famous man you're not likely to meet. (If you get a chance to meet him, however, go for it! Now that you've worked on your confidence and self-respect, you deserve him!) If you're determined and believe in yourself, nothing will stop you because you know exactly what you want, where you're going, and why. *Whew!* Big exercise for the ol' brain, but it works.

Be pro-active—take more interest in the world around you. Join groups. It doesn't cost much to know more. Take classes. Learn to paint, play music, dance, read faster, write, speak another language, decorate, garden, cook, fix cars . . . whatever you desire. When you become an interesting person, full of knowledge and exciting ideas, interesting, desirable men will be seeking you out.

Get rid of misdirected, shotgun criticism and negativity. They're your enemies. With practice, your mind can switch to positive thoughts at will instead of sloshing around in negative ones. In fact, it usually takes less effort. Cleanse yourself of that negative inner voice telling you that you're unworthy, useless, stupid, ugly, fat, et cetera. Say to yourself, "Gorgeous is as gorgeous does!"

In the event you get stuck on a negative, read something funny or uplifting. Call a witty, positive friend. (You can't cultivate too many of these!) Play some upbeat music and dance around the room. Take a walk around the block, breathe the fresh air, and smell a flower. Exercise. Go see a funny movie. Wash the windows, scrub the floors. Make yourself busy doing whatever works for you. But erase all negativity from your mind and replenish it with good, healthy, clean thoughts. (Good, healthy, dirty thoughts work, too!)

Never judge yourself by how you look in a miniskirt or whether you think men find you attractive. You don't need a man to tell you that you're beautiful. Know your assets and work hard to make them even better. Okay, so you don't look like the latest supermodel, film, or soap star. It's not important. You have your own uniqueness, your own great qualities. Cultivate an appreciation for who you are. Don't be your own pit bull. Replace *"attack, attack, attack"* with *"advance, advance, advance."*

You're living and breathing *now*, so create with the clay that God gave you, and mold yourself into a goddess. Be thankful that you have something to work with—great hair, great legs, great buttocks, great hands and feet, or whatever. And if you don't have 'em, build 'em, shape 'em, tone 'em, any way you want 'em. Have a romance with yourself. Think and feel that you're the best or that you can be the best. Then make yourself the *best*.

Take a few hours a week just for yourself. Pampering doesn't cost a lot of money. Draw up a bubble bath. Have a glass of champagne or wine. Light some incense and candles. Turn on your favorite music and surrender to the seduction of warm water and bubbles. Also, paint your toenails red, get a friend to massage your back and shoulders. Lie in the sun for fifteen minutes. A little vitamin D and sunshine will do wonders for your soul. Exercise and sweat all those toxins out of your system. I guarantee, you'll feel like the person you're supposed to be. Maybe ripe, juicy, red strawberries are in season, but you think they're too expensive. What's a little extravagance once in a blue moon? Enjoy a few of life's graces from time to time, and in the process *learn* to enjoy life in the here and now.

I like to use a character that I've named "Betty Can-Do" as an example: She's the epitome of a confident woman. No one can emulate Betty's confidence, because she reinvents herself as she goes along. Her presence, her aura, her magnetism can be mystifying to people. She climbs the ladder quickly, gets the man she wants, and has other women vying for her attention. Betty writes the book instead of following what's in it. She's a pioneer and a heroine in her own right. She's positive, she's curious, she's a motivator, she's a perpetual student, and she's honest with herself and her

fellowman. Betty doesn't have to trick, pretend, or ca-
jole, because she believes in herself and her accomplishments. She's creative and spontaneous in lovemaking.
She's not afraid to surrender to her man or her orgasm,
because she wants the best. What she doesn't know, she
learns. The magic that surrounds Betty arouses loyalty
and enthusiasm, and her appeal always finds her at the
center of attention. So why not create your own favorite
character. There's no reason why you can't do what
Betty Can-Do!

BODY TALK

*The academy has fought stoically to claim that they
named the Oscar. But of course I did. I named it after
the rear end of my husband!*

—BETTE DAVIS

Your body is perpetually dancing. It dances to the silent
sounds of your hands, heart, eyes, face, smile—and the
rest of your body parts. It may not chime in tune, but
you can be sure it's talking. It's show-me rather than
tell-me time. Even while making love, your body dances
with your beloved. Usually, he leads; sometimes you
lead. In love's embrace, organic rhythms are essential.

Now consider that most communication is nonverbal. At least two-thirds of the time you communicate
without words. Clearly, your body language should be
honed to convey subtle needs. After all, the language of
the body is a fine art and should be viewed as such. The
adept are never misunderstood in their communication.
Their intoxicating mind-body cocktail is communicated
to the high octane, the highbrow, and the in between.
Whereas the inept are always misunderstood, unclari-
fied, and unfinished—always strung out. Be aware that

your slightest movement is sending signals. Stay honest with your body-brain communication, and you're sure to find a relationship anchored in romanticism and respect.

For those of you who are bogged down in domesticity at home with nigh a farthing of sexual interest in your husband's eyes, you need to rekindle the spark and become that hot tamale he fell in love with many moons ago. But before you try to turn him on begin by turning yourself on. A turned-on woman is an exciting woman. Start by practicing an array of provocative poses in front of a mirror.

Marilyn Monroe used to do it. She would paint her lips with layers of lipstick and shiny gloss, then practice different ways of speaking while making her lips as sensual as possible. She cracked herself up before she turned herself on. Her lips were sending a silent, erotic message. She also practiced wiggling her derriere seductively enough to turn the mirror on! No wonder all those cameramen were falling over one another to snap a shot or catch a glimpse in between. All the effort certainly worked for Marilyn—why not you?

For scintillating ideas, thumb through an issue of *Playboy*, *Penthouse*, or other inspirational magazines and imitate how the girls position their faces, their bodies, their eyes—note what they're doing with their hands, fingers, lips, tongue, legs, derriere, breasts, and feet. In other words, see how their total being is talking. Notice how the suds from their bath sensually fall off their nipples or clitoris. Observe what they're wearing —jewelry, shoes, teddies, lingerie, street clothes, wet see-through blouses, shirts, and skirts. Which hairstyles and cosmetics are exciting to you? Try it! But take only the ideas that work for your particular body and attitude.

Did you know that centuries ago, long before the

advent of glossy magazines, women were using classical statues, portraits on canvas, or whatever the means of that time, as models to imitate sensual stances? They were posing seductively even then. Posing like the magazine models can get you started, but once you get into the mood and turn yourself on with your own inventiveness, I'm sure your man won't be able to unzip his trousers fast enough.

If you feel stupid and ridiculous strutting and posing, I suggest you do what feels natural to you. Maybe when you're dressing, bend over slightly while buckling your shoe and hold the position until you know he notices the unforbidden. Put your stockings on slowly so he can look at your beautiful legs being dressed in silk. Or put a string of pearls around your neck and a pair of high heels on your feet, then sit naked in front of your mirror, legs slightly parted while fixing your makeup and hair. Do what you do best, only do it in front of him. A word to the wise: don't do your sexual strutting while he's in the middle of an important sports event on television, or he'll have one eye on you and the other on the game.

Once, when I was guesting on a talk show, a very lovely lady was advocating that people make their time for sex by marking it on their calendars. That might be practicable for some, but I work twelve hours a day, and if I had to circle a day on my calendar for a sexual rendezvous with my man, I would feel silly. There's no need to mark your calendar for sex when you can turn whatever moment you choose into an erotic event with just your body language. Send loving nonverbal messages to him every day in one endearing way or another.

BODY BEAUTIFUL

To be born woman is to know—
Although they do not speak of it at school—
Women must labour to be beautiful.
—W. B. YEATS

You are what you truly believe you are! Begin with an honest evaluation of yourself by standing totally naked in front of a mirror. Don't be cruel, rather be constructive about areas you want to improve. Squint your eyes and imagine your fantasy shape. Looks good, huh? Feel proud and confident, because you want to remember *that* feeling. Your goal . . . creating "body beautiful," by you!

The human body is a magical instrument. It's breathtaking in its intricacy and, when well tuned, operates in a predictable manner which will respond to your commands. For example, imagine your body as a piece of clay and your mind as a tool. Direct it to eat only certain foods; direct it to exercise three times a week for at least thirty minutes; direct it to think positive thoughts; direct it to read, study, and learn. It will culminate in a beautiful, well-balanced shape—substantial from the inside and out. The power is yours. Claim it and make it your own!

Would you like to take off a few pounds and tone up? Almost everyone I know would like to lose a few. But just dropping weight is not the issue. Making yourself excited enough to create a better you is the issue. You can motivate yourself with proper focus, hard work, and discipline. That's the secret to success—and the path toward your lifelong goal of "body beautiful." See it, hold that vision, then become it. Leave notes and pictures around your home and workplace for encouragement. I have a poster of a terrific body with no face in my gym. Believe me, it works, especially when I feel lazy.

Have you ever noticed that the people you think are so beautiful are not really that beautiful if you look closely at their features? They are beautiful to you because they look healthy. Their hair and eyes shine. Their skin glows. Their cheeks and lips are rosy. They have confidence. And they have a wonderful smile—a magnetic smile. Healthy-looking people are like magnets. Everybody wants to be around them.

Health is *everything*. If you want to reap the benefits of a healthy body and a healthy mind, you need to sow the finest seeds. Eat well, sweat (which means putting yourself on an exercise program), and sleep. Get lots of sleep. If possible, get in a good eight hours a night, plus a fifteen-to-twenty-minute nap, appropriately called "beauty rest." I realize for most of you, this is an adaptive challenge, but it's worth striving for.

Finally . . . to complete the picture of a totally beautiful you, you need to nourish your mind—read, read, read with some sense of purpose. Educate yourself: get familiar with current events. Investigate. Listen to the news. Buy magazines that enlighten you. Take a class that you're interested in at a nearby adult school so you'll develop and have your own opinions. Every woman needs to have opinions that she genuinely feels, thinks, and believes.

A good man will respect your point of view even if he doesn't agree with it. He will support who you are and what you want to do in life. The wrong man will put you down at every turn, hold you back from attaining your goals, make you feel foolish for no reason, and stifle your creativity. If he doesn't get with the program . . . walk away.

EATING RIGHT

One of the best weight-loss exercises consists of placing both hands against the table edge and pushing away. That's definitely a secret to fitting into your clothes. But the greatest secret is: "You are what you eat." Period. True beauty is a by-product of good health. To look your best, you must eat nutritious foods.

Stop dieting! What a depressing word. To a woman, the word *diet* carries the same connotation as the word *commitment* to a man. Don't use the word, don't even think about it. Most fad diets are a waste of time and energy. And they serve to reinforce negative feelings. Instead, put yourself on a "program" of eating in a balanced way and exercising. But don't allow your world to revolve around food. That's not living. That's existing. Eat to live, don't live to eat. That's not who you are. You're not a hamburger and fries, cookies, or a quart of ice cream. You're a beautiful person with a lot to offer the world. Let's get on with the "eating right" program. The following is my basic eating pattern for breakfast, lunch, and dinner. It's filling, it's nutritious, it fuels my body and mind. The portions are always small but sturdy.

BREAKFAST

After awakening, I drink one or two eight-ounce glasses of water, walk around, read the paper, and generally get my body functioning before I begin work. Then I grind Vienna roast coffee beans and brew one cup of coffee (sometimes I have tea), adding half-and-half. If you like cream in your coffee and need to watch your calories, it's best to use low- or nonfat milk. Never drink coffee in abundance. A cup a day is OK—five is not. I avoid refined sugar and don't care for the taste of saccharin, so I use honey whenever I want something sweetened.

Almost every morning, I eat steel-cut oats (it's a heartier, more nutritious kind) with thin slices of either banana, papaya, apple, peach, or strawberries on top. When I get bored with oatmeal, I alternate with either one whole egg and one egg white, four egg whites scrambled, or an omelette with egg whites and spinach, and a piece of wheat toast—sometimes plain, sometimes with jam or honey. I drink freshly squeezed orange juice when I'm not too lazy to squeeze.

After I eat anything, I brush and floss my teeth. Then I'm less inclined to want anything sweet. It's a good habit for you, too! Try it!

And I also take vitamin and mineral supplements with my meals for better assimilation.

LUNCH

I teach ballet several mornings a week. On those days, I eat a heftier lunch consisting of baked or roasted chicken, or white tuna fish in water, accompanied by a green vegetable, carrots, and half a baked yam. On the other days, I eat sliced turkey and a fresh vegetable salad. When I'm writing a new book, I become so involved that I might just eat plain yogurt and fruit, or angel-hair pasta with sliced tomatoes, virgin olive oil, and lemon juice. When I'm in a work mode, I don't eat because I'm hungry; I eat because my brain needs the nutrition in order to concentrate and create. I feel nervous and tired without nutritious food.

"An apple a day keeps the doctor away" is the best advice I could give you for maintaining a regular digestive system. Also a few prunes a day are internally beneficial. These healthy items can be interspersed as a light snack to quell the midday appetite.

DINNER

I usually eat light in the evening—a spinach salad with hard-boiled egg whites and maybe white fish, shrimp, or salmon; or maybe plain yogurt with fresh fruit. Or, if I'm really tired, I'll have a bowl of wheat-grain cereal with raisins. And in summer, sometimes I just eat a huge slice of watermelon. Although it is most difficult, I try not to eat after seven o'clock in the evening.

ALCOHOL

One or two times a week, I drink a glass of wine or champagne. But I have gone for months without any alcoholic beverage while working long, grueling hours. During this time, I'm on a stringent schedule. Like a warrior—everything I eat, everything I do must feed my creative mind. I can't allow anything to slow my creative process, and even a glass of wine can make me sluggish the next morning. There is plenty of time to celebrate when I've finished the project.

Since too much alcohol can dry the skin and cause weight gain, you should be careful with your intake. If you must drink, a wine spritzer is refreshing and lower in calories.

The taste of a good wine or champagne is most welcome. One or two glasses now and then is both pleasurable and relaxing. My favorite champagne is Taittinger Rosé, but it's a luxury that my pocketbook frowns upon. However, on special occasions (my birthday, Christmas, or upon completing a project that I've slaved over for months), I buy a bottle and share it with good friends.

MEAT

Rarely do I eat red meat or organs, although liver and onions or a filet mignon gives me needed energy when I'm sluggish. For a real treat, I drive to the Apple Pan, a home-style diner, where I sit at the counter and order one of their delicious hamburgers with fries and a root beer. It makes me feel like I'm in high school again and adds to the emotional charge of the outing. But eating hamburgers is an *exception*. That's why it's a treat. Häagen-Dazs ice cream is another of my favorite treats. But a treat is a treat—a reward for something well done or a boost for a melancholic mood.

SWEETS

On candy, desserts, and snacks: Yes, I do eat a chocolate now and then (white chocolate is one of my passions). When I'm at a restaurant, I sometimes order lemon or fruit desserts—apple, berries, peaches, or whatever fruit is in season. I don't crave snacks because I drink eight to ten glasses of water a day. Water will cut down your appetite and you won't be as inclined to snack. Depending on the person and the climatic conditions, our bodies are composed of 94 percent to 97 percent water by weight. So it makes good sense to drink plenty of it, preferably bottled or tap free from contamination. If you must snack, dried fruits or freshly cut fruits and vegetables—carrots, cucumbers, apples—are a healthy choice.

SUPPLEMENTS

Vitamins and minerals are terribly misunderstood. They can be harmful when taken in excessive amounts or on an empty stomach. No one can tell you precisely how much to take because individual absorption rates vary widely. For best results, consult a nutritionist.

Remember that the human body cannot live on vitamins alone; it also needs good nutritious food to survive. Vitamins can never substitute for fresh food. Too many people make the mistake of trying to live on a severe diet of lettuce, water, and fifty vitamins. Your tendons, bones, and muscles will suffer.

I take a multitude of vitamins from time to time, but it's usually when I'm pumping iron, teaching, traveling, and working harder than I should. However, I always eat a variety of healthy foods with the addition of vitamins A, B complex, C, D, and E, calcium, iron, magnesium, and zinc. Magnesium is helpful for restless sleep, and the mineral chromium picolinate can cut down your craving for sugar and stimulate the activity of enzymes. I also pay heed to the fact that excessive alcohol, smoke, and caffeine contribute to bone loss in women.

The following foods are rich in vitamins and minerals:

BREADS: Whole wheat, kamut, spelt, rye, corn, oat, or any combination are rich in complex carbohydrates, vitamin B complex, vitamin E, potassium, magnesium, chromium, manganese, molybdenum, selenium, zinc, fiber, and unsaturated fatty acids.

CEREALS: (Same as breads.) The best are whole rice, rye, wheat, oat, and corn grains.

DAIRY: Unprocessed cheeses, milk, yogurt, cottage cheese, eggnog, goat milk and cheese, kefir, and ice cream are rich in protein, fats, vitamin D (fortified), calcium, vitamin B_1, B_2, B_6, and B_{12}.

EGGS: The highest protein of any food. The yolk is extremely nutritious and contains lecithin, which keeps cholesterol moving through the bloodstream. Eggs include vitamin A, vitamin B_1, B_2, and B_{12}, biotin, choline, pantothenic acid, vitamin K, iron, manganese, sulfur, and zinc.

FATS: Unsaturated oils such as corn, peanut, safflower, sesame, canola, soybean, sunflower, wheat germ, margarine, and mayonnaise fit this category.

FRUITS: Fresh, canned, frozen, and dried. Most fruits are rich in complex carbohydrates, vitamin A, vitamin C, bioflavonoids, chromium, cobalt, iron, manganese, potassium, and fiber.

SEAFOOD: Fresh, canned, and frozen. Most seafoods are rich in unsaturated fatty acids and trace minerals. Tuna is exceptionally rich in minerals, amino acids, proteins, unsaturated fatty acids, vitamin A, vitamins B_1 and B_{12}, biotin, choline, folic acid, pantothenic acid, vitamin D, copper, sulfur, vanadium, and zinc.

POULTRY: Chicken, turkey, pheasant, and their organ meats. These birds are rich in protein, vitamin B_1, niacin, cobalt, and iron.

MEATS: Lean cuts, wild game, and their organ meats. These animals are rich in protein, vitamin A (liver), B-complex vitamins, vitamin E, cobalt, iron, molybdenum, potassium, sulfur, and zinc.

NUTS AND SEEDS: All kinds are rich in unsaturated fats, vitamins B_1 and B_2, inositol, copper, magnesium, manganese, potassium, zinc, and fiber.

VEGETABLES AND LEGUMES: Fresh and frozen. Vegetables should be steamed or sautéed lightly to preserve the nutrients. Drink the liquid in which your vegetables are boiled. A lot of nutrients are in that liquid. Rich in complex carbohydrates, vitamin A, PABA, folic acid, vitamin C, vitamin E, vitamin K, cobalt, copper, iron, magnesium, manganese, molybdenum, potassium, and fiber.

Now that you know more about foods and their nutrients, eat well, drink plenty of water, and take a multivitamin.

FIT FOR LIFE

Women today want faces and bodies that reflect their inner strengths, and the most important part of looking good is being healthy and fit. The way you feel will most assuredly reflect in the way you look. This I know for certain because I'm athletic. I can't remember a time when I wasn't leaping through the air in a *pas jeté*, running track, hiking, pumping iron, or teaching yoga, aerobics, or ballet.

Although exercise is individual, every person needs to find a type of routine that works for her. Be it three times weekly or more, exercise should be as much a part of your life as eating or sleeping. You can't imagine how good stretching, sweating, and working your muscles are for your state of mind and the maintenance of your body, not to mention your emotional stability and confidence.

I see girls and women walking into ballet class as if they were carrying the load of the world on their shoulders. And they probably are. After an hour-long class, not only do they look better physically, but their attitude is more positive and inviting.

Also, I have my own theory that a woman carries around a lot of excess water in her system that most definitely affects the way she feels and thinks. A woman actually has more fat cells than a man, and fat cells hold water. Once the water is expelled through perspiration, the woman is a different person. I see it all the time, especially with the women that I train. They walk in my door cranky and bitchy, and after an hour of working out on the StairMaster and with light weights, they're smiling. They like themselves again. Their self-respect takes a giant leap.

Looking good is a consequence of feeling good. Exercise will increase body awareness, correct bad posture, add energy to life, bestow a more youthful appearance, enhance sleep, boost the immune system, and help the remodeling of bones, thereby warding off osteoporosis. Because of exercise and good food, my waistline measures the same now as it did in high school. I am without a doubt in the best shape I've ever been, both physically and mentally. My diet is better, and my cholesterol and my body fat are lower. I like my maturity and the wisdom of my years, and I'm certainly more confident. I strongly urge you to try what has worked for me!

I work out every day, but most people don't have the time. So I suggest at least three times weekly, thirty minutes to an hour during each session for noticeable results. If you have a regular routine of Jazzercise, dancing, tennis, fast walking, running, swimming, stationary bicycling, or climbing the StairMaster . . . good for you! You're already ahead of the pack in the game of life.

STRETCHING

Stretching is a natural exercise that should be practiced regularly—a *must*. Stretching increases both your energy and endurance levels. Once the energy is flowing through your body, you can begin your workout. A few reasons for stretching are: to stimulate circulation; to rid your body of stiffness; to relieve aches and pains; to loosen up ligaments, muscles, and joints; to increase coordination and suppleness; and most important—to prevent injury.

When you stretch your muscles, you make them long and limber. Your body movements will become more catlike. The way you walk and handle yourself will be more elegant. You'll have more flexibility and feel more confident. So don't even think about working out without stretching first. Okay? *Muy, muy, importante.* The first thing I do when I wake up is to stretch out like a cat. It feels good. Watch how a cat stretches sometime, then imitate him—stretch and then get out of bed.

Before you begin your exercises, *prepare* for stretching—walk around your area. Never stretch cold. Hold each stretching position about thirty seconds before you move on to another one. After you complete your exercises, cool down by walking around. I lift my legs up one at a time for several minutes while walking. I'm sure I look like a prancing show horse, but it works for me.

Of all the various exercises I've done and still do, I believe ballet to be the very best for my particular body. Not only does it create beautiful legs, a tight derriere, a small waist, and an erect posture, but it bestows immeasurable grace. The music is classical, romantic, and soothing. Classes are focused and disciplined and the result following the effort is a heightened sense of well-being. You can always spot a ballerina. The femininity is undeniable.

My training schedule begins at my ballet barre. I do pliés (gradual bending of the knees with the body erect) in counts of four (four down and four up) for about ten minutes or until I break a sweat and feel sufficiently warmed up.

I start with a demi-plié (or half bending of the knees), before graduating into a grand plié which is a full bending. When I am traveling, I use a chair or windowsill to hold on to. This exercise renders the joints and muscles soft and pliable and the tendons flexible and elastic. It develops a sense of balance, and it maintains your body's correct posture, which is to say straight and proud.

At the barre, I always make sure that I hold my stomach in tightly, tuck in my buttocks, roll my shoulder in a circle—forward, up, and back—and hold my head up straight and tall. This allows a full inflation of my lungs, facilitates my concentration, and helps me focus on my exercise regimen.

Create the mood you want with music. Use whatever sound you need for motivation. I work out to current hits and my old faithfuls Tina Turner, Prince, Donna Summer, Sting, LL Cool J, or Deep Forest for isometrics, weights, and stomach crunches. For stretching and ballet I prefer Chopin's nocturnes or Erik Satie's *gymnopédies*. A good rule to always remember: concentrate, don't force moves and don't jerk. Everything nice and slow and smooth. Tummy in, butt tight, shoulders back, and head up. The best time to exercise is one hour before you eat or two hours after a full meal. You can't work out in a dizzy or weakened state, so don't skip meals. You defeat your purpose. If you feel lethargic, eat a piece of fruit an hour before exercising for sustained energy. Carrot juice is also very stimulating. It's best to wait thirty to forty-five minutes after a workout before you eat. Your body needs to come down from the exercise.

Break your body in slowly. Your warm-up is just to get the blood flowing, nothing else. It gives your muscles time to adjust to their new activity. Be careful not to overdo. Being excited and motivated is great, but forgetting to warm up and doing too much too soon will definitely cause injury—perhaps a torn muscle or ligament. Caution is the key. Be sensible with your body and heed the motto "Train, Don't Strain!" The first few times, expect sore muscles. That means they're waking and growing. Soreness is a good sign. Soaking in a hot Epsom salt bath helps soothe soreness.

BREATHING
Don't forget to breathe! Inhale when your body is under the least amount of pressure, exhale when you have resistance. When there is any strain, breathe out. Deep, regular breathing helps your blood get its maximum supply of oxygen. Your exercises will be easier and you will feel better as a result of more oxygen flow in the blood. Breathing right will also keep your mind focused on your goal. Be aware of your body posture. Incorrect posture could restrict your breathing.

SKIN
Vitamins A and E and zinc and betacarotene are great for the skin. They help rejuvenate the skin cells. Don't neglect any body part. The skin on your body is just as important as the skin of your face or hands. It should be given equal attention. Moisturize every inch of your beautiful self.

The most effective time to moisten your skin is after a hot bath or shower when your pores are open and ready to receive nourishment. Your cells need rejuvenation—out with the old, in with the new. For youthful, satin skin, keep a brush or abrasive sponge in your shower or bath to scrub off the old cells and make room for the new.

For many years, I have lubricated my entire body with either Nivea cream or coconut butter. I brush the dead cells off my skin in the shower and immediately smooth on Nivea while I'm wet.

When I travel, I buy an organic product of the country. In Hawaii, I use coconut oil; in Tahiti, I use their tropical combination. And if I happen to be in a country where I can find an aloe vera plant, I manage to cut it and squeeze the juice all over my body and face. It's the best!

When I lived at the beach, my girlfriend Kristina would come over for a ten-mile run to the pier and back. One morning, we decided to try a natural moisturizer. It was seven o'clock A.M., and we didn't think anyone would see us, so we plastered honey all over our faces. I suggested we wrap our thighs in cellophane to sweat more. We did. All the way to the pier there was not a soul in sight, but on the way back . . . guess who we ran into with honey dripping down our shirts and stuck in our hair and cellophane hanging around our knees? Bruce Willis, who was taking his morning run. Totally embarrassed, we ran the rest of the way home looking down, trying to hide.

I no longer live at the beach, but I believe a few minutes of sun now and again supplies the skin with the necessary vitamin D conversion. It also relaxes the nerves and soothes your mind while the sun's rays caress and penetrate your being. The sun's healing power for the soul is one of God's luxuries that doesn't cost a dime. But if you abuse the gift and bake yourself, you could end up like a portrait of Dorian Gray, which is to say, much older than your years. Again, moderation is key. A little color is nice and healthy, too much color is asking for trouble.

Sunblock goes wherever I go. I never walk out my door without using sunblock on my face, neck, and hands. Have you ever noticed that a woman's neck and hands age quicker than any other body part? That's unfortunate, since we use our hands for everything and our neck is always visible. The skin loses collagen and elastin, the chief constituents of connective tissue. Their depletion leaves the skin looking dried and shriveled. Unless you protect your hands by wearing rubber gloves when you clean and frequently use moisturizer all through the day, your hands will look well beyond their years. Many men have told me that they can tell a woman's age by the condition of her hands. So a word to the wise: keep your hands protected and nourished.

Well-manicured hands and feet are so appealing, especially for those men with foot and hand fetishes. Treat yourself to a manicure and pedicure from time to time. Or do it yourself on a weekly basis. If you don't know how, learn from a professional. Since skin grows over the nail bed daily, soak your cuticles in warm water until they're soft enough to push back. Then oil them. For a healthier maintenance, file them in a square shape. (A natural product for the growth of healthy hair, bones, and nails is Alta Sill-X Silica.)

Treatment for my face consists of boiling a pot of water, adding a tablespoon of Swiss Kriss, which is a herbal blend that draws out impurities, putting a towel over my head for a more concentrated effect, and steaming for a few minutes. I remove the towel and splash my face several times with cold water to revitalize and close the pores.

For a mask, I use either egg whites, milk of magnesia, or cooked oatmeal. All three tighten the skin and draw out the impurities. Then I wash off with cool water.

Soap never touches my face. Instead, I use Ponds cleansing cream, Abolene liquefying cleanser (which can also be used for sex), cocoa butter, Noxzema, or Neutrogena to remove makeup and cleanse my face. Then I take a warm cloth and wipe again. For a moisturizer I use either Kiehl's, Elizabeth Arden, Oil of Olay, or Derma Centre, depending on how I feel, and I am always willing to try something that might be better. I always cleanse my face and use a moisturizer before going to bed at night. It's a rewarding habit that reaps great rewards over time.

Tiny wrinkles are called laugh lines when you're young and crow's-feet when you're older. Why, why do the eyes wrinkle? Because the skin is so thin and oftentimes dry. Without moisturizer and sunblock, it resembles a fish's scale. It's important to invest in a good eye cream. I have tried many brands, but La Prairie produces the best results for me. I must warn you, it is expensive. Lamentably, I can only afford it a few times a year, so in place of my favorite cream, I puncture a hole in a vitamin E capsule and spread it around my eyes. It's most effective. And speaking of E, I also use vitamin E oil in a bottle, 10,000 IUs for my breasts and neck, with remarkable results. Emulsified Vitamin E will penetrate the skin most effectively.

HAIR

Your hair is usually the first thing people see. It should be nourished and cared for; and having healthy and fit hair need not be a chore. Beautiful hair flows, is vibrant, and dances in light and shadow. After all, it's your crowning glory. However, you must wash it regularly and use a good conditioner, or it will end up being your worst nightmare.

My girlfriend Debbie changes the color and style of her hair more than she changes clothes. When she greets me at the door, I'm always surprised. One day she's a blonde, another day she's a brunette, and today, she's a redhead.

Last week, she came over crying. The color of her hair had three different shades of blond and the cut was . . . well, I could have done better blindfolded. Her hairstylist was having a bad day and Debbie's hair was the result. When I saw her baked and fried hair, I had to bite my lip to keep from laughing. It was cartoonish. But after hearing of her misery, I was upset, too.

We discussed several solutions to her problem, one being, do it herself. What did she have to lose? She was well on her way to a crew cut. Her cut was choppy, the color was disgusting, and her hair was brittle and dry. We drove to the nearest pharmacy, purchased a rich auburn color by Clairol, and drove home to apply it. I cut off the dead ends, applied the color, a Kolestral conditioner by Wella, and voilà—a miracle. She looked beautiful.

Instead of spending your paycheck on your hair every month, if you're not quite satisfied, do it yourself from time to time. You'd be surprised how adept you can be.

I don't particularly like going to hair salons. In fact, I've probably been inside one four or five times my entire life. I don't fancy someone I don't know cutting and pulling on my hair. Once I had a devastating experience. My friends recommended that I visit a famous stylist. I made an appointment. He asked me what I wanted. I said, "Trim it a few inches, that's all." My hair was down to my waist, so a few inches was nothing. I closed my eyes while he trimmed. When I thought he was almost finished, I looked into the mirror, aghast. The hair to my waist was suddenly hair touching my shoulders. I stood up, speechless, instinctively reaching to the floor to clutch the last vestiges of my womanly mane. I learned a valuable lesson. Needless to say, that was the last time that I have ever let anyone touch my hair without first knowing them well and trusting them completely.

Luckily, I found a man named Jimie whom I now entrust with my crowning glory. Here are a few tips for the maintenance of yours: Lightly shampoo and condition your hair every day; if you have extremely dry hair, then every few days. But the most important thing is to keep your roots as clean as possible. The roots need to breathe and they cannot breathe if they are not clean.

While there are many high-quality "designer label" hair products for sale in salons and beauty supply stores, you can also get excellent results from products on your grocery store shelves that are far less expensive. While in the shower, I apply Wella Kolestral. It leaves my hair shiny, rich-looking, and extremely manageable. After rinsing the Kolestral, I use a dab of Pantene conditioner to prevent tangling. Oftentimes, I soak my hair with mayonnaise, wrap cellophane around my head, and ride the StairMaster for thirty minutes. Then I rinse and wash with shampoo. Mayonnaise, without a doubt, is the best conditioner for the money that you'll ever find.

If you have a problem with dandruff, there can be three causes: oily scalp, dry scalp, or nerves. If you have flaking, find out if your hair is oily or dry. Purchase a shampoo for your type of hair. Use a dandruff shampoo twice a week until your condition has improved. And for those of you who are starting to lose hair, you might try using the herb rosemary. It worked for my neighbor Susie, who was losing her hair rapidly. She took several leaves from a rosemary bush and boiled them in water. Every time she washed and rinsed her hair, she poured the brew over her roots. Months later, she had healthy hair. Remember—your beauty is uniquely yours—and needs to be appreciated and cultivated.

Using color can be tricky. Henna is a natural color and will not harm your hair, but you should never use it on bleached, white, or gray hair. It will turn orange or some ghastly color. If you have blond hair, use lemon juice for highlights. It turns blonder in the sun.

Remember, when choosing a style or color for your hair, stay true to who you are. Emphasize the positive you. A cut should emphasize the better qualities of your face. Don't start changing your hair, makeup, and wardrobe to please another person. You must please yourself before you will ever be able to please anyone else. Never copy what you see in a magazine on a model if you don't look exactly like that model, because you may end up looking ridiculous and ruin what good points you do have.

MAKEUP

Makeup looks better when it's sparingly applied to a clean face. The idea is to see your face when you are finished. I see young girls and women coming into ballet class during the first few weeks of the season with little or no makeup, and they are quite beautiful. Then . . . they spot a cute guy, someone they want to impress, and a transformation occurs . . . out comes the heavy eyeliner, heavy blush, a new hair arrangement, and bright red lipstick. The problem with mixing cosmetics and exercise or lovemaking is that lipstick, mascara, eyeliner, and base makeup can smear, smudge, and disappear— on your face, his collar, or someone's pillow. Your man may wonder if the girl he fell in love with the night before wasn't left on the floor or bed in the drippings of sweat. The point I'm making is that you can still be the irresistible girl who turned him on hours before by heeding a few simple tips for lovemaking.

Skin: Spot your base with a brush only where it is most needed. If you need to conceal blemishes, scars, or whatever, use a cover-up or concealer stick. (One with a yellow base is usually best.) Then use a loose, light dusting of translucent powder, especially on the chin.

Eyes: Avoid raccoon eyes by using waterproof or liquid liner, not pencil. Then brush on a smoky smudge of brown that runs through the creases.

Lashes: Enhance lashes by curling and using single false ones because if they fall off, he'll think they are yours. If you use mascara, do so sparingly.

Cheeks: Blush rosy circles on apples of cheeks, then powder again.

Lips: Trace lips, then fill in the center with berry pencil. Follow with lipstick or dab with gloss. Kiss and bite a tissue and lock on color with powder. When you're drinking wine, discreetly lick your tongue over the rim where you sip and your lipstick won't stain the glass.

Nails: Keep nails functional in length, clean, and polished pink. Red is to give ourselves a boost or for those wanton, passionate nights.

For parties: To fire up the night, add a bit of gold lipstick or gloss on center of lower lip. Use a lighter-than-foundation shade between crease from nose to mouth and frown lines. Play up eyes by using a gold shadow on outer corners. Put a bit of pearly highlighter on collarbone, on highest part of cheekbone, and under brow. A pale mauve powder can enhance your complexion as it evens out the skin tone.

One of the world's top makeup artists, Francesca Tolot, often works on Cindy Crawford, Demi Moore, Michelle Pfeiffer, Elle Macpherson, and many others. Francesca says, "Less is more." She doesn't create a made-up look, she follows a woman's natural features. One thing she always notices is that many women wear a base that ends under their chin, and it's usually the wrong color. It looks like a face that belongs to somebody else.

For lips, Francesca's trick is putting a little of the same base you use on your face in the middle of your lips. It makes them look fuller. For the face, she often mixes three different colors in order to get the right tone and achieve a three-dimensional look. Using just one color makes the face look flat.

Let me leave you with this thought: Makeup is a tool to enhance rather than hide. Your goal is to look pretty and natural rather than phony and made-up . . . except when you are role-playing with your man and you turn into a femme fatale. Or if being excessively made-up makes you feel good from time to time, go for it.

DRESS

Dress and style help determine how you will be perceived by the world and the man you want to win. Woman to woman, the future is about personal style; and a woman today is not shy about playing with styles in order to find her individual look. The look is more inviting because it is so diversified—individual, fun, and comfortable, from the androgynous to the ultrafeminine, sensual and romantic. It's be-true-to-yourself time! Your clothes should be a celebration of you. That's what style is all about.

The real woman dresses with inspiration and strength. She wears her clothes rather than having her clothes wear her. She appears free, together, and confident. She seeks the link between inner and outer expression.

Now let's discuss the basic difference between fashion and fads. A fad is a momentary look—a temporary style for amusement. If you're very young and a fad looks good on you, go for it. But most fads only look good on tall, thin girls.

I enjoy browsing the shops on Melrose Avenue and Hollywood Boulevard when I want to see the latest fads. Most of the people are amusing in their black leather outfits, chains, tattoos, bright-colored hair, and rings twisted in parts of their anatomy.

One day, I saw an attractive girl walking down the street with purple-and-green hair, a ring in her nose, black lipstick, black gloves with the fingers cut out, fishnet stockings with holes, and a skirt exposing a bit of cheek. I stood there aghast wondering, "Does she really think she's pretty?"

Fashion is simply a mode of dress that is currently prevailing in society. Keeping pace with fashion will make you look young and together. Being in style needn't be costly.

Accessorize! It only takes a few items every season to update and enhance your wardrobe. A new belt, a new pair of shoes, purse, scarf, earrings or necklace, or the current-style blouse and skirt. There is no greater advice anyone could ever give you than to keep it simple!

Don't wear anything that doesn't complement your body. If you have large thighs, you certainly don't want to wear a miniskirt. Miniskirts are for very slender and well-tanned legs—not varicose veins, sagging skin, and cellulite. When you do expose yourself, make sure it's the most appealing part of your anatomy. Don't enhance a large waist with a flashy belt or a large bosom with lots of ruffles. Large breasts require a more simple neckline. Ruffles are great on a smaller-breasted woman because they enhance her femininity. Selecting clothes and colors to emphasize your assets demonstrates that you are a clever and wise woman. If you don't know the most flattering line of clothes to buy and you don't know what colors are best for you, ask someone you admire to help you. It could be a man or woman who knows what looks best on you individually. Or if you've been complimented on certain clothes by several people, make a mental note and stick to the style that receives the most compliments.

And please don't make yourself over for a man. Similar to the concept of dressing for success: the idea of changing your look to suit a man's taste is yesterday's news, unless he knows more than you about style, fashion, and the cut of a suit. In a current survey, 60 percent of the women felt that by using the right clothing and makeup, any woman can be attractive to a man.

If your fella liked you in the first place, he liked you for you. To change yourself completely and present another woman to him is ludicrous. Your natural beauty is probably what attracted him to you. So again, accentuate the positive, play down the negative, and keep it simple.

In a memorable and beautiful scene from the film *Sayonara*, Red Buttons was yelling at and berating Miyoshi Umeki, the Japanese woman with whom he had fallen in love, because he discovered that she wanted to change the shape of her eyes to please him. She had made an appointment with a doctor who could cut the top eyelid in such a way as to enlarge the eyes, making them look more occidental. He told her that he loved her exactly the way she was and he loved the shape of her eyes. Miscommunication. The moral to the story is: if a man loves you, he loves *YOU*, not some alteration!

COMMUNICATION

A person who has really known the heights and depths of ardent lovemaking manages to communicate what he or she knows about it not only with every word that's spoken afterwards but with every intonation of the voice, every glance of the eye, every slightest movement of the arm or leg. The message cannot really be kept a secret.

—STENDHAL

"Please, Please, *please*, baby, *please*, do we have to talk about our relationship *again*?" is the familiar refrain of the typical man when you try getting him to sit down and communicate. Right? Instantly, the color of his face changes from a vibrant peach to a reticent white. He starts to sweat. His eyes exude that familiar, "How long is this gonna take?" He puts his hands in his lap, looks down at the floor, and waits . . . bracing himself for the worst.

What pain this so-called communication must be for that poor man. Did you notice that he manifested the same physical symptoms when you talked about commitment? These two claustrophobic C words, *commitment* and *communication*, make him feel put upon —as in loss of independence. A functional equivalent would be your right leg crunching his crotch.

A man listens differently from a woman. When you say, "We need to talk!" he's hearing, "Let's be honest with each other." He's upset; he feels his integrity is being questioned. How dare you question his intentions. Your confrontation of his feelings makes him feel betrayed. Even if you are right and he is double-timing you, he still feels stifled. He feels the ol' commitment thing recurring—claws going into his skin, anxiety level reaching claustrophobic proportions. His independence is being imposed upon . . . his power stripped.

A man is an adventurer: he likes to look out over the horizon and dream about what he can conquer; what he can do that's new; what he can tackle that he hasn't experienced before; how many points he can score on the journey. He strays from the present a lot.

There is a sense of adventure about his future and its possibilities that will never die; unless, of course, his spirit dies.

For you, talking is a release, an aphrodisiac. For him, it may be a drain, almost an insult. He thinks, "Now she's gonna drag me around by the neck for a while. I'm losing control of my life here!" And *control* is his middle name. It's the only ground where he truly feels comfortable.

When a man loses control, he loses his sense of maleness, which, in turn, makes him feel insecure. And insecurity can bring out his worst. He doesn't mean to be nasty, and he certainly doesn't want to hurt your feelings. It's just that he would rather be Comet Shoemaker-Levy 9 crashing into Jupiter than discussing subjects at hand. He generally thrives on short questions and short answers. He's a short fuse and you're a long fuse. That's all. Remember the cavemen, "Ugh, ugh, ugh!" Modern men are bottom-liners. Their mottoes: "Say what's on your mind in three words or less and move on."

Henry Ward Beecher was noted for saying, "The older I grow, the more I listen to people who don't talk too much." Most men don't object to giving the subject of "Relationship" a few minutes now and then. What they do mind is that those talks take too long and are not fun. Once aware, you can learn to be sensitive to that distinction.

When Napoléon Bonaparte was asked how he handled both the affairs of state and his personal life, he replied, "I compartmentalize. I open one drawer, fix the problem, shut it, and go on to another drawer and so forth. I focus only on what I am doing at that moment." And you, ladies, are asking your man to focus on a subject that's not within his manly agenda. He would much prefer fixing the engine of his car, adding another room onto the house, pitching balls in the backyard, or playing the stock market on his computer.

Most men deal with life in the above manner. They like to set specific goals and then accomplish them. They deal in numbers and wins. They feel a sense of pride when they finish a task or excel at a sport. So when you ask, "Can we talk?" it sounds vague to him. He can't see, touch, feel, or smell it. So he thinks, "What's the point?" and feels pinned down like a bug in a display case.

A woman's territory is uncharted land for a man. In the Brazilian Amazon Rain Forest, there is a section of land into which even the natives don't venture. They believe it holds forbidden mysteries. It's the same with men and the female language. They don't speak the tongue; therefore, they don't fancy dallying too long with it. Anything over five minutes and they get an itch. They feel themselves out of their habitat like a fish out of the water. The only reason—and I do mean *only* reason—a man will sit still for long periods while you have "the talk" is that he wants to please you, either for love, lust, money, or sex.

Only when passing through the initial stages of your acquaintance does a man actually enjoy and engage in lengthy discussions. He wants you to understand him and his needs. At this stage he tries to be a good friend, enabling him to learn if you can be a good friend in turn. It's the "getting to know all about you" stage. And because he knows little about you in the early part of your relationship, everything becomes an intriguing challenge—he's in competition for your attention. Therefore, communicating with you makes him feel good and it also justifies that level of your relationship.

Then, months later, you say, "Let's eat out tonight." He *thinks*, "Great! We'll go to Chuck's Steak House." You see, he already knows where he wants to eat and exactly what he wants to order. So you *think*, "I remember seeing a quaint little restaurant about five miles down the road near that English-looking cottage with the rose garden in front." You get in the car and he politely asks, "Honey, where would you like to eat?" You reply, "Oh, it doesn't matter. Wherever you like." You don't mean it, and he doesn't mean it, but you are both trying to be courteous to the other. Okay, you're driving for a few minutes and you say, "Why don't we go to that little restaurant we passed on the way home last Saturday night?" Now it starts. "What restaurant?" he asks good-humoredly. "Oh, you know, the one about five miles from here near that little cottage," you say. "No, I don't know!" Now he's getting famished. All he can think about is that steak. "Honey, can you give me a better idea, so we don't have to drive around all night?" he pleads. You retort, "Just drive. I'll know it when I see it."

What we have here is a failure to communicate—a chronic dilemma. Thus begins the communication breakdown. Both parties become frustrated with the other. On one hand, we have a man who knows exactly what he wants to eat and where. On the other hand, a woman who knows only the general vicinity of the restaurant she wants. This, ladies, is the communication breakdown. He's focused. She's not. Her spectrum is broad and filled with intriguing nuances. His is staccato, spasmodic. He's the bass—boom, boom, boom—who, what, where, when, why, and how. She's the melody—the flute drawing air from the heavens and flowing through the universe.

A classic example of our male-female directional differences is humorously depicted in the beginning of the film *The Bridges of Madison County* when Clint

Eastwood drives up to the house of Meryl Streep and asks for directions to a certain bridge. As Meryl explains, the quizzical look and smile that crosses his face is a picture worth a thousand words. She finally decides to hop into the truck and guide him there. Great, great moment!

A woman wants novelty, excitement, and romance in her life, smelling the lilies and breathing in the fresh air. A man focuses on one thing at a time, mapping out his course in space and logic. But remember, your melody not only has a beginning and an end; it also has a focus besides giving beauty to the rhythm of his bass. So tune your thoughts. When he asks you where you want to go—be ready and say, "A quaint little restaurant that serves great Italian food, but let me direct you there." Be affirmative. Unequivocally state where you want to go. And he will drive you there. Being clear will not diminish your mystery, but it will greatly reduce his frustration.

The bottom line is this: learn his likes and dislikes and try not to tax his tolerance level. Be honest. If you take him shopping, tell him that you want to spend some time at the store browsing. Then, if he agrees, he will go knowing what to expect. That's good!

Be straight and up-front with your man. Be kind. Be flexible. He's trying. Give him credit. Respect his preferences and needs—and he'll open up his heart to you in time. You're not going to change him, but you can encourage him to grow.

True love involves negotiation and compromise. Make a friend, learn how to be still, and properly listen to his needs with your kind heart and disclose yours. Give him time to absorb it all. He'll get there if you're patient and gently lead the way, instead of forcing him with manipulation to be something that he's not.

In compromising, you must understand his field of

concerns. We've discussed his hobbies. And, of course, a man's job will always be a top priority: it's his first wife. You must learn to be the mistress at first. His work is an extension of who and what he is. The success at his job may be one of the reasons he's got you—the woman of his dreams. His success and ability to provide might have been one of the key points on *your* list.

Another compromise is in appreciating his need for male bonding, which translates into his time spent with "the boys." Obviously you are also a very big part of his world, but he needs to fraternize with his buddies from time to time. You must be sensitive to his moods . . . and to his compartmentalized way of thinking and living. You need your space—give him his.

Every relationship has three different entities— your life, his life, and both of your lives together. One, you need to have your own interests aside from his. Two, he usually has his separate interests. Three, you both have common interests, and ideally your relationship flourishes when you mutually explore new and inventive avenues together.

Men get bored quickly, so you'll need to keep your connection to each other alive, active, and interesting. Remember that communication takes place through many different channels, and you need to optimize each channel because each also has its limitations.

In communicating with your man, remember that he always hears "your music" much more than "your words." So *how* you say things is just as important as what you say. For example, "*Larry*, we need to *talk!*" As you stress the word *talk*, your body language, the tone of your voice, and your inflection may indicate to Larry that you're upset, uptight, and about to dish out unpleasantries, in which case he recoils and prepares himself for the onslaught. Now, let's take the same sentence and make it more inviting. "Larry, could I have five minutes of your time? I really need your advice about the food we're serving Friday night." As you ask the question, your body language is free and open, the tone of your voice is calm and collected, and your inflection is confident. Therefore, Larry is all ears. He wants to be of assistance because you've come to him with respect—you've opened the door to true *love*.

Your body language should be in unison with the tone of your voice and your actions. They complete your female symphony. Words coupled with appropriate body language and inflection are very powerful indeed. Without the complete chorus, it's analogous to a doughnut without a hole or a Twinkie without the filling. How you make use of each setting will determine whether or not you flourish in your relationship, in your job, in your life. Be consistent and unwavering in your attempts at "loving communication."

Once you accomplish this, he'll look forward to these little talks just as enthusiastically as he listens to his male friends.

A man needs to know that he can trust you no matter what. And his trust is hard to earn. So once you have earned it, take care not to lose it. Keeping your word is the foundation of good communication.

Couples communicate in many different ways. Some share every fleeting thought. Others, like Glenda, thirty, and Joel, forty-one, have a strong relationship because they *don't* share too much. Glenda said, "I'm something of a risk taker and Joel is not. But the fact that we're so different makes our marriage a challenge. Because of our jobs, we spend a lot of time apart. We both enjoy brain sex, teasing, challenges on the phone, and when we do come together, sparks fly. He thinks I'm mysterious and I like that. Everybody should have secrets. It adds spice to life. I continue to be the seductive individual my Joel was attracted to. And he continues to be the inquisitive scientist that I fell in love with. We don't feel the great necessity of long, drawn-out conversations. However, when something is bothering either of us, we come together and find a solution."

Whether you choose to share every thought or keep a bit of mystery in your relationship is your call. Some plants thrive in shady areas while others need direct sun. Every couple must find what degree of shade (mystery) or sunlight (openness) is the best environment for their relationship.

When out on a date with the hunk of your choice, delicately try to uncover the important aspects of his character. But do not, for your sake, launch an inquisition:

"How are your parents? Do you keep in touch?"

"How did they treat you growing up?"

"Do you have brothers or sisters, and are you in touch?"

"What kind of relationship did you have with your family?"

"How did the other kids at school treat you?"

"Did you have fun in high school?"

"What are your memories of growing up?"

"Were you tall/short and how did it make you feel?"

"When were you first attracted to girls?"

"Are you a late bloomer?"

Granted, these are good questions if you're sincere and you've known him for a while. However, if they're all on the first date, he may become suspicious that you're working an angle. Yes, you absolutely want the information. But it's much more effective if you make an effort to be charming and show him that your interest in him is genuine and lasting. Ask your man a *few* penetrating questions and he'll be flattered by your interest. Conduct a third degree and he'll think that you're nosy, insensitive, and rude. (And he'll be right.)

A common language on the subject of intimacy is still a mystery to both men and women. We approach it from all angles, but the feeling of warmth and caring that emanates is the same. So it's up to you to gain a better understanding of what your own intimate desires signify to you and what they mean to him. Then communicate what you want. Sometimes, a woman just needs a hug while she's cooking. Nothing more. Sometimes, a man thinks that a hug is a prelude to sex. If that's not the way you feel, tell him. He wants to please you. How will he know if you don't tell him? But don't just tell him. Explain why you are hurt—communicate. It's possible that he may be unaware as to how he disappointed you. Be patient in learning his ways while he's learning yours. And respect each other's differences—differences of gender, psyche, hormonal influence, and social background.

Males typically like to communicate about work, sports, craftlike hobbies, politics—physical or intellectual things. Women, on the other hand, gather their strength sharing intimate or emotional issues. So, ladies, initiate an open line of communication with your man by setting a few ground rules *in the beginning* of the relationship upon which you both agree. Set clear ground rules so he can please you better. Tell him what you want or don't want. Play by these rules and be happy. It takes two to tango, and sometimes one has to bend over backward to accommodate the other. Sometimes it's you, sometimes it's he who must master the art of bending.

If you begin by telling the truth about your feelings, it will lead to honest communication, thereby giving your man a better idea of who you really are. If he is craving Greek food, but you're dying to eat Thai, then suggest Thai. If he recommends a book for you to read, but you know in advance that you won't enjoy it, explain why. If he wants to see a certain movie, but you have either already seen it or you know for certain that it's not your type of film, say so. The point is stand up for yourself in a gentle, charming, and respectful way. Finally, it's good to know what you want, know when to ask for it, and also know when to give in to the moment at hand. Be open to give and take. This "dance of truth" will keep your relationship alive and real for as long as the two of you are willing to follow these steps.

COMMUNICATION TIPS

The Power of Words

A careless word may kindle strife;
A cruel word may wreck a life.
A bitter word may hate instill;
A brutal word may smite and kill.
A gracious word may smooth the way;
A joyous word may light the day.
A timely word may lessen stress;
A loving word may heal and bless.
                                        —Unknown

Listening is the first rule in good conversation. You learn very little by talking, especially about the man you're with. You can learn only when you *listen.* If you're interested, you become interesting.

Try to empathize and relate. If you get a chance, watch Larry King and Oprah Winfrey. Pay close attention to these interview experts—how they listen to their guests. They hear every word that's spoken and they are keenly attentive to body language. They appear to really care and relate to what their guest is saying and feeling. All the good talk-show hosts listen more than they talk. They also ask poignant questions that help bring out the true personality of the guest.

Eye contact is your greatest ally in communication. It will tell your partner everything he needs to know. Talk with your eyes. It's sexy, mysterious, and pro-voc-a-tive. Some of the greatest female stars on the silver screen spoke volumes with their eyes alone: Greta Garbo, Marlene Dietrich, Lauren Bacall, Bette Davis, Barbara Stanwyck, and Merle Oberon to name a few. Rent some of their films and watch carefully how expressively they talked with their eyes. You'll learn a lot. When you're at a party, on a date, or dining with friends, always maintain good eye contact. But please don't stare. That's rude. It makes a person uncomfortable, unless your goal is playing a Bacall with Bogart. Otherwise, make eye contact frequently while out with your partner and don't look over his shoulder at all the handsome hunks that grace the place. That's insecure behavior. If you don't want to be with a particular man, don't be with him!

Always, always share your *sense of humor*. If you can make a man laugh, he will open up to you in ways you never dreamed. Men adore women who can make them laugh. With laughter, they can relax, be themselves, and forget about performance anxiety. Haven't you ever noticed that most of the truly great men in the world are not with the most beautiful women? They seem to gravitate toward attractive, smart women who have good energy and a terrific sense of humor. Langston Hughes said, "Humor is what you haven't got when you ought to have it." How true it is.

But having a sense of humor is not enough if the

other person doesn't get it. Your humor must be transmitted by making your partner aware of it, either by word or by gesture. Laughter will be your friend at any time, any place. And keeping a sense of humor will get you through the night. Laughter is an aphrodisiac. It removes all darkness and brings in the light.

Be aware that everyone has a different sense of humor. I often watch Mary Matalin on CNBC and Jane Wallace on FX. I love their wit. Mary's is a bit cynical and dry. Jane's is hearty and robust. These ladies never fail to make me laugh whether the subject is politics, human interest, or the weather. Because of their humor, I'm more interested in their subject. You can gather more admirers with honey and humor than vinegar and sarcasm.

At a party: what to talk about. Parties are difficult at best, especially cocktail parties. I hate small talk. Don't you? It's boring, but one must learn a few essential conversation starters or be left in a corner . . . alone. First, look around the room and assess the crowd. Awareness . . . remember? See if you can spot a small group of people who look inviting rather than clannish or snobby. If you see a friendly few (or one will do), walk up and listen for a few minutes. Maybe a person with manners will try to bring you into the conversation. Otherwise, pick a key moment when you feel secure and confident to join the subject at hand, either by adding something pertinent or asking an intelligent question.

For example, if the group is talking about the hottest new movie, you might add what you found interesting about a certain scene, or if you haven't seen it, ask the group what they found interesting about it and why they think you should see it. It could be a discussion about a popular book. If you have read it, tell your point of view, and if you haven't, ask others to describe theirs. The same applies to a variety of subjects such as politics, real-estate, the arts, the stock market, and even business.

One of the best ways to coax a person into further conversation is to be genuinely interested. Demonstrate your sincere interest by asking follow-up questions. Then contribute an observation that shows you have been affected by what has been said. For example, I hear daily that someone is moving out of Los Angeles, and I usually know the reason. But I'm still curious and pursue the line of inquiry in order to advance the conversation. Oftentimes, answers that are expected become more interesting by sheer elaboration, but also each person has a different point of view on any given subject that I find quite stimulating.

Most all human beings have something engaging to offer, if you just give them a chance. And people, in general, love to talk. So don't be afraid to get the ball rolling. When you graciously supply any person with the opportunity to express himself, you will be *remembered*.

Chapter 2

●●●

What Men Want . . . And Don't

Licence my roving hands, and let them go
Behind, before, above, between, below.
    —JOHN DONNE,
       "TO HIS MISTRESS GOING TO BED"

WHAT MEN WANT

But I, being poor, have only my dreams;
I have spread my dreams under your feet;
Tread softly because you tread on my dreams.
  —W. B. YEATS,
    "HE WISHES FOR THE CLOTHS OF HEAVEN"

Usually what you think men want is not what they really want. In fact, what *they* think they want is not what they really want either. In the musical film *My Fair Lady*, Rex Harrison as Professor Higgins wonders why women (specifically, Eliza) can't be more like men (more specifically, and ideally, him). Higgins can understand men and their actions and their thinking, but he is genuinely perplexed by Audrey Hepburn's Eliza Doolittle, the woman with whom he has unexpectedly fallen in love.

On a bet and with Henry Higgins's instruction, Eliza turns into a beautiful, desirable, and educated woman. Suddenly, Professor Higgins's world is topsy-turvy. But she, too, has fallen in love with him and she wants more . . . a commitment. The metamorphosis is devastating to him. He wants everything to return to what it was before—when *he* was in total control and secure. It can't. Eliza has developed into a woman with her own independent mind; and he, therefore, must accept the change and take responsibility for their relationship. It's a tall order, but in the end, he matures, professes his devotion, and all is happy.

A man wants you to love him for who he really is and not a fantasy of what you want him to be. He's not perfect. Face it. Nobody is, but he is the same person you fell in love with and he can get close to some of your wishes if you only give him a chance. Make that a few chances, because it takes time for him to interpret your agenda.

Dispense with thoughts of your fella being insensitive and unloving. That's not true. He is sensitive; he is loving. He just expresses love differently from you—so differently that you might not be aware when he is expressing love.

We identify and respond in different styles, different dialects. If you didn't speak French, wouldn't you be hard put to understand when a Frenchman was desperately asking you to open the car door, because you just slammed it on his finger? You could obviously see that something was amiss, but you might not be able to see his finger in the door for the first few seconds. My neighbor Keith did it to his dog. The poor dog was wailing in pain before Keith realized that the dog's tail was caught in the closed door. In turn, a man just wants you to take a few minutes and try to read the interpretations before reacting critically to anything he does. For this, you need to become "bilingual"—fluent in his style of communicating and your own. You see, we've had this habit of miscommunicating for centuries; and now, we are finally making a conscious effort to improve at one another's language. There's a lot of hope in this possibility. It does work. But only if both partners are willing to spend the rest of their lives in so doing.

A man does not wish to be categorized with other men. He wants to be an individual. He wants you to appreciate that he's not like the man next door. Or your favorite movie stars. He doesn't have the body of Arnold Schwarzenegger, the face of Mel Gibson, the charm of Kevin Costner, the ruggedness of Clint Eastwood, the sensuality of Antonio Banderas, the style of Denzel Washington, or the humor of Billy Crystal—he's simply himself and wants to be appreciated *for* himself, that's all.

Calling a man a sexist—*just because*—is wrong. Maybe he appears to be a sexist outwardly, but that does not necessarily mean he is one. Because of a man's conditioning, he has a different outlook on life, habits that constitute who he is and what he thinks. He probably learned this behavior from his father (if, in fact, he had one when he was growing up) or an uncle, grandfather, or other major male figure. He may not know any better. So don't accuse him of being a sexist until you investigate the situation thoroughly.

It's unrealistic for a woman to expect a man to react to love and sex in the same way she does. His senses of seeing, touching, smelling, tasting, and hearing do not respond the same way yours do. To begin with, he sees things differently from you. His mind is more compartmentalized and geared more toward the visual, the mechanical, and the nuts and bolts of a thing and orienting an object in space. The two of you can look at the same object, and I can almost guarantee you will see it differently. You are more likely to notice subtle variations of color and texture, while he will tend to see its shape and size. If you share your observations, you will be surprised at how different they can be. You might even wonder if you and he were looking at the same object. Try it sometime. It's fun. But more important, you'll gain more insight into his character. *Observe!*

Second, his sense of touch is a bit more aggressive than yours. Even though he's gentle and tender, he may often seem more overtly assertive. (Testosterone, you know—that driving force!) Just observe the way the male gender plays with an infant. Different! I've seen my friend Andy toss his kid in the air and I nearly had a heart attack before that baby was back in his arms. Whew! What I thought was a close call was just daily behavior. Not all men play with their children in this way, but many do.

Smell and taste fall into similar categories—he may find certain things ravishing, while you may think they're rancid. It's almost as if men have different olfactory systems and palates installed. I've watched my fella drink milk that was, let's just say, past the date on the carton. He didn't even notice that the milk was a bit sour. He drank it anyway.

Furthermore, a man tends to hear dialogue in sound bites—in "bottom line" terminology. If you're going on and on explaining how your can opener works, he's thinking, "What's the point? Get to the point already!" That's his reaction to lengthy conversations that travel in circles.

Men also tend to speak unvaryingly, unwaveringly, without taking many pauses; and oftentimes, they get loud when expressing themselves. Their oversell is usually due to the sheer excitement of wanting to impress you, and you guessed it . . . testosterone! An example: I have a friend named Don, whom I dearly adore and would do anything for, but Don goes on so. He could be talking to a ficus bush for the little I contribute to the conversation. His enthusiasm tends to run unbridled, and once he gets on a roll, look out! I feel like a cheerleader again, "Go, Don, go! Go for the touchdown!" Since I care about him, I've suggested that he relax and breathe when he talks. He's a wonderful person; it's just that his enthusiasm is a bit overwhelming. He has taken my suggestions, and his communicative skills have improved immensely.

If you have a similar problem, explain to your man that you would understand him better if he would take

a few more pauses and lower his tone before continuing. And, in turn, you practice to be open and positive
when listening to him and trying to get your point
across. That's the key.

Women tend to speak in varying tones and take a
lot of pauses, usually asking, "Don't you think?" (I do
that one a lot!) "Isn't that right?" "You know what I'm
saying?" or "Shouldn't we?" Men, on the other hand,
use "umm" or "well" as a filler to formulate a thought.
Neither sex has the market cornered on filler phrases.
But men, categorically, may assume that you're either
looking for an answer or some kind of approval, when
actually you're just being nice by trying to involve them
in conversation.

We're not really asking a question with our spicy
phrases, do you think? We're speaking in female
tongue, using both sides of our brain. It's how we relate. It works. Why not use the same technique for the
opposite sex? Because it doesn't work, that's why. So,
bottom line: Men want us to make a conscious effort
to relate in their tongue when addressing them by
speaking a little more solidly. You know, the way they
do! Clarity of speech is a win for everyone.

These men obviously have a valid point: If you
want to be heard, you need to speak the male tongue.
It takes practice. When you wish to make a point, lower
your pitch, raise your volume, and stick with the topic
at hand. They'll love you for it; and, of course, they'll
hear you every time. Another sound practice is to praise
your man and give constructive advice on how to rem-
edy a situation. Think before you speak. Don't criticize.

Jerry, thirty-two, a bank clerk in a Boise, Idaho,
said, "I want a woman who can not only tell me what
she doesn't like, but who can also offer some good suggestions as to fixing the problem. I'm not a mind reader.
I can never come up with a solution that makes her

happy. I don't like being told that something's not working. Just tell me how to fix it."

Another bit of sound information toward relating: it's really hard for a man to sit and listen for long periods of time, unless you're entertaining him in a way he enjoys. For example, when I give talks to a group of men, I carefully observe their body language and the expression in their eyes and on their face. No matter how interesting you think your subject is, they may not. Even when the subject is fascinating, most men have a difficult time sitting still for too long. They start to fidget; then slump in their chairs; then yawn; then look around; then look at their watches; and then . . . you've lost them! Before it gets to slumping-in-the-chair time, I try to do and say something exciting to once again capture their attention. It usually works, but it's challenging to continually shift when they shift. It takes a lot of energy.

Once you are more aware of male-female styles, you can amend your behavior patterns to fit his—a natural talk mate will appear, seemingly like magic. We all have a different point of view on any given subject. So we must try harder to understand the other's point of view. By watching his body language and listening with trained ears, we will be on the road to a better understanding of the masculine sex.

Now, there are those few who will think anything you say or do is interesting and exciting. They will hang on every word you utter, every motion you make, believing every nuance makes perfect sense. Conversing will be like slicing butter. But that's uncommon. And bless those chosen few!

The language difference between men and women extends to the expression of humor as well. Male humor is generally a tad brash compared to the more gentle female humor. They don't mean to be offensive; they simply perceive the world differently from you. Their style of humor often involves teasing you verbally, kidding with you like kids play in the backyard, jostling—a few pokes in the ribs, an inoffensive shove, an elbow wherever it reaches. It's a man's way of showing acceptance. He likes you! (You might think, "Please don't like me so much, I need that shoulder!") And when he clamps down on your knee in jest with iron fingers that cause paralyzing pain, he's only kidding.

In their small talk, men prefer talking about external things—sports, politics, current events, late-night talk shows, or their job. Women prefer to tell funny stories or reveal something personal—maybe even a secret. When a man makes a remark that he obviously thinks is funny and you find somewhat odd—pause—reevaluate. Rather than responding angrily, recognize it for what it was meant to be and accept it. Smile and go on. Don't sweat the small stuff when there are greater things awaiting your attention.

So much of understanding another person involves the simple consideration of his point of view and his circumstance—turmoil included. Ronnie, forty-eight, a playwright living in Hoboken, said, "I want a woman who values my work. As a writer I might go for months without making any money. I can manage if I budget properly. I don't need a woman to make snide remarks when I'm out of work, put down my manhood, and make light of my profession. I may seem selfish and egotistical, but I love my work, and the amount of income it generates at a given moment is not the only measure of its value. I want a little respect for the hard work I do and loneliness that I must endure in order to succeed." He's obviously come into contact with too many women who measure a man's worth by the money he brings home. A woman of quality would understand that talent, integrity, discipline, and hard work are attributes to cherish and praise, and will most likely lead to stability and comfort.

Kenneth, twenty-six, an oil rigger from Santa Fe, had this to say: "I don't want my wife to make me responsible for her happiness, nor do I want her to tell me how much she's sacrificed for me and the kids. If I hear the word *sacrifice* one more time, I think I'll stay in Saudi Arabia and never come home. I do plenty of sacrificing, too. She doesn't realize that I hate being away all the time. Living on planes is no picnic. She shouldn't make me feel guilty for what I can't do. I can only do so much. There's nothing wrong with a little encouragement once in a while. It sure would help." What a shame that Kenneth's wife was so involved in her own situation that she failed to see and appreciate what a heavy load her husband was carrying. She should have been his greatest cheerleader, not his most vitriolic critic.

Mike, thirty-one, an insurance salesman from Chicago, declared, "My wife is always complaining that I don't bring home enough money. I do the best I can. Some months are slow. I come home to a dirty house most of the time—dishes in the sink, clothes all over the place. She could pitch in, too. Even if she took a temp job, it would help. If you love the other person, you do your part—whatever it takes, right? I mean, if I was playin' baseball all day, sure she'd have a right to complain, but I'm busting my ass on the street trying to solicit customers. Most of the time my feet are killing me and I'm dog tired. And what do you think she's doing when I get home? Painting her toenails and watching soaps, that's what she's doing!" Mike is frustrated that his wife isn't holding up her end of their partnership. They're in a rowboat together and she's not pulling her oar. Neither one of them will get where they want to go if she continues to behave like a passenger.

When one partner crosses over the line of what's right and what's wrong, what's fair and what's not, then the other one will eventually balk. "I've had enough!" So either you do something about it or you get out. It's essential to know that a relationship is a lot of give-and-take, but mostly giving. It's never fifty-fifty. Sometimes it's sixty-forty. Sometimes it's eighty-twenty. There will be times when you give more, and he takes more.

I know guys who only give forty percent all the time, and they actually think they're giving sixty or more. One spouse will always do more than the other. But people shouldn't "keep score." Keeping score erases love. Giving should be a joy and receiving a pleasure.

The more I listen to men today, the more I realize how hard they try to understand us and give us what we want, in their own way. They often appear like Forrest Gump bumbling around in a dark closet and coming out with one shoe, but how are they expected to know anything on the female level if nobody taught them?

A man's behavior patterns and training have been passed down through centuries. The manner in which he acts and reacts is spontaneous to his training and behavior patterns. And retraining involves a lot of time and patience on everyone's part—yours and his. Luckily, the willing men are getting the message, but they need time to absorb, filter, and process. Their masculine map-reading minds are busily at work investigating the puzzle of our female needs. They definitely deserve an A for effort because there are too many men who never have tested and never will test the waters. Consider your man exceptional if he has the desire to please, to investigate, to try. Bless his heart, his body, and his goodness!!

MALE PSYCHE—HOW MEN THINK AND WHY

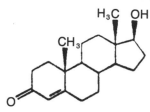

—chemical structure of testosterone

Ahhh . . . men!!! Why do you think men do what they do? What do you think makes a man behave in that foreign way that has eluded us for years? I've asked myself that question many times. After studying descriptions by psychiatrists, psychologists, physiologists, anthropologists, and social scientists who described the male psyche to the nth degree, I closed the books, sympathizing with Lord Byron when he complained, "I wish he would explain his explanation."

The information I found was so intricate and technical, I was more confused than ever. So I decided to write this chapter in fairly simple terms—partly because I was curious myself, and partly because I wanted you to understand your own man or the one you would like to have in your life.

Unraveling the male psyche and all the ingredients of his potent porridge—his fabric, texture, smell, smile, walk, talk, ups, downs, ins, and outs—will certainly add some titillating pleasure, but let's get real. The essential distinction between a man and a woman can—first, last, and always—be summed up in a single word: *testosterone*.

It's important to know that even among scientific experts much controversy exists about the specific behavioral effects of this hormone. No wonder we're confused! Classic theory relates aggression with excess testosterone. On the contrary, recent studies by endocrine scientists from U.C.L.A. suggest that male aggressiveness is actually related to a testosterone deficiency. I, along with many other experts, believe that it increases the sex drive and makes one physically stronger. But who knows what the truth really is?

Dr. Collins, a gynecologist in New York City, explains how this chemical influences and directs a man's behavior: "A man wants to deposit sperm wherever he can, to procreate the species. Now, I look at the body as being a survival machine for the genes' DNA. DNA's primary function is to duplicate itself, and over the billions of years that life has been on earth, the tissue around the genes are just machines which enable these genes to multiply and divide. As far as males are concerned, they seem to have one basic function and that is to deposit sperm. The main function of the female is to receive the sperm. To reproduce. Anything else is our conditioning, our culture. Even marriage is a blending into society. Polygamy or monogamy—there is nothing right or wrong about it. It depends on how you were brought up, where, and your attitude. Men, basically, when depositing sperm, don't care who they deposit it with!"

Now that we've identified man's primary hormonal driving force, let's look a little further into the composition of his personal symphony. Other than his mighty testosterone, he's tuned to an amalgam of the society in which he lives, his environment, his culture, male peer pressure, parental expectations, formative nurturing, subjective goals, and, of course, let's not forget, his genes.

This concoction is directed by guideposts he uses throughout his maturing stages. Early in life he develops heroes, living or dead, that provide guidance for his growth. As he matures, the intensity of his aspirations does not change. It merely orients itself to more worldly events. Deep inside, he imagines his role in gallant, chivalrous ways. He lifts his goddess onto a marble pedestal and adores her. He sees her as perfect, wants her to be perfect, and places her image on the hood of his car, boat, plane, or spacecraft. He writes, sculpts, makes music, poetry, or just dances, or makes plain loud noises, with her as his inspiration. He carries her image in his wallet, his mind, and heart, and he tries to imagine how life would be in her company.

So he strives throughout his adolescence and manhood to grow, to learn, to be successful, to conquer it all, and then put it at the feet of this strange creature he loves—his ideal woman. But it's a struggle. He knows he has to mature and succeed first. All through that process of growing and striving for success, his relationships with women are very rocky, filled with ups and downs, with momentary successes and fleeting failures. If he does something right and succeeds, he wants to be close to her. If he has setbacks or failures, he pulls away in despair and solitude. Women should recognize these deep, inner aspirations instead of regarding them as unstable thought patterns. In so doing, she can provide the steady companionship that will foster his hopes and nurture them into a mature reality within a solid relationship.

Setting aside some of his deeper fantasies, you can begin to understand a man by discerning his distinctly male attitude toward life. There are several fundamental aspects to consider, but the most salient needs of a man are *RECOGNITION* and *ACCEPTANCE*. All the rest will fit into these two main categories.

A man must have recognition to feel that he's part of society. When he gains recognition, he needs to know that his family will affirm his credibility. These days, it's much more difficult than it was years ago. Then, the road to recognition was easier. It was more prevalent for both father and mother, working as a unit, to guide their son into a useful profession. Role models began at home in that less fragmented era.

Today, parents still influence their children, but innumerable divorces have loosened the foundation of family structure. Suffice it to say, there are an increasing number of obstacles involved in the happy integration of males into society. But given certain inherent aptitudes, a man can gear himself toward success at something—with one of his main motivators being the acquisition of recognition—even if that means role-playing.

If his true vocation coincides with the role, then he is whole and happy. But if he has geared himself toward a profession that is not attuned to his true self, he gains success and recognition, but then realizes sometime later in life that there is another self inside crying out for fulfillment. It's safe to assume that most men, in one way or another, are playing a role. They display two characters: one on the inside and one on the outside. The real person underneath will always be there, but he plays a role when confronting society. This may explain the seeming anomaly of the proverbial physicist who plays the violin, the architect who wields chessmen, and the statesman who strokes his paintbrush at the easel. They all have artistic impulses and inclinations which they've had to suppress in order to become successful professionals driven by a need for recognition.

So today's male plays a successful, professional role on the outside and for each friend, and for himself; thus becoming the complex triad of characters as explained before—the one he shows others, the one he thinks he is, and the one he really is.

Okay, ladies, here's where you come in. When a woman falls in love with her man and gives him acceptance, she gets under his skin. He feels and appreciates that she cares. Now you can see why the marrying woman doesn't have to be a sex bomb. She only needs to know how to please her man. She laughs at his jokes, even if she's heard them a hundred times; she *sometimes* fakes orgasms (as long as she has the real ones often enough), she coos on the phone when he calls, and sings his praises, saying, "Oh, how great, how intelligent." He feels accepted and loved. He needs it. Every man needs that acceptance. Every present he brings her she praises. If he brings one rose, she puts it in a vase, shows it off, smells it. She makes a big deal of his small gift and then the next time, he brings a bouquet of them. He feels accepted. He feels that he's done something right, so he makes progressively greater gestures. He does what he can to feel accepted.

And so, we see the same pattern within his social role. He studies whatever is required to be somebody —anything to be recognized. Then, after the recognition he needs acceptance. The potential trap is the acquisition of one without the other. There are many famous and well-to-do people, instantly recognizable, but totally miserable because they don't feel genuinely accepted.

What comes of this recognition and acceptance? It gives a man his *self-esteem*. There exists a harmonious integration of all three of these states that blossoms fully in the well-adjusted man. If you as a woman can understand that a man needs to feel good within himself, you will foster his self-esteem. This is the glue that helps bind your marriage. A woman of encouragement might say, "Look, it's going to be fine. You're striving.

I love you. We'll work it out." If she makes him feel good about himself, he should succeed.

However, even if a woman loves a man, but constantly nags at him ("Oh, you're wrong. Look at the neighbors. They're doing better than we are. Why can't we have a swimming pool?"), she chips away at his self-esteem. And that can trigger highly destructive behavior.

So if you're clever and caring and can bolster the self-esteem in your man by telling him "You're my hero," "I love you just the way you are," "Look how nicely you're dressed," "I like the way you smell" (or whatever else you find desirable and attractive about him), you make him feel good about himself and help raise his level of self-esteem.

A man needs to know that his heroine is standing in the wings watching him—doting on him when he comes offstage. She needs to praise him, to encourage positively: "You were great!" And when she's routinely not there, he eventually will find acceptance elsewhere. Please understand that helping your mate is in no way demeaning. His potency—physical, mental, and material—is directly related to yours. Your rewards are as great as his. And what wouldn't you do for your best friend in life?

Having examined healthy aspects of the male psyche—the need for recognition, approval, and self-esteem—let's explore some of the less savory aspects in order to recognize telltale signs, so that positive and timely action may be taken to ward off unwanted consequences.

The need to be right, even when wrong (très important): Consider the usual sequence of events at an automobile accident. Usually, regardless of fault, each party will accuse the other. Two people will get out of their cars and start yelling about the other's fault—not recognizing their own. "Look what you made me do! Your fidgeting distracted me and now I've hit a telephone pole!" The perpetrator knows he's wrong, but will still fight to accuse the other person. This behavior finds its way into contemporary battles when a lawyer offers the best defense in the form of offense, regardless of justice. This type of mentality is ancient—seeing the speck in his brother's eye when a plank is lodged in his own. So, girls, keep your eyes open! He'll be certain to appreciate the one woman in the world with eyesight good enough to see that he's right when everybody else thinks he's wrong.

The propensity to make false claims and/or coopt others' work (importare): In his continuing quest for acceptance and recognition, a man can brag undeservedly about accomplishments that are not his own. "Fish stories" are legendary. He falsely expands the day's catch from a few bluegills to a bag full of prize-winning trout. He can turn personal losses at a Las Vegas outing into an armful of blue chips. My girlfriend's husband boasted that he had shot an eight-point buck while hunting in Montana, but we discovered that he didn't even see one! Do you think my girlfriend let her husband know that she knew? Not a chance.

If a man buys something in the market, brings it home, doctors it up, and exclaims, "Look what I cooked!" he only wants to be your "hot fudge sundae" with a little admiration and acceptance sprinkled on top. Granted, many men who invent a life full of half-truths are bad eggs, but there are quite a few lovable ones who just don't know any better. My uncle, for example, was a portrait painter and jazz musician who never left Mississippi, but he told great stories of adventures that took him around the globe, and those stories gave joy to my aunt and the rest of us. Who cares that they weren't strictly (or even approximately) true?

A terrific example of coopting another man's heroics that you can visually enjoy is in the film *True Lies*. It was beautifully enacted by the actor Bill Paxton, who was trying to win the affections of Jamie Lee Curtis. He drove a red Corvette, imitating the real heroics of her husband Arnold Schwarzenegger, but his clever antics were humorously uncovered.

The distorted need for power (muy importante): Society is replete with examples of excess and abuse of power. Too many men are obsessed with a pathological need to control and/or "win." Remember the film *Dangerous Liaisons*, when John Malkovich dueled with Keanu Reeves over a mindless matter? This winning obsession was certainly not worth a life. But with the flick of a blade . . . finito.

Even when the results aren't fatal, these abuses can ruin reputations and careers as the stakes rise. In certain criminal circles . . . *whack*, your man may lose his "humdinger," or his life! Extreme examples, I agree, yet they can and do happen. So be sure to keep a close eye on your man and his manhood. Even when it's not in danger, it's worth watching.

The lack of humor, aka the inability to take a joke: A relationship with a man who lacks a sense of humor takes an extraordinary amount of hard work. Take some time to evaluate whether he's worth all that trouble before you take him on. A man who lacks humor may be unsure of himself or even clinically paranoid. If the paranoia is deep-seated, it may be unalterable. However, most men are less damaged and you can gently lead them to the lighter side of life by your own example. Inspire your man by taking your motto from Rabelais: "For all your ills I give you laughter," or simply, "If your man needs a smile, give him one of yours." Smiles can be as contagious as yawns, so share them.

Having reviewed some of the negatives of the male

psyche, it's important to realize that each of these de-fects manifests a need—a need to believe he's made the right decisions and taken the right actions in life; a need to be congratulated for his accomplishments (small ones as well as big); and a need to know you are aware of and even honor his male potency. I don't think that's asking too much as a price for lasting relationships, do you?

After all, don't they do as much for us? They'll even go so far as to pretend to not only admire but also follow our own eating fads. A while ago on a late night talk show, I once heard Alec Baldwin, the incredibly handsome, funny, and bright actor, admit that he some-times "fakes about food" for his gorgeous wife. She's a vegetarian; so is he (except that once in a while, he gobbles down a few McDonald's hamburgers). Richard Gere, another terrific-looking and sexy actor, says that he has often played a similar gallant role with women: "If *she wanted* me to be a vegetarian, I *was* vegetarian. If she wanted me to eat meat, I ate meat. I would do anything to woo her. Then I would hide in my room and smoke cigars and go out with the boys for beer and steak." You see, we all extend ourselves to please one another, if we feel the prize is worth it.

Be careful here that you don't let your desire to please lead you to disguise, distort, or mutilate your own character and personality. In the long run, if you do not display your true colors, you run the risk of his falling in love with your disguise and not you.

For your part, study your man! Find out all you can about his good and bad traits. Look at them real-istically and decide if you can live with his psychological makeup exactly as it is. Don't count on his changing. People never really change, they only alter a few habits—sometimes for the better, sometimes not. When you fall in love with a man, make certain you can accept his faults as much as you do his accomplishments. Because you will be living with both of them.

Once you've decided that you *can* live with his faults, don't emasculate him at home or anywhere else. Every time something goes wrong in the house—such as the plumbing, electricity, or construction—and he tries to fix it, let him! Keep your sense of humor, smile, and say to yourself, "I never did mind about the little things."

Remember that your fella wants to be your hero. So don't be too quick to call in the professionals. It's embarrassing for him and it's his house, too! Never sacrifice his ego for your desire to have things "perfect." For some reason, we tolerate atrocities from perfect strangers, pay more than eighty dollars an hour for aggravating incompetence, but refuse to endure inabilities in the man we love. Sound familiar?

If you love your man, back him up at all times. Protect him, praise him, and give him the respect he deserves. Respect his individuality, his privacy, his silence, his small victories, his mind, and traces of his soul that he leaves in all the "little things." Remember that he is emotionally fragile and he thinks of you as stronger even in your weakest moments. If you withdraw your support, he may, in his despair, begin to seek help elsewhere. And you know exactly what I mean!

LAST THOUGHTS
The evolution of a true romance is like an adventure. At the beginning there is almost a dreamlike state. The middle of an adventure is challenge and discovery. And at the end of this journey . . . elevated happiness. For a man, romance is the spirit of adventure. On the Barbara Walters show even the great John Wayne admitted to being a romantic. Men just need a little encouragement in this area.

Your man wants to be your Don Juan. It's a role where he is allowed to become more dramatic, more wondrous, more heroic, more chivalrous. It's also the most divine intersection where a man and a woman may find true union; where they may vibrate to the promise of the extraordinary. But unfortunately, a woman believes him the least in this dance of romance. Half the time, she thinks he's faking to get her into bed. Not true! That's just who he is. He's being romantic in the only way he knows how. Stay tuned in to him because he's anxiously waiting for the words: "Go slay a few dragons for me, baby!"

CLASSIC TURNOFFS

If you think you're outclassed, you are; you've got to think high to rise. You've just got to be sure of yourself—before you can win the prize.

—UNKNOWN

There are many women who are wealthy in assets and poor in love. Their days and nights are rife with disappointments—married men, men who disappear, men who are stalled in their careers or stalling in their commitments, men who tell tales and weave webs of deceit.

Why do you think these women live in misery and sabotage their own happiness for the wrong man? Either they don't like themselves and project an unattainable ideal onto the wrong man; or in their enthusiasm to turn him on, they inevitably turn him off. Wanting to please a man you like is natural, but turning every encounter into an event is a bit unnatural and a desperate approach.

Pause . . . take a deep breath—question your old approach—and be willing to change your old way of thinking. It may be time to take stock of your approach, attitudes, and behavior. See if any of the comments below sound familiar.

Never do the following to catch a man:

1. correct his grammar
2. do drugs with him
3. get breast implants
4. follow him
5. be too available
6. call him at all hours and hang up
7. criticize him
8. lie about how many men want you
9. change your appearance
10. try to appear smart while making him feel stupid
11. after a few dates, tell him you've stopped seeing others
12. sleep with him on the first date
13. starve yourself
14. spend all your money refurbishing your wardrobe
15. give yes and no answers to his questions
16. lose your identity
17. pretend to be something you're not

Simple don'ts:

1. Don't be like Glenn Close in *Fatal Attraction*. Michael Douglas was in serious lust until he realized she was nuts about him.
2. Don't be like Bonnie Bedelia in *Judicial Consent*. When she became suspicious of her husband, she fell into the arms of Billy Wirth, the first young, attractive man who chased her.

TYPES OF WOMEN MEN HATE

Winnie the Whiner

Motto: "I don't eat anything—I don't know why I'm so fat. My nose is too large, my hair is thin, I burned the dinner, and I have PMS!"

- is extremely insecure
- nothing is ever right
- complains for the sake of complaining
- finds fault with everything
- wants attention all the time
- is always depressed
- can't find a good man
- sends her dinner back, often
- always puts down other people
- thinks the world owes her a living
- can't make a decision
- blames everybody for her misfortunes
- puts herself down all the time
- looks for the easy way out
- doesn't want to work
- can't keep a job

Jane the Jealous

Motto: "She's a star because she's had plastic surgery done to every part of her body and she's married to the producer!"

- thinks she deserves the best without working for it
- is usually conceited
- whatever you've got, she wants
- can't stand to hear good news about another
- must be the center of attention
- is seriously insecure
- doesn't really like anybody, not even herself

- always compares herself to others and invariably wants what they have
- puts down anybody who is successful at anything
- is a real downer most of the time
- never trusts anyone, especially her man
- is suspicious of every woman and every man
- imagines the worst
- is overly possessive
- is usually phobic

Polly the Pleaser
Motto: "I know it's 3 A.M. and all the stores are closed, but I'll find you a chocolate bar somewhere if I have to drive to the next county!"

- is the first to volunteer
- is wishy-washy
- thinks she's boring
- allows her man to walk all over her
- is generous to a fault
- makes excuses for everything
- usually pays the check
- gives until it hurts without asking for anything
- lets the spotlight shine on everyone but herself
- is obsessed with doing good
- can't make a decision
- doesn't know where she stands on political issues or even if she liked a movie
- finds only men who take
- fools herself
- is a do-gooder
- is passive
- never argues or expresses her point of view
- doesn't know her point of view

Betty the Bitch

Motto: "Just watch me. I'll take her husband away from her without even trying!"

- is selfish
- is sarcastic
- puts everybody and everything down
- has an overblown sense of entitlement
- is always frustrated
- believes everyone should think like her
- can often be downright nasty
- takes over every conversation
- has a snide remark for every occasion
- thinks she's better than anyone
- is very angry
- will do anything to succeed—anything
- tries to change everyone
- fights, complains, blames
- is destructive
- is abrasive
- usually has no dignity or pride
- will do anything to look good
- demands a lot, usually does little in return

Cybil the Cynic

Motto: "Oh, yeah, right, he's really gonna go to the moon!"

- finds the worst in every situation
- thinks the world and all the people in it are doomed
- is pessimistic
- is sarcastic
- is always afraid
- has a sour outlook on life

- makes negative remarks
- is usually a hypochondriac
- is a frightened little girl inside
- invents reasons why she's rejected
- gives up too easily

May the Manipulator
Motto: "Look how I sacrificed for you and never asked for anything in return!" (just your life . . .)

- uses charm to manipulate
- cons everyone into doing what she wants
- inventories everyone's emotional buttons for later use
- pretends good deeds are for you, but it's always for her
- is a control freak
- needs to know everyone's business
- gives presents for entrapment
- does everything with a string attached
- tries to run everyone's life
- suffocates loved ones under the guise of love
- has fits of hysteria
- has no sense of humor
- is extremely jealous
- always does her good deeds for a price
- gossips big-time
- makes loved ones feel guilty if they don't do what she wants
- marries a man she can boss
- tries to run her children's lives

If you recognize yourself in any of the above when faced with a difficult situation, overcome the frustration, anger, or rage with constructive resolutions: recall the goals that you originally set for yourself. Think hard about what you really want. Close your eyes and picture yourself a winner—say, "I can," "I will . . ." And maintain your sense of pride by quickly doing something positive—take a walk and fill your lungs with fresh air; call a trusted friend; take five or ten minutes to reel off a few affirmations to yourself; read a pleasant passage, note card, or line of poetry that brings you harmony; play music that makes you smile; sing a song; exercise; speak lovingly to yourself: "I am a good person," "I will attract good, loving, and caring people," "I respect myself because I have accomplished a lot with hard work," "I deserve good things—a good man, a good job, a good life," "I will achieve my goals because I am focused and disciplined."

Women who are needy, anxious, and desperate to find Mr. Right are usually hearing their biological clocks running overtime; or they're lonely; or they want financial support. They're existing in an unlived life with an unrealized self-image. They need to apply emotional cosmetics by discovering values that have meaning for them, interests that involve activity, and enthusiasm for things outside their own egos. They need to find things to do by themselves and for themselves. That very neediness or anxiety or desperation to find a man communicates itself to a man as fear does to a dog. Just as a dog who senses your fear will be inclined to attack, a man who senses your anxiety and neediness will likely be turned off and run. And you will be brushing off the dust from his quick exit.

ROMANCE

A true love never tires or wanes but is with us always, like our blood, like our breath. I shall never weary of that brow nor those grey, wistful eyes.

—ABELARD TO HÉLOÏSE

More and more, men and women are returning to romance. Technological advancement, deterioration of the environment, deadly communicable disease, and ignorance of reality have catapulted us into a lonely, confused, valueless, and alienated state. We don't communicate enough on a human level anymore, so we turn to fantasy, romance, and surrealism as a substitute.

Look around. We are immersing ourselves in mechanistic fantasies and communication systems which distance us from reality. We're inundated with PCs, CDs, VCRs, TVs, CD-ROMs, cyberspace, cyber sex, virtual reality. Wow! Listen to those words! And now we've got interactive TV—talking to your television. How stimulating! Just turn on your tube for thirty minutes and channel-surf. You'll see that we have so numbed ourselves, nothing less than a stun gun to our heads will make us feel.

Today, we live out our relationships on talk shows and soaps. Beepers and car phones have taken the place of face-to-face relationships. There's rarely peace of mind. Someone is always beeping us on our cellular car phone or digital pager. We read less, we ponder less, and we interact with others less. We're surrounded and absorbed by the mechanical rather than the natural. We are slowly bankrupting our spirits as we rush to meet the future, expanding goals of technological "progress."

It's sad, but even our ability to distinguish right from wrong is eroding. In a *Los Angeles Times* interview, filmmaker-actor Robert Redford lamented: "There used to be a thing called ethics. And there was a thing called shame. It doesn't exist anymore, because corruption has become a way of life."

Of course, our modern tragedy is that we're losing our true purpose in life: living and loving, being honest and kind to each other, and tending the better angels of our nature. As we lose the awareness and practice of relating to one another, we turn to the illusory aspects of heroes and heroines, gods and goddesses—the fantastic, the mythic, and the beautiful. Lacking the human touch, we live vicariously through the symbols of media imagery, always longing and searching for the beauty of sweet romance—that realm of magic that transports us into the spiritual world where goodness, love, and hope reign supreme, forever bathed in human affection.

But what are we really searching for? Is it infatuation, romantic love, real love . . . or ourselves? That is the question. I thoroughly believe the answer lies in the happy combination of *all* these aspects of love. The attainment of true love in its highest form involves a natural progression which begins with infatuation, travels through a star-crossed romance, and culminates in real love. And along the way, we just may be fortunate enough to find the true essence of ourselves.

And yet, the road begins simply . . . with infatuation. Infatuation in itself is a trifling state. In fact, *infatuation* is defined as "a state of foolishness." But there's much more involved; it includes not only illusion and fantasy, but hope and a promise for the future.

A man gives you a glance. Hmmm . . . you've intrigued him. You're titillated, too! It progresses into good positive communication, and then . . . he asks you for a date. Yes! Finally! The moment arrives—he prepares himself nicely—he brings you a considerate little gift. He surprises you with a well-thought-out evening.

If the date goes well, he invites you on another one, or you invite him to a picnic or the theater. You soon discover that you are compatible—and sparks begin to fly!

The courtship commences with true and positive feelings, with no ulterior motives. You're just getting to know each other, finding out your likes and dislikes, your dos and don'ts. You give each other music, books, flowers, food, notes, candy, cards, tickets to special events—tokens of your affection as your relationship grows.

It leads to real commitment. As long as both of you grow in the same direction, it will develop into true love. Be sure to tell your man in a subtle and charming way what your feelings are. He can't possibly know if you don't tell him. Most men are not visionaries. So when your man brings you something thoughtful, express your appreciation, even if it's not exactly your cup of tea. It's important to encourage the romance in him. You need to show him that what he does is pleasing to you. That way you'll command the attention of *all* parts of him!

Now let's look at what we all love about love . . . romance. Romance is as old as time itself and is a form of behavior that can be traced from biblical times up to the present. The medieval era was especially noted for the celebration of "courtly love"—a chivalrous form of devotion that had its basis in the spiritual rather than the physical. Knights wooed their ladies by fulfilling service, worship, obedience, and idealization, but always from afar—always full of proper intention. They were never to suggest anything intimate or sexual; they could feel passion, but never consummate it. In this realm of the presumed ideal, love was never ordinary —always ethereal, self-effacing, calling for discipline, courage, and generosity. The fuel of the imagination was thus fed, giving rise to tales of legend, adventure, and chivalry. To this day we anoint our icons with the

Arthurian mantle. The Kennedy White House, steeped in elegance, culture, and grace, came to be known as "Camelot." Noble love has been the inspiration of literature for centuries, as evidenced by the following romantic verses:

Abelard to Héloïse: "Would that I love my God as I do you!"

Tristan to Iseult: "We shall go together to a fortunate land from which none return. There rises a castle of white marble; at each of its thousand windows burns a lighted candle; at each, a minstrel plays and sings a melody without end . . . what does death matter? You call me, you want me, I come!"

Romeo to Juliet: "Ah dear Juliet, why art thou yet so fair? Shall I believe that unsubstantial Death is amorous, and that the lean abhorred monster keeps thee here in dark to be his paramour? For fear of that, I still will stay with thee, and never from this palace of dim night depart again."

The power of the pen has amazing capacity. It can induce laughter or tears, praise or consolation. It is one of the richest allies of communication, just as beautiful Héloïse described to her lover: "What cannot letters inspire? They have souls; they can speak; they have in them all that force which expresses the transport of the heart; they have all the fire of our passions!"

It is fortunate for us that despite their innate delicacy, letters have endured. How many of us can be transported instantly to another time through a letter? Long after a conversation has dimmed, we can recapture the full blush of feelings by rereading our letters . . . or those of our predecessors. Family chests are full of such treasures. My own chest is filled with love letters from my mentor, the late sage and writer Henry Miller.

As an avid letter writer myself, I urge you to pick up your pen and communicate with your loved one or sit down at your computer and send him an E-mail. If you prefer, confide your thoughts to your own diary. You will be able to communicate feeling and thoughts that you could not or would not do on the phone or in person. Not only can you enlighten, persuade, console, compliment, fantasize, and love, but you can also turn an average affair into one of passion and romance.

With all its heroism and inspiration, the "fairy-tale" romance, steeped in fantasy, is destined to fail. Overwhelming lust and haunting passion remain unreal unless two lovers can accept one another as individuals and want what is best for the other without selfishly clinging. And what is best oftentimes means parting. Unfortunately, our attachments often latch on so tightly that they suck the living breath from both parties as they run wild and unbridled, straight into disaster. The intensity of their passion is enough to make them believe in a life of eternal ecstasy with no peace, no sleep, no food, and no thoughts that aren't of one another. These lovers would rather die than be apart for one moment. This is selfish love. When separated, they have no patience to wait. In true love, people can be separated by war, disease, or death, and wait years and years or a lifetime for each other.

Yes, it is wonderful to journey into "fantasy love," as long as you know that romantic novels, romantic stories, and romantic movies are a beautiful escape— not a reality. Most mythical lovers were "in love with love," not necessarily with each other. I've certainly been "in love with love" before I was actually in love with the man himself—flaws, foibles, and all. Haven't you? It's great for the very young, but it goes nowhere.

It can't; it's not real love. Only real love can last for an eternity—imaginary love is simply an idealistic projection.

When you're in fantasy and you think you're in reality, you're actually in confusion. A wise woman knows the difference and uses fantasy to color her world, not to confuse it. Your key is knowing the difference.

A strong caveat: *Beware the romantic user!* The romantic user will provide you with plenty of fantasy, but he will use your romantic sensibilities for his own needs. He will always be attracted by the thing he doesn't have, the place he hasn't been, the girl he hasn't met. Once he wins you over, he becomes bored, and off he goes to the next conquest. Sound familiar? He's a parasitic evil knight looking for a new paramour; and the wide-eyed innocent, longing for love and romance, is the one he will mark for his prey.

The "too good to be true" romantic man will take you to parts of your brain you have never visited and make you feel as though you were having a religious experience—a divine ecstasy that excites your molecules and titillates your rosebud. When this same "too good to be true" romantic man sweeps you into his arms and carries you up the steps of his marble castle, with melodious music filling the air and white candles lighting the way, he is spinning his magic spell by intoxicating your every sense. You are temporarily invited into a dream where he reigns supreme. He will put you on a pedestal and worship you as his queen—until you wake from your dreamlike trance and seek a commitment. Then he'll be hitting the high road to China.

Only the most hardened woman would fail to succumb to such pure magic. The way he describes a restaurant, a day, the weather, a particular event is colored with spectacular flair. He beguiles you. You wait, breath bated, until the moment he will occupy the same space with you. He learned the art of romance from every woman he encountered because he pays attention; that's his job. He captivates the emptiness of your soul with his mysterious images, his attentive charm, his colorful conversation, his transformation of the ordinary into the extraordinary. His "magic wand" perfumes the air with drama (and enlivens the bedroom with irresistible alchemy!).

He *is* your knight in shining armor, if only temporarily. He fills your vacuum with vision, but he usually lacks soul and substance to back it up. He's simply a figment of your imagination—a projection.

And because it's a selfish love, it can only destroy. So a comedy of errors ensues: a lack of commitment, empty promises, canceled dates. You know the rest.

He takes his leave of you, tramples on your love, and flits to another ingenue who yearns to lose herself in his elusive advances. He's a one-man show; a pro at dealing fantasy and illusion. And by living in fantasy alone, he's unable to graduate to a level of maturity. His relationships remain mysterious and childlike, which is fun for a while, but they cannot last. Inevitably he leaves you with a broken heart and plenty of self-doubt.

So if you happen to fall "in love with love," and with a man who takes you on a magic carpet ride of unrealistic visual beauty . . . don't stop to think, *run*! This man is unable to reveal his true self, because the "self" is missing. The actor in him is a superlative and opulent delight, but the man is an emotional retard.

No one can maintain insatiable passion, devout charm, and intense adoration for too long. Intense emotions at a fever pitch are unnatural. But they can lead to love if you guide them properly. If a man is true, his romantic endeavors will be directed toward commitment and a lasting relationship. All of his actions will make good sense. He will have forgiveness, understanding, care, concern, and compassion. He will look beyond the externals and see only the beauty and goodness in you—for he is your "knight in shining armor."

To avoid getting caught in an illusory web woven by an "evil knight," you must respect yourself, even if that means redefining your values and changing your old patterns. *Don't deceive yourself!* Infatuation without an afterlife is a lonely life.

Ask yourself the big question: "Is he gonna be there when the going gets tough?" Hard times are getting harder. You must stay away from that endless journey toward the perfect man, the perfect relationship, the perfect marriage, the perfect friendship, the perfect job, the perfect diet, the perfect table setting, and the perfect penis. Because perfect means entirely without fault— flawless. I certainly don't know anyone without a defect. Do you? In fact, defects can actually be charming. Think of Clark Gable's large ears. It added to his strength of character and made him appear more manly. Sly Stallone's lazy bottom lip does not prevent him from being a great kisser, as Sharon Stone will attest.

The point I'm making is don't be blinded by outward beauty and brawn. Look to a good man who is worthy of your devotion. Search for someone who's at home—his door open, his smile inviting, and his fireplace crackling with the fresh smell of real wood to warm your hands and ease your heart.

Yes, life should include passion, a positive attitude, and a vivid and active imagination. And I will strongly encourage hopes and dreams and fantasies. We desperately need them. But it is unhealthy to live only in your imagination. You need to experience the beauty of life with a complete person who can give love as well as receive.

There are men who instinctively know the art of true and meaningful romance, but they are uncommon. If you find one, nurture the relationship. Never lose your own sense of giving, caring, and romance—moonlight, candlelight, champagne, roses, little thoughtful gifts, poetry, music, lovely scents, sensual foods, eroticism, a walk on the beach holding hands, sitting on a mountain watching the sunset, sharing an ice-cream cone, or appreciating nature together. You can keep real love alive long after the initial infatuation and heated passions fade.

Here are some off-the-cuff romantic notions:

- writing love letters and love notes
- kissing the nape of the neck and shoulders
- getting caught in a snowstorm
- a late supper of cheese and champagne
- leaving love and sex notes in a trail to the bed
- sharing hors d'oeuvres and desserts
- sleeping nude
- erotic lingerie
- a feel under the table at a divine restaurant
- outdoor comfortable sex
- a garden café
- a bunch of handpicked wildflowers
- falling asleep spoon fashion
- surprise gifts (a book, CD, music box)
- flirtatious looks across a crowded room
- slow dancing
- walking in the rain
- waiting a long time for sex
- wearing a part of his clothing
- a marriage proposal

- long, lingering, seductive kisses—anywhere, everywhere
- a warm hug
- touching your face tenderly
- phone calls just because
- thoughtful gestures
- inventiveness—ingenuity to make something unexpected out of nothing.

Remember: age has no bearing on romance—on the enjoyment of things shared. These experiences should be nourished and cultivated. Romance is a simple way of celebrating the beautification of the senses—seeing, touching, smelling, tasting, and hearing.

True love: What does "true love" mean to you? Saint Paul, who is not generally thought of as a romantic figure, had a real handle on the subject. We learn from him that love is unconditional; patient and kind; never jealous; never boastful or conceited; never selfish or rude; never offensive or resentful; ready to excuse, to trust, to hope, to support, to endure whatever, and will last forever.

Eighteen centuries later, Elizabeth Barrett Browning gave us a feminine perspective:

How do I love thee? Let me count the ways.
I love thee to the depth and breadth and height
My soul can reach, when feeling out of sight
For the ends of Being and ideal Grace.
I love thee to the level of everyday's
Most quiet need, by sun and candle-light.
I love thee freely, as men strive for Right;
I love thee purely, as they turn from Praise.
I love thee with the passion put to use
In my old griefs, and with my childhood's faith.

I love thee with a love I seemed to lose
With my lost saints.—I love thee with the breath,
Smiles, tears, of all my life!—and, if God choose,
I shall but love thee better after death.

Love is the sunshine of the soul. Without giving
love or being loved, we grow old and bitter. Love colors
the world in vibrant hues and gives us a reason to be
happy. It sweetens distasteful experiences and softens
jealousy and selfishness that is also intrinsic in human
nature.

When true love guides your actions, the ego is not
important; the well-being and protection of the other
person is. We value and honor their worth as a human
being, are considerate of them, care for them, and support them for who and what they are.

Love inspires loyalty. Henry Miller, writer and
sage, used to say: "Love is complete and utter surrender. That's a big word, *surrender*. It doesn't mean letting people walk all over you, take advantage of you.
It's when we surrender control, let go of our egos, that
all the love in the world is there waiting for us. Love is
not a game, it's a state of being."

In conclusion here is one of the most profound and
beautiful expressions that any man could ever give to a
woman. I cherish this letter from Henry and share it
with you in the hope that you will understand what it
meant and still means to me.

May 29, 1980

And now, . . . madly in love with a young woman
who writes me the most extraordinary letters, who loves
me to death, who keeps me alive and in love (a perfect love
for the first time), who writes me such profound and
touching thoughts that I am joyous and confused as only

a teenager could be. But more than that—grateful, thankful, lucky. Do I really deserve all the beautiful praises you heap on me? You cause me to wonder exactly who I am, do I really know who and what I am? You leave me swimming in mystery. For that I love you all the more. I get down on my knees, I pray for you, I bless you with what little sainthood is in me. May you fare well, dearest Brenda, and never regret this romance in the midst of your young life. We have been both blessed. We are not of this world. We are of the stars and the universe beyond.

Long live Brenda Venus!

God give her joy and fulfillment and love eternal!

Henry

Chapter 3

....

*How to
Get Started*

SETTING THE STAGE FOR SEX

She walks in beauty, like the night
Of cloudless climes and starry skies;
And all that's best of dark and bright
Meet in her aspect and her eyes.
　　　　　　　　　　—LORD BYRON

Napoléon Bonaparte is the greatest conqueror of all time, but do you know who conquered him long before Waterloo? The exotic Josephine. Do you know how? By using the art of seduction, flair, panache, intelligence, and an eye attentive to detail, Josephine beguiled Napoléon's senses. No other woman had captured both his heart and male member quite so passionately—and for that, he crowned her empress.

One thing we can say about Josephine . . . she was *prepared*! Preparation for their lovemaking was a lavish production. She made it her business to find out all of Napoléon's likes and dislikes. Her choices were his choices. She planned the romantic interlude using all of *his* favorite objects, which appealed to *his* senses. Doing it for herself would have defeated her purpose.

When Napoléon arrived for an evening, she would have his favorite incense smoldering through the air, perfume generously sprayed onto chaise longues, candles burning in chandeliers and throughout the house. Rivers of flowers strewn from the front door, up the staircase, into her bedroom, and finally covering the bed where they lay. His favorite champagne iced in solid silver served in fine crystal glasses. The powerful aphrodisiac of music could be heard from a concealed room where several musicians played the music of his choice during the entire rendezvous. Erotic books were cleverly placed within view. Of course, food for his palate was on display everywhere his fingers could reach. Napoléon was famous for soaking in a tepid tub for hours, and Josephine would always have one ready—just the right temperature—filled with exotic oils and bubbles.

The final touch was Josephine, herself. While Napoléon soaked, Josephine would dance. Wearing only Napoléon's gifts . . . rare jewels, silks, and satins, she displayed her naked body for his pleasure. She screened her velvet skin with transparent, diaphanous fabrics while she seduced. Her breath, sweet like the nectar of succulent fruit, laced their conversation with compliments, witty remarks, news of the day, courtly humorous gossip, and always comments on his winning strategy in battle. She praised his efforts, she lifted his worn spirits, she bathed him, massaged his aching body with soothing oils, and loved his manhood on her sensual satin sheets. She treated him like an emperor long before he took the throne. That's how Josephine got Napoléon!

Cleopatra, queen of the Nile, was a little more risqué. For her true love Mark Antony, she contrived new ways to win his favors. Always swathed in the finest fabrics, finest fragrance, finest jewels, Cleopatra tantalized his imagination and his senses not only with her own divine beauty but also with a bevy of the most beautiful girls.

While lounging in her famous Titian pose, she would summon the pageantry to begin with a clap of her hands. And what followed was bloodred wine from her queendom to intoxicate Mark Antony's mind; plus a variety of exquisite-tasting foods from various countries, carried to the dining hall by muscular servants scantily clad in mere leather straps. Mixed in with these delicacies were other feminine lovelies, wearing only strawberries on their nipples and grapes on their fur. While dining, Cleopatra used her wit and cleverness to affect Mark Antony's ego. During the feast, a flood of highly sexual and erotic dances were performed with ecstatic energy. The exhibition began subtly, and built to a haunting frenzy. With plenty of spirits for his head, food for his stomach, eroticism for his eyes, and music for his ears, Mark Antony's senses had fallen madly in love with the ethereal lady.

My point in telling these tales is that one of the ways to a man's soul is through his senses—all of them: sight, smell, taste, touch, and hearing. Research his favorite tastes. Microscopically study his likes and dislikes. Maybe what you like doesn't appeal to his senses. The key is to make him feel comfortable and at home. Without prying, ask subtle questions about these particulars and pay close attention to what he doesn't say. The most important point: set the scene for *him*, not yourself.

The *right mood* can make an evening. The wrong mood can end in disaster. Color and lighting should be your first concern. Inquire about his favorite colors. If he finds certain colors offensive, don't wear them. A good rule to remember is that men tend to like whatever reminds them of nature. Colors like red, orange, and yellow remind a man of fire. The "language of love" is embroidered with the theme of fire—hot, passionate, smoldering, sizzling, burning. Fire is alive, dangerous, mysterious—the burning of embers . . . dazzling—forever changing a lover's mood. One of the most erotic nights of my life was in front of a blazing hearth. Bodies and faces look more attractive in the glow of firelight, candlelight . . . moonlight.

Creating a mood does not cost money. You need imagination and a few trade secrets: candles, music, exotic oils, delicacies for the palate, champagne or wine, and your sexy self. With little effort, parasols, rattan screens, sheer curtains, artistic pictures, and plants can also create a dramatic effect.

Even though many men often say their favorite color is blue, blue lighting is not flattering when setting a romantic mood. For romance, your skin should look like a *Playboy* photo. The photographers at *Playboy* make the girls look gorgeous by using orange filters over their cameras. You can manipulate the same effect for your skin by buying orange filters and putting them over your lamps. You'll be amazed how the flaws disappear. Or if you prefer candlelight, put all shapes of candles in your living space. (Don't depend on a single candle to light your face.)

Soft lighting, in general, is flattering to the face; red lighting casts a sexy, decadent effect; floor lighting sets a theatrical mood; and dim lighting behind a palm tree is seductive. If you're making love under a full moon in a secluded garden or your own backyard, nothing else is needed. The moon creates its own mystique.

After appropriate lighting, you need appropriate sound. What about his sense of hearing? Does he enjoy silence or music? Although music is a powerful tool for seduction, use your intuition to gauge his momentary needs. Maybe he has a clambering headache from the noise at work and all he wants to hear is silence and the music of your voice.

Music, on the other hand, has the potency of a mind-altering drug for many people. The Institute for Advanced Study of Human Sexuality in San Francisco, California, rated music the highest of aphrodisiacs. Romantic music is certainly individual. That's why you need to know his taste. To your ears Edith Piaf's "La Vie en Rose" may be the sexiest ever, but to his ears it may sound like fingernails raking across a blackboard.

Without knowing his personal likes and dislikes in music, you can only go so far. However, I'll give you a starting place to look for the music that will excite him. If you know his approximate age, try out the romantic songs that were popular when he was in his high school and college years. More often than not, he'll find them very evocative. Also, music from his cultural and social background is a good bet. Test it sometime.

Watch your favorite romantic movie and observe. Maybe it's *An Affair to Remember* with Cary Grant and Deborah Kerr, *Gone with the Wind* with Clark Gable and Vivien Leigh, *Romeo and Juliet* with the young Leonard Whiting and Olivia Hussey, or *The Age of Innocence* with Daniel Day-Lewis and Michelle Pfieffer. Turn the sound off and watch without the grandiose themes. Pretty bland, huh?

Think of creating a movie scene to please your lover. What he hears in the background while making love to you can either enrich his senses or distract them; and you don't want any distractions while trying to win his affections. So research the kind of music and the artists he listens to, especially his more sensual favorites. During lovemaking you want seductive and sultry sounds, not heavy metal, rock and roll, or rap.

Eliminate other background noises—telephones ringing, message machines clicking on and off, and a television blaring—while you're trying to win his heart.

The sense of smell is an erotic channel. Fragrant aromas can work romantic wonders on the olfactory receptors. I've noticed that more men comment on a woman's perfume nonverbally. When a lovely-looking, great-smelling lady passes by, a man's head automatically turns in her direction—following her with his eyes long after she's gone, while the scent of her perfume permeates his mind. Try putting a few drops of your perfume or favorite oil on a lit lamp bulb. The heat will disperse its fragrance over the entire room, right into his memory. I spray my perfume over my sheets hours before my man arrives, because men hate anything laden with heavy perfume and scents.

You must be very careful not to overdo. That can be distracting, too. I know the sweetest woman, named Addie, who believes that she once lived in the eighteenth century. Her house is filled with incense, scented oils, scented soaps, scented candles, and her scented self to the point where it is nauseating. She's thirty-eight and wants to marry, but unfortunately can't seem to find a man willing to tolerate the abundance of fragrance. Maybe she'll get lucky and find a man with an obstructed nasal airway. Don't overwhelm your fella with too much of a good thing.

Most men tend to like the smell of the outdoors. Fresh-cut flowers, plants, clean hair, and a freshly scrubbed body will turn him on (a dab of your favorite perfume on you and parts of your clothes). But whatever your choice, keep it moderate. When I was preparing a romantic packet for lovers for QVC, I included massage oils and lotions, soaps, incense, candles, robes, music, my S.O.S. book, and other items. Since it was a universal package, I tested hundreds of men's olfactory senses. Almost all of them preferred the less fragrant scents, the more natural-smelling ones. The richer smells seemed to make them grimace. But that doesn't apply to all men. So I suggest that you visit a bath-and-body shop with your fella and select scents that you both enjoy.

Your man's sense of taste should not be overlooked. Eating together is one of the greatest pleasures in life. It can be both sensual and seductive, depending on what you serve. First, find out what foods he likes and what foods he cannot digest. Some men have serious problems with indigestion. Take that into consideration when you display your delicious delicacies on a silver or glass tray. I don't know a man alive who doesn't enjoy a good home-cooked meal.

I spent several months in Iran once and came to understand the words of the medieval Persian poet Omar Khayyám, who gave us his romantic guide. "Here with a loaf of bread beneath the bough, a flask of wine, a book of verse, and thou beside me singing in the wilderness." Ask your man if he likes champagne and what his favorite vintages might be. Inquire about his taste in red and white wines, beer, brandy, and liquor. Some men only like dry martinis, others find the taste of fine champagne intoxicating, while some don't drink at all. In that case, you need to be inventive and serve him chilled and interesting mineral waters, sodas, or unusual fruit juices. Whatever you serve him, make sure it's what he likes.

The sense of touch can stimulate the release of endorphins—chemicals that change your moods. If he's as tense and nervous from a draining day at work as you are, mutually exchanged massages to the temples, neck, and shoulders will do wonders for you both! Use your fingers to relax his body and his mind. Try doing it rhythmically. The right rhythm can be hypnotic.

A complete body massage is heavenly. It's also a prelude to lovemaking and I will share techniques popular with seductresses and love goddesses in the next chapter.

The sense of sight is arguably the most significant erotic channel. Gazing into each other's eyes is so sensual. To appeal to his tender sight, you need visual stimuli in your home and on your body. For example: the book *Erotic Spirituality: The Vision of Konarak* is a healthy start. Each page is a wonder of sexual appetites and it's acceptable decor for your coffee table. Anyone who appreciates great art and hasn't previously viewed its pages is in for a treat.

Other sensual books by certain well-known photographers can also be a contribution to your scene-setting mood. Erotic statuettes strewn throughout your home stir attention. Mirrors in carefully chosen places are highly sexual. Subtle but provocative art hanging on your walls, fresh-cut flowers or roses in a vase, lit candles, a warm bubble bath, a large bed with lots of pillows and turned-down soft sheets are spicy for a night to remember. Be aware that there are a few extremely shy men out there. Insofar as possible, display your fine arts with his tastes in mind. You don't want to shock, you want to *please*.

Now for your person. You know he likes to look at you because you like to look at him. So give the hungry warrior something to look at. Dress with clothes that you feel comfortable wearing, but also keep in mind that they should feel sensual to his touch and be pleasing to his erotic eye. Whatever your assets, let them peek out but not fall out. Falling will come later.

Most men love stockings and garter belts, lace bras, tight or flowing dresses, clean shiny hair and body, well-kept fingernails and toenails (some men like red, some don't), a sweet mouth with no chewing gum or smoke in it (you can do that when you're alone)—in general, healthy-looking women who radiate happiness, and confidence.

If your man doesn't feel freer, more relaxed, rejuvenated, and turned on after all your consideration and fanfare, then he must be an alien!

WHERE TO FIND MEN

I do want to get rich but I never want to do what there is to do to get rich!
—GERTRUDE STEIN

Soul mate searching? He's out there. You may not even realize it, but he may be working with you side by side, or in the car next to you at a stoplight, or in a record store, or walking down the street headed in your direction. Don't be surprised. It happens! I was in Albuquerque, New Mexico, walking up a steep hill with my girlfriend Loretta, looking for some obscure restaurant that served good food. As Loretta spotted the restaurant, the most beautiful pair of sky blue eyes that I had ever seen walked out the door straight in our direction. I couldn't breathe or move. He stared at me, I stared at him, and we both felt like a bolt of lightning had suddenly hit us. Call it fate, destiny, karma, kismet, or whatever you believe. It does happen. Not very often, granted, but then it wouldn't be dynamic if it happened every day. Would it?

Your soul mate may even be the man next door whom you tease unmercifully, but because he falls short of your fantasy, you never open your heart to him. Take another look around you. By putting your mind back into your body, observing and paying attention to the little things, whoever and wherever *he* is, you'll soon see him. Maybe he's the guy who looks a little nerdy and wears glasses. Well, remember Superman? He acted a little nerdy and wore glasses. Look what happened when he took off his street clothes. *Mamma mia!*

My thirty-two-year-old friend Jamie, a cinematic art director, told me recently that she had fallen madly in love with a writer-director she worked with intermittently for four years. She said, "I never took him seriously, until we were working closely on the same film. Every morning we would find ourselves sipping coffee and laughing uproariously. He was so funny, my days passed in humor. We quickly discovered that we had a lot in common—the same sense of humor, artistic interests, music appreciation, and sensibilities. Coffee led to lunch, lunch led to dinner, dinner led to bed!"

Now they are blissfully intertwined. He asked her to marry him.

The bottom line is keep an open mind, be spontaneous, and maintain your positive attitude. When you need a pair of pliers urgently, rush off to the hardware store. You never know where he's lurking. Most fellas need hardware items. And so do you! Browse around auto supply stores and learn about your own car (how to change the oil, fix a flat tire, or enhance your car's physical appearance). Just ask some available hunk.

I met my man in an art gallery. We both appreciate art, so we had a lot to talk about. There are several art openings throughout the year usually listed in the local paper. Just put yourself together and go. You will always find someone interested in discussing art. It might be *him*.

Bookstores are definitely in fashion, even if you're not a great reader. There is always a good book you can find that will pique your interest. The library is an intriguing place for those of you who like to investigate. There is something very erotic about meeting a man in a library among all that time-honored knowledge.

I was primarily raised in the "rag" business and have watched people's behavior patterns while they shopped. For those of you who love to dress, you could easily meet the man who shares your fashion sense in a men's clothing store.

There are some women who love sports. Innumerable men hang out around athletic stores or places where baseball memorabilia is sold. Hobby and specialty stores in general cater to a variety of interests. You will find not only browsers, but hard-core collectors. And if you are interested, there is no better way to start a conversation than to ask a question. I happen to love old movies. A movie memorabilia store is a fun place to meet men interested in that subject. Men who are true collectors tend to be obsessed about their hobby. I have found that they are enthusiastic about discussing any aspect of their specific interest.

A while ago I enrolled in a computer class where I met several highly intelligent men. If you are computer oriented, then join a class. Computers are changing more rapidly than I can type. By the time you learn or buy the latest, you discover that an even more efficient system is on the market. Computers and software are endless, and you will find endless personalities from all walks of life who deal with these machines. Almost every person today either knows a bit about them or is an expert on the subject. Ask questions and learn from the lucky male.

Are you interested in gourmet food? It's amazing how many men are good cooks, many of whom enroll in cooking classes (probably looking for women friends!). I'm usually an average cook, except when I'm in love, and then I am exceptional. How about you? Doesn't love bring out the creative juices in all of us? As you know, food can be erotic and sensual. And obviously we need to eat, so why not make your gourmet delight for him?

Men involved with the preparation of fine foods are usually very sensual men. I've known a lot of professional men who are great cooks, but I've also known a lot of nonprofessional men who are superb cooks. The choice is yours. Walk through kitchen supply stores to buy your utensils. There is nothing more appealing and important than a variety of good, sharp knives in the kitchen. A kitchen without good knives is a kitchen without a good cook. Men who cook seem to be extraordinarily knowledgeable on the subject of knives. So when you see that "certain man" wandering around in the supply store, what better line of communication than to ask his advice on the best peeling knife? We all need one.

In health food stores, you will usually find healthy men. If you happen to meet a friendly face in the produce section, then make an inspiring comment about nutrition or ask a question concerning natural foods, juices, et cetera. Get the ball rolling down the aisles. Also, the same information applies at the larger supermarkets. Whether you're standing in line at the checkout stand or strolling your basket through the aisles, if you spot someone who captures your fancy, think fast. Say something innocent but clever.

Looking for a pet lover? We know women love pets, but so do most men. Men tend to love their dogs, especially the larger breeds. It's more fun for a man to roughhouse with a dog half his size than a toy-sized terrier. They can both playfully unload their aggressions. If you own a pet, you will obviously need supplies from time to time, right? Plan on spending more time than necessary at the pet store some day.

What about the Laundromat? I can't tell you how many young actors and actresses, secretaries and businessmen, musicians and music lovers, doctors, lawyers, and Indian chiefs meet at the Laundromat. You can tell a lot about a guy when you watch how he does laundry. How he folds or throws his clothes in the basket. The type of clothes he wears. Yes, indeed, you can tell a lot about a person at the Laundromat, if you're so inclined.

When I eat out alone I often take a seat at the

counter. If you are not in a hurry, eating counters are intimate and fun because there are usually other interesting people dining at the same counter. The same applies to sushi bars. I have noticed that men in general prefer eating at the counter than sitting at a table, especially during breakfast or lunch. So if you want to meet a beauty, don't stick a book in your face while you're nibbling. How is he gonna see your beautiful face when it's buried in a book?

Nowadays there are more men jogging on tracks and at parks, especially on the weekends or early mornings. I've jogged most of my life and can attest that a track surface is easier on your joints than the pavement. If you're a jogger, I don't need to tell you anything you don't already know. If you're not, and you want to meet a fellow that's fit, then put on your shorts and sneakers and start running toward that piece of passion that you can't resist. A word to the wise: don't wear jewelry and a lot of makeup. That turns the athletic type off.

I taught aerobics classes a few years ago, and I usually had more men than women in my classes. But if you don't find what you're looking for there, wander through the gym into the weight room where all the Herculean types congregate. If you're not familiar with weights, get one of the gym regulars to show you. Heavy weights are very dangerous, so please stay away from those grunting gorillas until they are resting between sets. Only then will they notice your loveliness. When they're training, they're working. And when they're working, they're focused. But as you know, a man must breathe. It's a biological fact. Shine your prettiest smile in the direction of his breath.

On ski slopes it is hard to miss single men. In the lift lines they seem to be looking for you. The more often you ride the lifts, the more your chance for conversation. In fact, you could wear your sexy ski clothes and ride the lifts all day!

Stadiums of all kinds are loaded with single, available men. Even though you may not be the athletic type, force yourself to go to baseball, football, and hockey games, tennis matches, golf tournaments, and marathon races. Try anything that deals with sports. It's also healthy for your head. Bowling is close to golf in popularity, so check it out if you want to have plenty of opportunities. You are likely to come up with a prize.

Magazine stands are raging with single male hormones. I have yet to stop by for a paper or magazine and not see several men hovering around auto, mechanic, or provocative mags. You'll find them there on Friday or Saturday nights, especially if they don't have dates. People who are interested in world events or who just like to keep abreast of the latest whatever will always pick up something to read on their way home from work.

You're going to hate this, but financial seminars are occupied with mostly men. Men who want to enrich their lives learning about the stock market, investments, bonds, and so on. And in our poor economy where foreclosures abound, not only will you have your choice of well-wishers, but you might also learn something beneficial for your own future. And that ain't bad.

Don't be embarrassed by singles gatherings. If you don't have success at some of the locales, then check it out. There's certainly no harm in it, and you might come out with a gem in jeans.

Let's not forget *home improvement* stores. Tim Allen is a current television star for a reason. Men definitely have a huge ego about their homes—all men. It's territorial pride. Whether or not they are adept at making improvements isn't an issue. The fact is they *will* try. Their adrenaline surge is fabulously infectious when they succeed at fixing something. You will always find mucho hombres at home improvement stores. I guarantee. The same for lumber yards. There are many manly construction workers buying lumber for their jobs. There are several well-known and successful actresses either married to or dating construction hunks. Talk about a *real man*! Um-hummm . . .

While you're inspecting the merchandise, do not lose sight of the true reason why you want a man in your life. You want a partner; a friend; a good man who will enhance your life; a companion with whom you can grow, create, laugh, love, and have incredible nights of irresistible sex. Keep all of this in mind when your eyes lock with his and your heart flip-flops to the tune of "Please help me, I'm falling!"

THE MALE OF THE SPECIES

Snips and snails, and puppy dogs' tails! That's what little boys are made of!

—ANONYMOUS

Before we talk about dating in general, let's become acquainted with a few qualities in good men. Age has nothing to do with a man's goodness. I've known men at thirty who have experienced all of Job's tragedies and come out winners. I've known other men fifty-five and older who haven't a clue and probably never will. You can't judge a good man by his age, and you can't judge a good man by the amount of crisp new hundred-dollar bills he unrolls. You can, however, consider the following:

He should be emotionally healthy, having learned positive views from life's lessons. He does not blame anyone for his misjudgments or mistakes. In other words, he takes control of his life and responsibility for himself.

He should have strong moral values, conviction, integrity, and a sense of honor; he does the right thing regardless of how tough it seems.

He should be able to endure emotional upheaval (perhaps he already has)—a tragedy, a personal loss, perhaps even a sick or disabled parent or child. Through the ordeal he gains perception, sensitivity, and concern. Without any of life's calamities, his character doesn't have a chance to grow.

He should be above narcissism. I was out to dinner one evening with a want-to-be charmer, but I had the feeling that he was addressing an audience of thousands seated behind me. Every inflection, every turn of the head, every hand gesture, or every glance was choreographed to seduce his public. Beware if he looks in the mirror more than you!

He should be detached from drugs and/or excessive alcohol.

Finally, he should genuinely like women. Some men have a subconscious disdain for women. If your intuition tells you that he does, close the door.

Let's explore other prototypes of certain men you may find:

MR. PARTICULAR

Mr. Particular carries the image of a specific woman in his mind. Terry, a forty-two-year-old Washington, D.C., lobbyist said, "I have always preferred blue-eyed blondes, usually five feet eight inches tall, 126 pounds, in their late twenties or early thirties. I know I'm looking for the perfect woman because every time I go on a date, I get this feeling that she may not measure up. I mean, what if I marry the girl I'm having a relationship with and then later meet my dream woman? I'll begin resenting my wife." Mr. Particular is obviously afraid of commitment, so he devises defense mechanisms to avoid marriage at any cost. He will isolate himself if need be and color or slant a situation to fit his framework.

MR. RUNAROUND

Mr. Runaround loves to date, *period*! He is charming, handsome, inventive, and plans everything down to the appropriate mineral water at dinner. At dinner, each date and outing is perfectly orchestrated—the most divine Italian restaurant with Pavarotti singing in the background, the best wine, the best food, the best ambience, the best of everything—or perhaps it's a wonderful night of jazz under the stars at the Hollywood Bowl complete with great seats, a perfectly prepared basket of food, wine, fruit, cheese, coffee, cognac, and dessert; a blanket if it gets cold; and a pillow for your precious buns. When you return to the car, he plays a CD of the music you just heard.

How appropriate, how prepared, how romantic, how thoughtful. How dangerous to fall in love with Mr. Runaround. He will be so elusive, so controlling, so incapable of committing to you. Let's give him his due. He *is* a great date! He's just not looking for the intimacy of a deep ongoing relationship to nurture. Next!

MR. CONVENIENCE

I know a man who was the Don Juan of Los Angeles, California. He's fiftyish, and until recently his entire life had been dedicated to his art and women. He never wanted marriage for himself. He simply had no desire. Nothing's wrong with that. Each person marches to the beat of a different drummer. That is Mr. Convenience. Oddly, though, things can change. One day, he met

Ann. They worked together on a project. She had a lot of qualities on his wish list. They dated for a while—and then married. A natural harmony has developed, as well as a family. Perhaps it was timing. It often is.

MEN AND AGE

Men's attitudes concerning dating and marriage, in general, do change at various stages. Although it's difficult to generalize, there are certain characteristics you'll find at various ages and stages of development. For example, a man in his late teens and twenties is primarily controlled by his raging hormones—our old friend testosterone. Testosterone gives a male youth a voracious sex drive, unharnessed energy, and ephemeral qualities. Without a clear head and strong convictions, he can easily be led astray. But he can also mature in fine fashion by setting certain goals for himself and seeing them to completion.

Men in their twenties also desire a lot of sexual gratification. And if it doesn't materialize after a few dates, they often move on to another potential conquest. From my interviews, I have discovered that men in their twenties still engage in a diversity of sexual partners, but most of them use condoms.

Also in this age category are some exceptional young men—rare and few—who have decided to settle down with a wife and work toward being a good provider. A woman has a better chance of teaching and shaping a man in this particular age group, because he's still impressionable, ready, willing, and able to be molded with the right words, the right touch, the right care, and the right love. And he's ohhh so willing to let her guide him through whatever stages of sex that she desires. Whether it's playing games, dressing up, or exchanging roles, he's happy to penetrate in the forest, in the ocean, in a plane, or in a tree. Remember, he's still learning. And testosterone's symphony won't often allow him to say no to anything you ask concerning the ol' in-and-out.

Men in their thirties are quite wonderful in another way. They have newly discovered sensibilities. The look of maturity finally arrives and they're usually more accepting of themselves. They're beginning to relax with what God gave them—mentally and physically. Oh yes! They still crave satisfaction just as frequently, but a new hue of growth is added to the horizon—a rich red. According to Phil, thirty-four, an internist and friend of mine, "I was dating an actress who makes karate films and I was crazy about her, to say the least; but I discovered after eight months of dating that she lied often, was insincere and just not the type of woman that I would want to raise my children. I finally got the message that she was money hungry. Now I'm dating a woman with an honest and good heart. Sex with the karate girl was incredible, but sex with my new lady is even better because I know she really loves me."

Men in this age group are usually either getting ready for marriage and a family, or they've been through a divorce. If you happen to date a divorced thirty-something, you need to find out if he learned from the marital experience and its breakup or if he's carrying baggage with "blame" written all over it. So watch his body language carefully when he speaks: Does he appear laid-back most of the time, but prone to sudden profanities when an incapable driver rudely pulls in front of him? Does he act like a poor, vulnerable puppy, or does he confess his mistakes with conviction? If your instinct tells you that this man is consistent, then believe it! Your instinct doesn't lie. Take a moment and really listen.

There are two categories of men who turn forty. I adore the ones who seem to be in touch with themselves—feeling comfortable, satisfied, and glad to be forty for all the wisdom they've acquired. They like themselves. The key is *like*. However, the reverse is also true. Many men at forty look in the mirror and cannot recognize their reflection. Instead of feeling joy and pride, they feel like failures whose time has run out and whose mortality has become self-evident. They evaluate their lives, their jobs, their bodies, their wives and families. Quickly, they try to change everything to mimic their adventurous, fun, and sexy days in high school and college. And you know what that means—a cute, tight-bodied Playmate look-alike. So look out if you have a menopausal male, because he'll need a lot of care, caressing, attention, love, and consideration while going through it. And unfortunately, it may be a few years on the steep face of the Matterhorn.

In a man's desperate attempt to regain his lost youth, he's capable of changing his job, wardrobe, hairstyle, or diet. He may begin an exercise program, drop old habits, take a new lover, or, quite possibly, get a divorce—all to convince himself that he's still a contender. In general, he will race Father Time by challenging his strength, his stamina, and his sex appeal. He simply wants to know if he's still desirable.

On this "proving" ground many men hurt themselves. Harry Bloomingdale reputedly had a cardiac arrest when sharing his masculinity with a girl a fraction of his age. In Tennessee Williams's play, *Cat on a Hot Tin Roof*, the aging Brick drives out to his high school football field one night and tries to jump hurdles just to test his once-great athleticism. He falls and breaks his leg during the drunken escapade. His mind remembers the routine, but his body forgets.

Accepting change is very difficult for these gentlemen. They want desperately to hold on to a certain part of their youth. But it's impossible. And yet, if a man takes exceptional care of himself—a lot of exercise, appropriate sleep, good food, and a positive attitude with a nurturing woman, he can look and feel surprisingly young for quite a while.

Wouldn't it be ideal if your man could move gracefully through each new year with a maturing ease and self-assurance, growing ever more beautiful. Unfortunately, that's asking far too much from the suffering midlife searchers. If the forty-somethings could only understand what a man named Joe Kogel has figured out, they would find peace within themselves: "The worst thing in your life may contain seeds of the best. When you can see crisis as an opportunity, your life becomes not easier, but more satisfying." See, it's attitude all over again.

Now, for the fifties and over: Ted Turner, Clint Eastwood, Sean Connery, Tommy Lee Jones, Warren Beatty, Bob Dole, Charlie Rose, and Jack Kemp are but a few great examples of men who have passed the half-century mark and not only look terrific, but maintain a positive attitude while continuing to work, create, and strive toward their vision. They seem sincerely satisfied with themselves and this stage of their life. If you're so inclined, this is a wonderful age group to date and to marry, if you happen to find one who is not already married.

A man over fifty has done it, seen it, been it, had it, loved it, lost it, felt it, and for better or worse knows what he wants. The good news is that his menopause is over (or it should be). He is much more in tune with the rhythms of life. And when he dates, it's usually a woman with whom he shares a common interest and who is closer to his age. He's not likely to go surfing in Malibu in the dead of winter to prove he's a man. It was said of Jacqueline Kennedy Onassis that she found great happiness with Maurice Sempleton, an older gentleman who shared his life with her. He was good to her, helped her with her finances, and was by her side through her decline. A lot can be said of a man who sticks with you! There are so few.

Of course the fifty-somethings and beyond still have fantasies. I hope they always will. Fantasies excite the adrenaline and keep a person invigorated. But do they react to the fantasy? Usually not. They are too wise and comfortable with themselves to waste precious and valuable time chasing an illusion. They want the real thing—to love, to hold, to feel, and to enjoy the different seasons of nature. They like dependability and affection. And much like a woman, they go for substance, stability, and sustenance.

It's only natural to look at and enjoy the vision of a pretty, attractive woman, but these men no longer swing from the trees beating their chest to get a young girl's attention. Tarzan simply prefers sitting in his tree house with his Jane watching the sun rise and set, enjoying a good meal, a good glass of brandy, a good book, a good joke, and good sex from time to time. He's earned his bowl of cherries. He closes his eyes with a smile and a warm feeling of contentment in his heart.

Dating is much more appreciated and never taken for granted by this group of men, partly because they realize that special moments are finite, and partly because they know exactly what pleases them.

DATING—ANXIETY 101

Man is young as long as he can repeat his emotions, woman as long as she can inspire them.

—OSCAR WILDE

No matter what your age, dating is like taking a class in Anxiety 101. And it's important to know that you are dreadfully like other people, men included. Everybody, and I do mean everybody, feels anxious and insecure when they go out on a date, especially a first date. Your sense of inner security has everything to do with your romantic success.

Examine what you really want when you meet a man who appeals to you. A lot of women flirt, tease, and come on to a guy to get him interested, and then reject him. Why? Because she may feel threatened, resentful, and uncertain about being able to fulfill his needs—sexual or otherwise. Fearing physical contact or feeling desperate to have a man in your life will absolutely jump-start anxiety and ruin what could potentially be an exciting romance. Some women flirt by rote, for no reason at all. But, when the man responds —she jumps off because she is not prepared for a relationship.

So if you like men and really want to have *a relationship*, be prepared, be confident, and you will find a man with whom you can share a mutual love. As Katharine Hepburn said, "The trick in life is not getting what you want, it's wanting it after you get it!" To avoid this particular trap, know in advance exactly what you want, lighten up, and open up. And don't make every man you date feel as though he must walk down the aisle with you . . . tonight. You certainly won't be a hit; you're more likely to remain a miss.

Know in your mind that to be a success you don't have to have the face of Venus, the brains of Minerva, the grace of Terpsichore, or the figure of Juno. In other words, you don't have to be a brain surgeon, climb mountains, and wear a G-string. It's much more important to be approachable, to show a man a little encouragement. The right smile from across the room can spark his fire. Or a little flirtatious eye contact now and again will give him something to shoot for.

So it worked! He's walking in your direction. Ahh, he stops and engages you in conversation. Good girl. Now, don't sit there and give him yes and no answers. *Think!* Notice something about his person that you can compliment. Maybe his haircut. Or if he's wearing a suit and you like his tie, then tell him so. Men love it when you compliment their ties. Or maybe you notice the cut of his suit, the style of his shoes, and so forth. Maybe he's wearing a great pair of jeans and a fabulous black leather jacket. Compliment the color or whatever feature you notice first. Fortunately, in jeans, you can be fairly sure of the shape of his legs and his buns, right? Unless they're two sizes too large and he's into the latest fad that hangs rather than fits.

After a while, ask him about himself, but be careful not to get too personal or pry into intimate subjects. If you appear to be curious about his salary or his investments, he'll think you're after a loan rather than his charms. Mark, forty, a financial broker in Los Angeles confided, "I've dated a couple of women who on the first date had the audacity to ask me how much money I made." I find asking such questions supremely tacky. That kind of intimacy is likely to come later if the two of you are serious about one other.

You should never go on a date with a man if you're only interested in his bank account. Life's too short for such hypocrisy. I know several women who married men for their money only, and they're pitifully empty, sad, and lonely inside. They also have dead eyes. But if you happen to fall in love with a man who happens to have a thick wallet, lucky you! And yes, it is just as easy to fall in love with a rich man as it is a poor man. Just be sure it's the *man* you're in love with and *not* the size of his wallet.

The key to engaging the man you want is to find a common ground of interest. If he's reticent and shy, then tell him a bit about yourself. Share your interest —something current that impressed you—maybe a hot new movie, an experimental theater, the latest popular book, a recent sports event, or the newest number one CD. But whatever the topic, keep it light, flirtatious, and friendly.

Always listen in a way that will make him feel relaxed and special. Place all your attention on him when he's talking. Don't dart your eyes around the room muttering, "Yeah," or "Uh-huh," because that's not involved. No matter who the person, with a little subtle investigating you may hit on a subject he likes. Then watch his eyes light up. When you hit a home run, communicating will be fun.

I don't know if you've seen Vice President Al Gore being interviewed on Larry King, but this exceptional talk-show host expertly brought out the intriguing and funny side of Mr. Gore's personality. After watching him blush, laugh, and make fun of himself, you would think the wooden jokes that have been repeated about him are ludicrous. Mr. King has learned to draw out the best from even the most difficult guest, mainly because he is sensitive to nuances of conversation and asks pertinent and interesting questions. In different ways, Barbara Walters, Phil Donahue, and Charlie Rose share the same gift. We could all take lessons from their style. The key is finding out what turns a person on. And you can only do this by listening and paying close attention to the answers along with his body language, then asking the right questions.

During conversation, also remember that guys hate a serious, romantic link too soon. It scares them away. Just be yourself and keep your feminine mystery intact.

Communication is the fertilizer for the flowering of

a relationship. You must let him know your preferences as well. Don't be afraid to communicate your preferences regarding ambience, and activities you enjoy. The place and type of dress needed for the date must be broached before he comes to fetch you. You needn't ask him what you should wear, but you should ask if it's casual or dressy. And there's no harm inquiring about his dress. You must communicate or else one of you will be miserable.

I happen to love surprises, but . . . I make it a point to communicate the type of surprises that turn me on. Once a man understands a variety of things you like, he can please you with unbridled creativity and inventiveness. Otherwise, the surprise could be unpleasant. I want to share one of my unfortunate episodes involving a surprise brunch. For about a year, a fellow actress-girlfriend named Sally wanted me to date her husband's best buddy, Jerry, a very witty and attractive director. We met. He made me laugh and I thoroughly enjoyed his company. He asked me out. I agreed to brunch. It was a beautiful Sunday morning. I took my usual morning run and dressed for what I thought would be a posh hotel brunch—pearls, stockings, high heels—the works.

He arrived in his Land Rover ready for a rendezvous at the beach or the mountains. Anyway, my feminine self hopped into his truck and I told myself to give him a chance. He described a charming restaurant overlooking the beach where we could dine. Well . . . we drove and drove and drove—on the freeways, up the mountains, along the ocean, while I slowly watched brunch turn into lunch. The bright morning light had evolved into the noonday sun before we reached our destination. We parked. He opened my door and we walked up to a closed restaurant. Yes, *closed*! I was tired, starved, frustrated, and angry. He suggested another restaurant down the road. We drove once again, but never did find an open restaurant. I firmly asked him to turn in to the first grocery store we passed. We shopped for takeout food and actually made a quick picnic. Then we drove across the street to a private section of beach, sat down, and gobbled the food. I don't think I said two words to him during the meal or the drive back. Jerry is a wonderful man. It's just that we are not on the same communicative wavelength. Hopefully this experience won't happen to you, because it was dreadfully disappointing.

A good rule in the art of the chase: think of the men that you have been attracted to in the past. Aren't they the ones who like you, but keep you wondering, rather than the ones who call you all the time and are always available? Most people want what they can't get. If a woman is too easy, a man doesn't feel as though he has won a prize. But don't make it too difficult, either. He may pass over you for a woman who acts more interested in him. Be honest, but be reserved. Always hold back a little. In the end, it will pay off. Let him discover your essence as slowly as perfumed petals open on a rose. Discovery is the beauty of a relationship.

During the discovery phase, engage your two feminine forces—teasing and flirting. You need these allies as part of playing and having fun with the love game —lust, love, and romance. But there are two distinctively different types of teasing and flirting: the playful, feminine, and fun kind, which you will find in Scarlett O'Hara from *Gone with the Wind*; or the insincere and frivolous kind depicted in Geena Davis's character from *Thelma and Louise*. You may recall that Thelma became severely intoxicated, then began flirting with, teasing, and rubbing herself all over some country stranger. The more Louise warned her to stop, the more Thelma drank, and the more provocative with the stranger she became, until . . . they walked outside, he pinned her facedown against a truck, ripped off her panties, unzipped his own pants, and took liberties. When you tease the wrong man, you could very well end up in some dark-alley circumstance. Please be careful.

Now take the same erotic, seductive body rubbing, lip licking, finger touching, and toe teasing and turn it toward your true man. *Whooaah, Nelly!* That hot stuff should be for your fella only. Teasing is beyond flirting. Flirting is playing at love, acting a bit coquettish—a twinkling of the eyes, a toss of the hair, a girlish smile and blush, a subtle crossing of the legs, a movement of your body in his direction, or a touching of his arm to feel his muscles. Whereas teasing is a more serious form of foreplay. It's a calculated physical action—a mindset to achieve something. When your stockinged foot rubs his leg under the table, or when your fingers find a bundle of goodies in his trousers while at dinner . . . that's teasing! It's fun and exciting when it's your man that you're teasing.

At dinner, don't play the jealousy bit. It shows insecurity. Just as you hate hearing about his exes, he hates hearing about your past conquests. Instigating jealousy is futile. There's absolutely no point in making him turn pea green with envy. It will only lace the air with negative energy instead of positive fanfare. Besides, a divine seductress does not need her ego massaged in this way. There are other, more direct, and sexually erotic methods for ego inflation.

Also, forget about his *potential*. I know more women who like a guy for what he's going to do, or the job he's going to get, or how much money he's going to make, ad nauseam. *Now* is who and what he is —not tomorrow and not next year. You can only intuit his development. That, too, is like looking into a crystal ball and seeing the future. Hmmm . . . Impossible? One can never tell, but it will be a long, arduous wait until he matures into the man you envision. If, in fact, you are dissatisfied with him at present, don't expect to be satisfied with him in the future. He is what he is!

Like your man for himself. Like him for the manner in which he adds to your life, or find a man who has already developed his potential. You don't need to be nurturing someone else's possibilities; you need to be nurturing your own. Time goes by so quickly. It's all a snapshot . . . snap, snap, snap! One day, you look in the mirror and *say what*? What are all those charming, characteristic tracks of life doing on *my* face? At which time, if your man still hasn't developed into the fantasy of who you think he is, you will not only resent everything he stands for, but you will also hate him for not fulfilling your expectations. Happens every time!

To avoid deceiving yourself, take a good, long look at the whole picture before you start spending your precious time on a man's potential. I was in love with the illusion, once. The lesson cost me my entire savings and a few precious years. Guess what? The man is still full of undeveloped potential. That's when I realized a woman has two choices: either be happy with the man himself, flaws and all, or show yourself to the door . . . *Leave*! Tomorrow is just a state of mind, nothing more.

Now that we know you're in love with the real man and not his potential, let's snap into action. Do you want him to ache with lust? Of course you do! Well, you can dazzle that darling with your sultry voice, simmering glances, an innocent brush or two of your hand over a piece of his clothing, an intoxicating whisper in his ear at dinner, or a stance close enough for him to inhale your perfume . . . always close, but not too close; a slight brush, not a solid touch. It certainly won't be a secret when the hot coals of attraction are forcing both of your energies together. It's in the senses.

You simultaneously see it, smell it, taste it, hear it, and the two of you are craving to touch it. It's hard to hold back, if you catch my drift.

You know in your heart that the man is profoundly physically and sexually interested—wanting to be closer than is humanly possible. So the only thing you need to do is . . . *wait*! Yes, wait. I know you would like to tear his shirt off and devour every inch of his divine flesh, but it's in your best interest not to rush the lust. Delay the inevitable moment. It's not going away, not when so strong a desire and passion are the precursors.

So far, it's been a delicious date with seductive thoughts of kissing, touching, embracing, and slipping into the Sargasso Sea with pieces of his landscape. Why complicate the night? Keep it nice and easy and he will be relieved that you made him wait. It's *you* and no one else he wants. Stir his rich palate of emotion. Never give in too soon or too easily. Orchestrate the level of heat and harmony.

Remember: men always want what they can't have. Get to know him better. His character is just as important as his touch. This brings to mind an unforgettable moment in the Martin Scorcese film *The Age of Innocence* when Daniel Day-Lewis is in a moving carriage with Michelle Pfeiffer. After not having seen her for many months, he takes her gloved hand and holds it as delicately as he would fine porcelain, and with slow suggestive caresses his two fingers begin to open each button, gently peeling back the cloth to undress her vulnerable flesh. With wanton desire, his burning lips kiss her exposed wrist with a soft but consuming passion. Her body shivers. Her searching mouth surrenders in reckless abandon. That one action displays the intense power of lust combined with the truest love. You'll know when he loves you. There's no mistaking it. It's in his eyes, his touch, his actions.

In contrast, there is a scene in *The Godfather* that is more about lust than about love. Remember the early wedding sequence where the bride's (married) brother Sonny made off with one of the bridesmaids? Well, that short scene in the film was much more fully developed and described in Mario Puzo's novel. The scene as written was worthy of several reads—volcanic, to say the least. I highly recommend you get hold of the book and read it yourself.

A word to the wise: if this pure primeval electricity falls upon you, don't fool yourself into believing it's love. It's not! However, if the two of you are available and you really like and respect what each other is capable of giving, then you have a tremendous chance for a loving relationship to blossom.

TO KISS OR NOT TO KISS

A kiss, when all is said, what is it?
. . . a rosy dot
Placed on the "I" in loving; 'tis a secret
Told to the mouth instead of to the ear.
—CYRANO DE BERGERAC

After he brings you home, the next burning question remains—to kiss or not to kiss? At the moment his face nears your lips and your heart jumps into your throat, if the evening has tasted of strawberry parfait and the conversation has had the effervescence of champagne, then absolutely yes! Absolutely, positively yes! But if all is not copacetic and there were a few red lights of warning throughout the course of the evening, then you'd best be prudent. There's not a more intoxicating, romantic, or enduring symbol of love than *the kiss*. So be careful on whom you bestow such sublime enchantment.

I asked several guys to describe the best kisses they've ever had. Collin, a thirty-nine-year-old college professor from Scottsdale, Arizona, gladly responded with: "I don't want to feel like I'm doing all the work. I prefer a meeting of the tongues. But not a tense and insistent tongue that makes me feel as if she hasn't kissed in years. That's the tongue that strikes into my mouth like a cobra. And I don't like mushy or passive kisses."

Jack, forty, a cowboy in Billings, Montana said, "I think a kiss should be soft and slow and very moist, but I don't want to have to wipe my face on her shoulder from all the drooling. I also like it when a girl puts her arms around my neck and touches my face while she's kissing me."

Kevin Costner's character in the film *Bull Durham* deliciously expressed his views on kissing: "I believe in the soul, the cock, the pussy, the small of a woman's back . . . the sweet spot, soft-core pornography . . . and I believe in long, slow, deep, soft wet kisses that last three days!"

Anyone can learn to kiss, whatever their endowment—small lips, big lips, long tongue, short tongue, large teeth, or no teeth. It's all in the attitude and the approach—the feeling behind what you're doing and whom you're doing it with.

As Marlowe's Doctor Faustus said, "Sweet Helen, make me immortal with a kiss. Her lips suck forth my soul; see where it flies!" To be able to suck forth your man's soul and make it fly, begin with a relaxed mind and relaxed jaw. Then with parted lips edging toward his mouth, your laser-beam eyes at half-mast sending silent signals of how much you want his sex, greet his lips ever so gently with a tender hello kiss. After he feels your soft display, open your mouth a little wider to explore his essence—breathe his breath, smell his skin, taste his essence. He may give you his tongue partially. Touch it slightly with yours as though you were sipping a fine brandy for the first time—not too much too soon. To tease is to please.

With slow movements a natural familiarity will slide into rhythm. When he offers a bit more, you give a bit more, until a tango of the tongues ensues. Then with the point of your tongue delicately circle his lips. After he gives you a broader, longer, deeper stroke of his muscle, respond by gently sucking on it a few times. For more titillation, cover your teeth with your lips and carefully bite down on his tongue. Then rhythmically suck on it again with the intention of giving him fellatio. It'll drive him mad. The soft sounds of nibbling, biting, and sucking on his lips from time to time are also erotic.

You can spend hours exploring each other's senses with your lips, breath and tongue. A few sincere moans and groans are extremely sensual. And with grace and direction, your pointed instrument can circle around his teeth. Simply from an erotic and gentle kiss you can learn more about him than he probably knows about himself. Your confidence and creativity will torch his soul if he's a sensual being.

If the kissee does not respond in kind, perhaps it's because he doesn't know how. Maybe he's never experienced a woman who really loved him. Only you can decide if you care enough to show him the way. Some men learn quickly and others need more time. Take it slowly, be patient, and impart your knowledge with loving care. If this is the man who's captured your heart, then he is definitely worth the wait.

A full oral, erotic kiss is exquisitely intimate and can arouse untamable passion. It's akin to intercourse.

The mouth is constructed from similar components as the vagina—membranes, juices, and muscles. So, this masterful game of love play will ignite his unyielding weapon in the direction of your perfume garden. Steal his mouth with your best kiss and you will steal his heart, too.

FOODS FOR LOVE

A good cook is like a sorceress who dispenses happiness.

—ELSA SHIAPARELLI

Do you have enough *juice* in your love? Is your relationship dripping with *moisture* and *succulence*? Does your lover call you *ripe, luscious, mature*? If not, you may want to add the ultimate spice to your life—*aphrodisiacs*.

Just listen to that word—*aphrodisiac*. It conjures up images of the goddess Aphrodite, her nude form rising out of the seashell. We recall the ancient Greeks, teasing their concubines with stems of bursting cherry-red grapes; the Arabs and Egyptian pharaohs swallowing salty seawater to enhance their sexual powers and stamina; the gods themselves imbibing ambrosia, the elixir of love and wild abandon. Speaking of ambrosia, in the South we make a dessert of several mixed fruits, topped off with freshly shredded coconut and maraschino cherries. And once you start eating it, you simply cannot stop. That's probably why it's appropriately called ambrosia, the food of the gods.

Foods, spices, and herbs have been used for centuries by both men and women to stimulate their partners into more passionate and fulfilling lovemaking. In this section, we will take a closer look at some of the more popular aphrodisiacs.

A smart woman knows that the fastest way to a man's heart is through his stomach. But in her zeal to feed her beloved beast, she needs to remember the principle of moderation. Sometimes, in her determination to demonstrate her culinary skills, she is too successful— and her man ends up with a potbelly, love handles, or even a spare tire! A light meal can either be foreplay or afterplay; but it needs to fire a man's lust, not put him to sleep. You want his belly to be happy, yet with room left over for dessert . . . *you*!

The world of food itself is sensual with delicacies that delight the eye and please the mouth. Some of these foods of arousal, for example chocolate, contain a natural substance called phenylethylamine which is thought to be a true aphrodisiac with "love" molecules. This fact is strangely ironic since the act of being in love can cause the body to manufacture its own phenylethylamine. So the one aphrodisiac that lovers truly need is each other's company with a bar of Hershey's for a quick fix. Their closeness causes them to generate their own "love" molecules.

Now let's venture into Mother Nature's cupboard of liquid aphrodisiacs—potions of love. The brilliant advice of Shakespeare reminds us, "It [alcoholic beverage] provokes the desire, but it takes away the performance." There is nothing more gracious than being a charming hostess and offering your man some liquid refreshment for his tired weary throat. But don't offer too much too soon!

Science is not quick to acknowledge the efficacy of aphrodisiacs. Many scientists feel that aphrodisiacs are a placebo—or perhaps a man is deficient in certain nutrients and when these nutrients are replenished, voilà —the long-awaited "whopper"! However, there is one

aphrodisiac that has a confirmed mechanism of action
—the legendary Spanish fly. It is a fluid found in Meloid
beetles, blister beetles. When alarmed, these beetles exude dangerous fluid from their knee joints. When ingested
by humans, Spanish fly acts as a urinary tract irritant
that indirectly stimulates the genitals. The painful burning of the genitals was once considered a sign of lust.
The Marquis de Sade was famous for using Spanish fly
on himself and on those he wished to seduce. Unfortunately, it's a poison so toxic that as little as a tenth
of a milligram can blister and burn the skin and in high
doses it is lethal. So beware of this potent potion of
nature. Pain is definitely not the same as eroticism.

Rumors abound that ginseng, a nutritious herb
from the bark of the yohimbé tree found in Korea, Rus-
sia, and China, not only calms the nervous system, but
also gives a thrust to virility. I know people who swear
that ginseng has straightened many a loose tool. There
are hundreds of foods and herbs that are used around
the world to awaken the sleepyhead. The Japanese believe that raw eel excites and restores the powers of
potency. For sexual warfare medieval women used the
leaves of myrtle soaked in wine. In modern times, aromatherapy offers the same enrichment. However, in
place of wine, diluted brandy or natural vegetable glyc-
erin is substituted.

Many Arabs, Europeans, and Chinese advocate the
consumption of eggs, which are rich in proteins, but
also symbolic of fertility. In the Mayan brothels, cacao
beans were choice payment for a night of bliss. Mon-
tezuma, the Aztec emperor, conspicuously consumed
several cups of the cacao beverage before entering his
harem.

The cacao bean has a long, exciting history. It is, of
course, the raw ingredient of chocolate, and was introduced to Europe centuries ago by the explorer Cortés,

perhaps because of its satisfying richness and sensual texture, perhaps because of its love hormone ingredient phenylethylamine. Or perhaps because of a combination of all these factors, chocolate has been a favorite bedroom delicacy for generations.

Another treat reported to have special power is the black truffle, which contains an androgenic substance similar to male hormones. This musky substance is often used in perfumes. Can you imagine why?

Of course the sensual is not strictly earthbound. Aphrodite's emergence from the seashell depicted most famously in Botticelli's *Birth of Venus* reminds us that anything coming from the sea is endowed with her sexual magic and scent—fish, shellfish, turtles, seaweed, caviar, roe, lobster—seawater itself is reminiscent of the salty taste of semen. And what about oysters?

The great lover Casanova was said to have eaten dozens of oysters daily. I'm sure he needed the protein and minerals from the oysters to replenish his own lost sperm. Ah, yes. A healthy man with a healthy appetite and hundreds of women to vouch for it. Oysters have a smooth, moist texture and a delicate aroma that can be very erotic. They go down so easily that they are affectionately dubbed "sliders."

American Indians ate bear and buffalo for strength, but reserved deer for virility. Today, in many health food stores, deer antler is one of the most popular potions. For the red-blooded male, rare beef comes highly recommended as a potent sexual stimulant. Body parts and intestines of certain animals are still traditional tonics. Rhinoceros horns are used in the East as aphrodisiacs.

Other favorite erotic entrées are fruits such as figs, pears, mangoes, peaches, strawberries, burgundy grapes, bananas, kiwis, plums, pomegranates, kumquats, and maraschino cherries.

For the more creative types, watermelon can be titillating, fun. My girlfriend Sandy made a surprise picnic
lunch for her husband, George. It seemed that sex had
become lackadaisical and she wanted to hold a sexual
pep rally. She decided on a secluded field and unfolded
her goodies under a big oak tree. She promptly took
out a book and began reading a seductive poem aloud,
while George pleased his palate. Then came dessert. The
sultry summer day was ideal for Sandy's watermelon
display waiting on ice. As soon as George sliced the
melon, Sandy dug her anxious fingers into its heart. She
slurped a large red clump into her mouth while letting
its sweet divine juice drip down her chin, neck, and fall
over her breast. She took another slice and rubbed it
over her erect nipples, down her belly to her silken
peach panties already moist with dew. She rubbed her
legs with yet another piece and touched her own erection. George was aghast! Taking advantage, she slid her
own large piece into his mouth. He lost himself in her
freedom, while she doused melon juice over his exposed
engorgement. Sandy jump-started their marital intima-
cies, all in a splendidly concocted afternoon.

In choosing to smear on foods and then lick them
off, be innovative. For sex play, you may want to consider whipped cream, honey, peanut butter, fruit pre-
serves, chocolate eclairs, fudge, caramel, butterscotch
sauces, Popsicles, bananas, and any Jell-O substance.
Also just plain water can be the most sensuous experience of all—still, dripping, flowing, running, splashing,
or raining.

For more heated pleasure, you may add a red-hot
sensuous video. *9½ Weeks* is a good choice. Mickey
Rourke and Kim Basinger are at their erotic best while
making an art out of edible delights. To view another
example of "eating sexy," rent *Tom Jones*, starring Al-
bert Finney. In a movie that was famous for sexiness,

the most provocative scene was of Tom sharing a meal with a woman of loose morals. Their delight in the food and in each other was more expressive and erotic than most scenes that show naked couples kissing!

But whatever your preference, the secret to successful food sex is to let improvisation be your guiding light. Who knows, maybe he wants to decorate your anatomy with vanilla ice cream, strawberry cream cheese, or lemon icebox pie, and lick it off . . . slowly. Then again, he may tantalize your nipples or your clitoris with ice cubes!

Talking about the thrill of the chill, you can also rub an ice cube all over his body, over your body, and into your vagina. Several love partners are purchasing penis-testicle molds. They fill the mold with water, freeze it, and then use the design for love play. The ice design becomes the size of an erect penis, at which point the ice can be pushed into the vagina until the inevitable heat melts it down.

The master of all nature is freedom. Let go. Be adventurous. Serve the law of love in play, in all of your multiplicity. Pleasure is the real delight of existence— the secret flame of rapture. Let your wildest fantasies become reality. Who knows, maybe you'll write the definitive book on the power of aphrodisiacs!

Chapter 4

••••••••••••••••••••••••••••••••••••••

Acts of Love

*The more knowledge is inherent in a thing,
the greater the love. . . . Anyone who imagines
that all fruits ripen at the same time as
the strawberries knows nothing about grapes.*

—PARACELSUS

THE SEX ORGANS

The object in life is not to be the best of the best. It's to be the only one who can do what you do!
—JERRY GARCIA

Making love is an art. Before an artist can sail into inspired creativity, she must spend time learning about the physical tools of her art and how to use them. For example, a painter must know how to stretch canvases and mix colors; a musician must know how to handle and care for his instrument; a dancer must take classes and discern elements of music; a gourmet cook must know how to choose and operate cooking utensils as well as how to select delicious foods; a wine connoisseur must study vintages and possess a fine palate, and a love goddess extraordinaire must know herself and every nuance of her man.

All of this knowledge must be in place before you can paint a portrait, perform a sonata, dance a duet, prepare a culinary delight, choose a great wine, or become a magnificent seductress. That is . . . if you aspire to a *superior* level of achievement. To become a magnificent seductress, you must know and understand the tools of your art—the sexual organs. Wholly understanding both sexes allows you to give your lover absolute pleasure.

Too often (perhaps because of ignorance or fear) our own sexual organs are an unknown quantity or, worse—the object of a smutty joke or, much, much worse—an expletive used to express anger or contempt. But you're smarter than most. You read and learn. You understand that the sexual organs are the essential tools with which you will create your masterpiece. To make magic, you will need to know the what, where, and how of his sexual organs as well as your own. Learn all about them, especially how to use them to your—and his—greatest advantage.

Now let's move on to the mechanics and mystery of sexual anatomy. In the early stages of fetal development, a penis forms in the male from the same tissue that develops into a clitoris in the female. Structures or tissues derived from the same tissue are called homologues. The penis is the homologue of the clitoris; the testicles are homologues of the ovaries; and the scrotum is the homologue of the labia majora (outer vaginal lips). Even the male sex hormone, testosterone, is existent in small amounts in every woman, just as men produce a bit of estrogen.

HIS

Let's start with the basics—the penis, which consists of a shaft and a head. Inside the shaft is his urethra (the tube that carries his urine and semen and opens outside his body through a tiny slit in the top of his mushroom head). A man's penis contains no muscle or bone. That's astonishing when you think of how rock hard it can get. It's actually composed of three rods of erectile tissue, each encased in a strong fibrous sheath underneath his thin, delicate skin (which is also expandable and slides up and down); the rods become firm and responsive when stimulated. Erection occurs when feelings of arousal are processed in his brain and relayed through the nervous system straight to his penis. Although we'd like to think that it's the presence of beautiful, wonderful us that's inciting this vertical miracle, in truth, the cause can be constriction from tight pants or even vibrations from riding in a car or truck. When the penis is filled with a lot of pressure as a result of blood buildup, the valves close off to sustain his erection.

An average erect penis is 4 to 6 inches (most are 5⅜ inches). Under 4 inches is short, and over 6 inches is long. Fewer than ten percent of men have penises longer than 6½ inches. The longest penis ever documented was 13 inches! The blue whale penis exceeds those of all Homo sapiens, measuring 10 feet long. Imagine that! No wonder most men claim an extra inch or two for their penis. But remember, it's not the meat; it's the motion! And during lovemaking, you can make a whale of a difference with your skillful hands and mouth.

Also, don't be fooled by the two basic states—flaccid (soft) and erect (hard). The size of a flaccid penis may not necessarily correlate to the size of an erect penis. For example, a small flaccid penis may grow to be enormous when erect. Again, the opposite may be true. It's all individual. Plus, there is absolutely no relation between a man's penis size and other body parts. So stop looking at hands, feet, and noses for clues. The only clue you'll get is when you're hugging. You'll know by the mountain growing on your stomach when you're kissing. Needless to say, that's a *big* clue!

The circumference of, or thickness around, his penis can be narrow like a hot dog, medium like a banana, or wide like a cucumber. Then there's the matter of inclination and shape. It can be straight, curved upward or downward (the way a banana is curved), or narrow at the base and thicker near the top. This particular shape can sometimes be up to three times as wide at the tip as opposed to the base—so the head stands out in comparison, making the man "top-heavy."

Now that you know all about his penis, let's take a look at the scrotum. You're familiar with the sac beneath his penis, right? The one that holds his testicles? His scrotal skin is thin, loose, and stretchable with a thin layer of muscle. When he becomes sexually stimulated, exposed to the cold or physical exercise, the muscles of his scrotum contract, pulling the testicles inside the scrotum closer to his body. I actually think they're sexier when contracted. It enhances the artistic picture of a solid erection and a tight scrotum. It's so dramatic!

The main reason the testicles hang outside the body is that sperm can only be produced at a temperature lower than body temperature. The testicles are responsible for the production of various male hormones, as well as the sperm cells themselves. Most men like to have their balls touched, licked, and massaged. However, many men don't. It may irritate him when you dance with his dynamic duo, so take care!

It's time to move from the general to the specific. The next time you're making love, really observe the fundamentals. In subtle yet important ways each male organ is different from any other. Study its shape, color, texture, skin tone, shadings, veins, ridges. When he's erect, you can actually see a bulging ridge running through the center of his penis. This ridge is the projection of the uretha, which carries semen or urine.

Watch closely as it rises in stages from its dormancy. It also has a pulse you can feel that beats in the same rhythm as his heart. Observe every nuance. Houdini or David Copperfield could never invent anything as miraculous as what your man can do when he decides to change from a limp piece of warm licorice into a pulsating, penetrating piece of steel with the robust roar of a "Lion King"!

Don't just look. Touch! When stroked, it throbs in the tenderness of your hands; and, at an unexpected moment, like a cuttlefish, it will squirt a milky warm liquid in the place you designate.

Don't stop with looking and touching—smell! taste! hear! (Admittedly, penises don't make much noise, but that's no reason for you not to have all your senses working at full throttle to take in information.) Are you worried that your man will resent all this attention being lavished on his penis? No way, José!

A man loves his "objet d'art" more than any other body part. He tends it, fondles it, protects it, talks to it, admires it, pees with it, and takes great pride in it. His penis is a monument to his manhood; the very thing he spends the most time trying to satisfy, even when he's not thinking about it. He gives it endearing nicknames such as: Little Pete, Little Henry, Brutus, the Big Man, the Mighty Sword, King Cobra, Lightning Rod, John Thomas, Big Bad Ben, Red Rooster—take your pick.

So, ladies, you might as well make friends with it, too, and give it the same importance that he does . . . *enjoy his toys.*

YOURS

Women's sex organs are shrouded in much more mystery not only are they a puzzle to men, but also to many women who know less about their own organs than they do a man's. There are various reasons for this. First, women's organs are less accessible. Men are exposed to other men in locker-room situations after sports play from childhood on, but women, for the most part, are not. A woman can't even see her own genitalia by merely looking down at it the way a man can. In general, women do not buy pornographic material displaying other women's genitalia. So, your lack of basic information is understandable. Face it, womanhood is mystifying even to *women*. And finding that G-spot? Goodness me! We need a road map, a flashlight, a mirror, and literally hands-on exploration and experimentation to locate our own bodily bliss.

Before you spread your legs wide and get acquainted with your sexual self, know that just as each man has a unique penis, you have unique internal and external genitalia. The vulva—your external genitalia —is camouflaged in sexual fleece. The little mound over your pubic bone in Latin is called mons veneris, or "mound of Venus," from the Roman goddess of love. See, your feminine parts are all about love and the quest therefor.

Next, the labia majora extend from the mound of Venus tapering below the vaginal opening. These folds of skin involve nerve endings, oil and sweat glands, and fatty tissue. They also feel sexy when sucked or gently tugged on.

For your information, the labia can have many folds or they can be smooth. One side can be smaller or larger than the other. The labia can look closed or open and vary in color or odor during sexual arousal. Also, the inner lips (labia minora) can fit inside the outer ones, or they can protrude. Whatever design God gave you, their ability to receive pleasure is infinite.

Now, try squatting over a mirror to glimpse your labia minora flesh—pink, glistening with moisture, and delicately appearing devoid of skin. Your lips extend from directly above the clitoral head to the vaginal opening. These matching folds of hairless skin are not only lacking fatty tissue, but they also have more nerve endings than their outer sisters, making them ultrasensitive. So take care to treat them with gentleness. The color varies from pink or red to purple or black. All these colors are perfectly normal and when you become aroused and excited, the color may change to their formal sex color which is a bright red. Think about it! Everything changes when you become sexually activated.

Let's talk about the female penis, aka the clitoris, which (you remember) develops from the same tissue as the penis and has a similar response. Unlike the penis, it doesn't have a hole or urethra running through it. During my interviews, a number of women were shocked to find out that their clitoris did not expel urine. I'm talking about ladies of all ages. For those of you who want the truth: your urinary opening (urethral meatus) is about 1½ centimeters or ½ inch *below* your clitoris.

Your clitoris is located just below the top where the lips meet. It has a tiny glans and a little hood or foreskin called the prepuce, which is a body of loose tissue. Most of it is inside and not visible. Maybe that explains why most men don't know how to find your clitoris. Either they don't know female anatomy at all, or perhaps they're not interested enough to find out, in which case, you may want to subtly take his finger and place it on your sensitive spot. Show him how to touch the delicate delight by massaging it at your heartbeat rhythm or whatever stimulation you prefer. Keep this thought in mind: direct stimulation on the open love bud is not only uncomfortable, it can also be painful.

When you push your hood upward, you'll see what I am referring to as your love bud. It's that pink root jutting out that's comparable to a tiny button or green pea. That's your clitoris, the most sensitive part of your entire genitalia. It's filled with hundreds of nerve endings. Like a man's penis, it swells when stimulated and becomes firm and responsive. What was Freud's hypothesis? That women have penis envy? Please . . . we have an awesome little pink bud that only receives pleasure and will *never* know performance anxiety.

Located just below the urethral meatus is the entrance (introitus) to the largest tube in your female genitalia—the vagina. It's three to four inches long, flexible, and made of folded muscle. The inside walls are covered with mucus membrane. In fact, the texture, warmth, and wetness of the vagina are similar to that of the mouth, which may be one of the triggering reasons why a sexy French kiss can cause an immediate erection from either sex. French-kissing is the bridge between our mouth and genitalia. You can also French-kiss the genitalia, but we will discuss that topic later.

During arousal, your vaginal walls lubricate, producing a slippery liquid that helps guide and accommodate any size hose for the watering of your lush landscape. If you want to look at your fertile land, I strongly recommend buying a speculum. You can buy a plastic one for about three dollars and have entrance to the gates of heaven.

What's next? The cervix—Latin for "neck." Your cervix is connected to and protrudes into the innermost end of the vagina. Just an aside, but during intercourse, providing your man's endowment is praiseworthy, he can feel your cervix and he will know with your unsolicited screams that Elvis has entered the building! Obviously this does not feel good!

There's a little hole in the center of the cervix called an *os*, which means "mouth" in Latin. Your menstrual flow is like Dorothy journeying to the Emerald City, passing from the uterus to the vagina through the os. The os is the gateway either into or out of the uterus. It's also what your man's sperm must swim through (from the vagina into the uterus) in its race to find your egg.

Picture a juicy ripe pear—turned upside down— wide at the top and tapering at the bottom with the stem hanging downward. That's your uterus or womb.

It's a hollow organ about three inches long and two inches wide that will expand to fit a newborn.

All right, we've discussed vagina, cervix, and uterus. Next in line and adjacent to your luscious red womb are two white ovaries (each about the size of a grape), which produce eggs and sex hormones. Each ovary contains about two hundred thousand immature eggs, and each egg is encased in a thin tissue called a follicle.

Your fallopian tubes are the horns of the uterus. Each attaches at one end to the top of the uterus, with their other end hanging near the ovary. When your ovaries release an egg it must travel through one of the fallopian tubes to reach the uterus. When that occurs, the stage is set for conception. When your man shoots his sperm into your vagina, some sperm goes through the os into the uterus. You can feel this warm glow of love caressing all of your internal genitals. However, it takes at least fifteen minutes for this lovin' feelin' to occur after ejaculation.

BOTH OF YOU

The most powerful sex organ which the two of you share is the brain, the place where you experience arousal, emotional foreplay, and the acme of love-making—orgasm. It produces thoughts and fantasies and helps enable you to achieve orgasmic release. We usually only orgasm in a state of fantasy—a state of virtual reality within our own brains, a belief in the fantasy so powerful that we step out of our ordinary world and enter into the orgasmic world of fantasy. Although it's possible to orgasm using fantasy alone, it is rare. Even Masters and Johnson did not find one person in five hundred cases who could achieve this feat, but they believed it to be true.

The brain orchestrates our whole sex program,

producing endorphins and enkephalins, which cause the ovaries and testes to produce hormones. They also cause the entire sex cycle. So you see, you can control the quality of your sex life by properly programming your brain. It's your call. You can have the will to be mighty, to be divine, to have any orgasm you choose—minor, major, or volcanic.

Speaking of hormones, generally women who produce high levels of the male hormone testosterone are more sexually active or wish to be. They may enjoy sex more than their sisters who produce a normal amount. Certain women who produce ten times more testosterone than other women tend to do most of the riding, positioning, and coming during amorous adventures. The body produces its highest levels of testosterone at the middle of your menstrual cycle, which explains why women become so disturbingly beautiful at that time.

Here's a little secret: when you ovulate, and your corpus luteum (an encasement on the ovary) breaks, it not only discharges a ripe egg; it also discharges more testosterone and also pheromones (the sexual organic molecule that exudes from your skin revealing to males that you're fertile). The testosterone makes us become more sexy; it is a compelling aphrodisiac. The pheromones attract men to you as a female deer attracts lusty bucks when she drops her scent of musk along the fertile trail.

For rhapsodic lovemaking, your brain and sexual organs must work in unison. But start slow. Employ all of your talents and then some. As the gorgeous Brad Pitt said, "Only you know what you got in you!" To teach your man to be a hot lover, you will need to slow him down by your example. Begin with the art of arousal and bathe yourselves in foreplay.

THE ART OF AROUSAL

As long as you know that most men are like children, you know everything!

—COCO CHANEL

Arousal is a game you play with your brain. Although some might consider arousal to be synonymous with foreplay, foreplay ends with intercourse, while arousal can be a continuous state of mind. Don't be afraid to stimulate your mind, to challenge yourself, and to knock Mr. Gorgeous unconscious!

What really feels good to you? What makes your eyes shine and your clitoris chime? What makes your mouth water and sugar walls glisten with nectar? What shameful sounds alert your ears? What lubricates your brain? You don't have to tell anyone. It can be your secret.

Wouldn't it be wonderful if your man knew exactly what buttons to push to keep you perpetually aroused? Realistically, no one can push all the right buttons all the time. Our sexual energy is like the tide. Sometimes it's in, sometimes it's out.

Let's imagine that you're with the perfect lover. Benevolently speaking, it's not fair to put the absolute burden of sexual arousal on his shoulders every time. Sometimes you need to take responsibility for arousing him and yourself. We asked for equality. We certainly have it in this arena. Coming to your lovemaking sessions already turned on is a supreme aphrodisiac for him—much better than banana cream pie.

How can you do it? Take a tip from my friend Mary Ann, a thirty-three-year-old copywriter from Chicago, Illinois, who confides, "I had such hang-ups about my body, about receiving an orgasm, about pleasing a man, until I turned thirty-three years old. For my birthday I took a trip to Big Sur, California, alone. I had an unforgettable experience on the patio of my Ventanna Inn suite listening to the music of Frank Sinatra while the sun penetrated my naked body. Breathing in the natural smells of my surroundings, I unconsciously began touching my own personal natural surroundings—my thighs, breasts, face, and hair. While exploring my womanhood in front of God, I imagined that my fingers were "his"—the man of my dreams—caressing every area of my body in rhythm with the music. Before I knew it, I had goose bumps from head to toe, then tiny spasms. I thought my brain was contracting or hallucinating. The world disappeared for a brief moment. Without warning, a flood of warm wet liquid ran down my thigh. I leaned over the balcony and let loose a yell that would have beckoned Tarzan himself."

The bottom line is, if your man does not arouse you to the point of surrender, do it yourself! If you arrive at that wonderful place, what difference does it make who gets the credit?

Just as an actor prepares for a role, you can prepare for lovemaking by doing things to keep your erotic mind fueled. Remember to treat your libido as a living thing to be nourished and nurtured. Don't neglect it. It's sure to dry and die like a plant that you forgot to water. (Don't you just *hate* it when that happens?) But the good news is: while your plants can die from too much water, your libido only grows stronger and healthier with more encouragement. And you stay younger longer, because the testosterone, pheromones, endorphins, enkephalins, et cetera, generated at that time are exactly the same organic molecules that help rejuvenate your beautiful body. That's a fact!

Now that your motor is humming, what are you going to do for his? Remember that arousal can be inspired by sights, sounds, words, smells, touch—the power of suggestion—anything. And you don't have to look too far to find sources of inspiration. It's not for nothin' that million-dollar industries keep us interminably aroused. We love it. We feed off it. *Stimulate! Stimulate! Stimulate!*

Romantic novels written for women jump off the bookstore shelves. Magazines for men continue to grow in popularity. How different can one woman look from another? Every month they keep finding new interpretations and men ride with the tide. Different is exciting. Different is enticing. But you may ask: how do I keep his aroused energy focused on me?

Since you are the gatekeeper of your jewels, you can—in all propriety—promote an incident in public that will leave him with wide-eyed fascination. Actually, anywhere you sense the tactile tigress taking over, just go for it! You only live once, but check it out first, and do be careful.

Here's an idea. If you're sitting opposite your lover in a restaurant, take your stockinged foot and massage his crotch with your toes; or if you're sitting side by side, let your fingers talk to "Lucky Chuckie" under the table or take your man's hand and put it on your wet tulip. The presence of other people in the restaurant and the danger of discovery will add more than a dash of spice to the proceedings.

For sheer provocation, wear a bra with the nipples cut out. This can lead to arousal for both of you—the feel of the fabric rubbing against your erect nipples will keep you perpetually stimulated while the sight of their protrusion should have a salubrious effect on him.

Throughout the evening, consider bending over to give him a glimpse of your cleavage. If you don't have ample cleavage, buy a Wonder Bra. They're great. Or cross and uncross your legs to let Adonis peek up your thighs. I wouldn't suggest playing the room. Pick your moments. But always be a lady who gives her gentleman a few private diversions. After all, seduction is about anticipation. He needs to look forward to what lies ahead. Or didn't you know that anticipation is extremely arousing? *Anticipation* is the key that unlocks the door of desire. So make him wait!

Flirt! Flirting is intriguing when done with sincerity and charm. Always flirt with the man you love. It keeps the embers stoked. If he has encyclopedic knowledge, stare deep into his eyes with genuine admiration. A knowledgeable gent certainly gives my libido a wake-up call. If he's working on an interesting project, ask him all about it. Let him talk while you listen with adoration. He'll feel a mounting sense of well-being and think he's discovered gold, which he has—you.

Make him feel that whatever realm he's chosen, you are impressed. He's the basis of the earth's core. Be sincere. Be perceptive. Be sensitive. Maybe you have something he can fix. Or a project he can help you finish. Allow him to be manly. That masculine specimen will defend you, protect you, and hold you forever dear in his protective, strong hands.

Also, if you have a flair for humor and know a few provocatively funny jokes or stories, tell him. Remember to keep them amusing, not crude. You don't want to sound like one of the boys in the locker room. Use your humor with aplomb and panache. It will always be one of your greatest allies. There's nothing better than a hearty laugh from the gut to open up a fella. When a man is happy, stimulated, and in love, he will bring you the Holy Grail. Keep it light! Keep it fun!

What about sounds? Is there a singer or a song that turns him on? Find out! You *need* to know these things. Aural foreplay enhances anticipation. Call him at work or leave a message on his machine using sexual double entendres. Whisper a fantasy in his ear, preferably one that excites both of you. He'll get the picture.

Most men love to read erotica. So do most women, for that matter. Only our choices are a bit dissimilar. Give him something artistic, yet suggestive, as a gift or let him "accidentally" come across some of your erotic spirituality and encourage him to thumb through it.

I can't begin to tell you how alluring soft, silky fabrics are to a man's touch. Why do you think lingerie is a billion-dollar business? It's the feel of the fabric against your femininity. Wear them often and position your anatomy in ways that entice his fingers to wander into your wanton zones.

Nonchalantly, ask him to feel the silkiness of your satin blouse, the softness of your cashmere sweater, or the texture of the fine cotton, crepe, rayon, jersey, acetate, or other slinky materials you happen to be wearing at the time. Whatever fabric you choose, as long as it's soft and sensual, it will increase his desire.

If you have no objections, let him run his fingers through your hair. Men love the smell and feel of a woman's clean hair. It's intoxicating to them. Try not to be too concerned about your hairdo, but more concerned for his enjoyment. Now, if you're dashing to the theater, concert, or a sophisticated dinner, that's a different matter. I'm sure he can wait, if you charmingly communicate.

About smells: why do you think we spend so much money and time on perfumes, scented powders, and body lotions? For ourselves? Of course! But also, for our man. I love it when my man inhales the fragrance of my body, whether the clean smell of soap straight from a shower or my tried and true perfume. A suggestion: if your fella responds strongly to a certain fragrance, make a mental note. And when you see him again, wear it. Smell is a central part of arousal and seduction.

Another endearing and inviting smell is the aroma of succulent food cooking in your kitchen. As he walks through your door, the smell of cooking food will seduce his stomach and send his senses to fond memories. My grandmother (who was the best cook in New Orleans) repeatedly said, "The best way to a man's heart is through his stomach!" (I know my grandmother's not the only or even the first one to say it. These sayings become proverbial because they are true.) The hunger for good-tasting, fresh food is another kind of sexy desire. Of course, there are many other feminine wiles, but Grandma's way is tried and true, provided you're a *good* cook. If you're not, beguile him with your other specialties.

Before we withdraw from the smell sense, I'll leave you with the biggest turn-on of all—pheromones—the musky scent which emanates from your vagina and his scrotal skin at certain times. In other words, your natural juices. (These pheromones are different from the ones mentioned above.) When he inhales your pheromones, his gears shift from first to fifth in milliseconds. Presto . . . an erection! It's also a signal that you're turned on, too, and knowing *that* is even more exciting to him than your perfume. It's the domino effect! He gets delirious because you're enthusiastic. Let him savor the scent. You know how testosterone loves estrogen.

Okay, now that you're both aroused, let's experience a potent one-two—emotional as well as tangible foreplay. The necessary stimulation you so deservedly crave before intercourse. And if everything goes well, orgasms for everyone.

FOREPLAY

Don't ever let me catch you singing like that again, without enthusiasm. You're nothing if you aren't excited by what you are doing.
—FRANK SINATRA TO HIS SON, FRANK, JR.

Foreplay is a delicious and exciting activity, usually (but not always) precedent to intercourse. Before we get too involved with the details of how, I want to remind you that engaging in foreplay does not oblige you to conclude with intercourse. You still have the right to stop and say no. I think it's also important to remind you that activities involved in foreplay that don't conclude with intercourse can still result in the transmission of serious illness. I don't want to spoil your fun, but I do want you to be around to enjoy life and your dream man for many years to come, so please heed my warning.

Although matters of sex should always be fun, there is a certain amount of responsibility that never should be abdicated, such as the intimate discussion of sexually transmitted diseases (STDs). Taking appropriate precautions (condoms and regular testing for STDs) is a necessary part of responsible lovemaking. It's wise to have this delicate conversation before you enter into foreplay. Of course, I know you will broach the topic with considerable tact and charm, right? Then exchange proof that both of you are healthy. If he will not go along with the program, he's a cad, he's definitely not living in the real world . . . drop him!

Onward with foreplay. You may be under the impression that men don't need or don't like foreplay. *Wrong!!* During my interviews, I asked the question, "Would you like to be sexually pampered by the woman you love?" Answer: "Oh yeah! Why not? Except I'd have to trust her first, and feel comfortable!"

Ladies, it's time to call forth your consummate womanly wiles—knowledge, imagination, skills, erotic paraphernalia, and other inventive resources. You don't want to be a memory, unless of course it's the kind of memory that Travis Tritt pines over in a song—*the one he can't forget!* Yes, you want to be the woman he will die for, the woman he will never leave, the woman he can't get out of his mind and the slightest thought of whom brings on a "grand erection." To be this woman, you need yet another ally—foreplay—the skill of feel.

Remember that his ability and desire to enjoy foreplay are no less than yours. Be gentle but purposeful. If you've come this far, begin to assess his shape through his clothes to give scope to the preparation of your masterpiece. With your sensitivity and acute awareness, every ounce of his body will be in full cooperation. As you slide your fingertips over his pectorals, feel *his* erect nipples. How naturally his body responds to your touch! Slowly continue to run your fingertips up and down the length of his anatomy. Take your time. Give him a sense of security. Now, use your hands to squeeze sections of his flesh a bit more firmly. At this point, he should be comfortable enough for you to proceed with the complete undressing.

Undress your man with finesse. After you fondle and caress him through his clothes, after he accepts your pre-massage, it's time for more serious and meaningful stimulation.

While you're kissing his lips and massaging the front of his chest, you could begin to unbutton the front of his shirt or, if it's a T-shirt, with your sensitive, nimble fingers slip it over his head. It's not imperative to begin at the top, especially for a man. He may think you're never heading for the gold. And that's precisely the root of his excitement. The *wait*! The *tease*! The *anticipation*! As you open his shirt, make a trail of kisses over all exposed areas. If he has a hairy chest, nuzzle your face in it, smell it, play with it. If his chest is bare, kiss and lick his smooth skin. Whatever he's got, enjoy.

The key to undressing yourself in front of him or undressing him is: take your time with each item of clothing. As you remove each part of his clothing, make love to that uncovered part. In undressing him slowly, you're showing him how you want him to undress you; now it's up to you whether you leave parts of his clothing on or undress him completely. Remember: different moods and surroundings dictate different actions. Act accordingly.

Ahh, so you've decided to undress him completely! Good! Now that he's naked, you can begin to paint his picture. Think of him as the canvas and yourself as the brush and paint combined. Use your exquisitely sensitive fingertips and far-reaching toes to trace a design. Bring your lips and tongue into play to add color and depth. Nuzzle some of those hard-to-reach crevices with your nose and eyelashes. Cover large areas with your soft breasts and hard nipples. Let your silky hair brush all over him. Use every inch of yourself to caress every inch of him. His entire body is an erogenous zone waiting and longing for the immortal touch that only you can bestow.

Your artistry and patience should inspire him to reciprocate in kind. In fact, don't be surprised if he's eager to do so. And then you can fly to Never Never Land on Aladdin's magic carpet—*together*. Moreover, after you please him completely, he'll be the clay for your Rodin. He'll fantasize, hope, and dream for an encore of celebration. In the interim, I'm sure he'll do whatever is humanly possible to make you happy both in bed and out.

Since every man has a different libido, the road to foreplay has no rules—no right or wrong. The guide to your inamorato's erogenous zones lies dormant—waiting anxiously for you to step up to the podium to commence the inauguration. My, my, what power you have. But never forget: you're only as powerful as your sensitivities and acute awareness. Without awareness, your intelligence and artistry are wasted. Your tango can be smooth as silk or rough as burlap. It's your assignment to discover through grace and subtlety exactly what areas delight him most. What touch—how light or firm, where and when he feels comfortable being stroked. His sounds, body movement, and hands will guide you. Pay close attention!

He will have places of pleasure and responses that no other man has. And when you locate the precise place, keep it your secret. If you talk about it or tell anybody, you will lose your magic. Magic cannot survive mistrust.

Don't be impatient. Exactitude rarely happens on the first take. Opening up is a slow and somewhat arduous process, especially for a man. Nonetheless, you might get lucky. Make experimenting on his bodily reactions your life's mission. Finding his turn-ons could be a joy. One day it might be one thing, another day, something else. Since turnabout's fair play, allow him to explore your turn-ons.

Always remember that the *brain* is the engine that drives all erogenous zones. Your allure must run deeper than your killer looks. To really turn him on you must first relax his mind. Expel his negativity and anxiety-ridden thoughts. Instill fun, positive musings such as exchanging provocatively humorous experiences that you've both had, heard, or read. Stimulate his senses with photos, videos, music, or a striptease . . . *anything* enticing. Just free his mind!

Indulge his whims with a bit of role-playing—act out a fantasy. But make sure it's fun for you, too. Project yourself into an imaginary situation, dress the part, and act out the role. Ideally, plan ahead so he can anticipate. Eat light. Be spanking clean. Set the desired mood. Take the phone off the hook and hide the beeper. Use pillows, silk scarves, oils, lotions, incense, sexy foods for sex play; inspire aural foreplay with tempting naughty talk. Take your time and relax with a glass of champagne, wine, juice, or whatever you prefer. The key is to let go of inhibitions. Sometimes roleplaying can free both partners' inhibitions.

ROLES
You can be a cheerleader and he the football hero. *Encourage him!* You can be a slave girl and he can be your lord and master. *Please him!* You can be the femme fatale and he can be the innocent farm boy you're initiating into the mysteries of sex. *Seduce him!* He can be the teacher and you can be the little girl who's getting a spanking. An erotic spanking with the right words, the right pressure, the right hand, the right place on your buttocks while you're lying over his lap with your panties partly down, can release a lot of juices. He'll probably tell you how bad you've been while he makes you even badder. Talk about libidinous!

Now that you've opened the door to your imagination, keep exploring that territory. You play the lovely Guinevere who is rescued by the handsome knight Sir Lancelot. *Show your gratitude!* He is the powerful Viking, Erik the Red, and you are his captive. Struggle for a while, then *surrender unconditionally.* Another time, switch roles. You are Captain Hook, the most feared pirate in the South Seas, and you've captured both his ship and his men. Command him to surrender all of his weapons. Tie him to the mast and blindfold him. If he so much as whimpers while you undress him, simultaneously tickle his naked body with a feather and spank his bottom. Maybe with more than your hand. And if he refuses to submit, threaten to throw him overboard, where the sharks will have a banquet with his delicacies. He's your prisoner—do as you will!

Some men really like this type of sport. Ali, a thirty-four-year-old lawyer said, "I love playing the submissive role with my wife, Tina. She dresses in fishnet stockings, a bustier, and six-inch black leather heels. She wears a choker, a mask, and sometimes carries a whip or a feather. She does things to my body that excite me to the point where I get so turned on that I feel silly. She never laughs. She just continues my fantasy. That's why I love her so much. The following week, I'm the party in control and command her to masturbate herself while I watch. Afterwards, I use a few toys and vibrators to excite her to multiple orgasms."

Silly-for-love is not a bad place for anyone to be. But never do anything that makes you feel bad or uncomfortable. Lovers must have fun in their own way, their own style.

Different men have different styles of expressing their erotic side. Some men revel in submission, some men rejoice in domination, some men relish both. There are men who handle women, handle wild horses, and handle life with a certain savage but tender and romantic flair. The classic American lover. But whatever his deepest desires, you won't know until you investigate his inner soul.

MORE MALE ROLES

Playboy, TV anchorman, Chippendale dancer, hair-
dresser, famous athlete, psychiatrist, truck driver,
sultan, gynecologist, politician, movie star, gigolo, prisoner, Mafia don, traveling salesman, starving artist,
cowboy, porno movie producer, rich sugar daddy, pizza
delivery boy, rock star, surfer, serious musician, big-
game hunter, policeman, stranger, Batman, Dracula,
Don Juan, Valentino.

MORE FEMALE ROLES

Lawyer, nun, model, movie star, airline stewardess, li-
brarian, housewife, debutante, sex therapist, jungle
queen, groupie, prison guard, princess, professor, harem
dancing girl, stripper, tax collector, mechanic, waitress,
real estate broker, singer, interviewer, rich socialite, best
friend's girl, carhop, judge, cowgirl, Southern belle, far-
mer's daughter, saleswoman, dentist, highly paid lady
of the night.

Imagination is such a dynamic tool for great sex. My
friend Katie, a thirty-year-old real estate broker who's
married with two children, knows how to make good
use of her imagination. "After twelve years of marriage,
my husband, Don, and I still make love at least three
times a week or more. I wear sexy lingerie and costumes
that I put together for his amusement—crotchless panties, pasties on my nipples, fishnet body suits, a nurse's
uniform, a school girl's uniform with a black garter belt
and stockings underneath and high heels or boots,
whatever mood strikes me at the time. I keep things
exciting, not only for Don; being sexually aggressive
and playing different roles stimulates me, too. Sometimes I wear a particularly sexy dress when we go out
to dinner or a party. During the entire evening, I flirt
and tease, but I never touch him. I just appear as if I'm

about to and it makes him really hot. By the time we get home, I'm ready to devour him. Kneeling on the floor of the kitchen, I unzip his pants and perform oral sex."

Katie and her husband have learned the important lesson that anything is possible in an atmosphere of trust and deep, deep caring. They indulge each other's fantasies in a fun-loving environment while reaping rich rewards.

USE YOUR HANDS

Now both of you are engaged in the process, you're both aroused, both willin', wantin', and waitin' with anticipation. At this point, use everything available to you. You can't find enough ways to use your hands in the art of making him feel good. Mae West certainly used her tactile assets. Take the last scene in her movie *She Done Him Wrong*. Cary Grant (who turned out to be an undercover cop) produced a pair of handcuffs by which he intended to take Mae into custody. She looked at him dubiously and protested, "I ain't never worn a pair of them things." Cary responded knowingly, "A lot of men might have been safer if you had!" From the glint in his eye, I don't doubt that Mae's mouth and fingers strummed a few bars on Cary's instrument. Hmmmmm, hmmmmm, that's a very sexy woman.

Like Mae West, after you've had your expert hands all over his anatomy, he'll be in seventh heaven. If you're sensitive, imaginative, and a bit courageous, he'll consider you and your hands "dangerous." The sexy side of dangerous—butterflies in the stomach, a quickened heartbeat, a juicy mouth, flushed cheeks, can't eat, can't sleep. And does your main man deserve anything less than magic? I think not.

Speaking of hands, who can forget that wonderful scene in the movie *Ghost* where Demi Moore is working at the pottery wheel? I could see strength and artistic expression flow from her hands while she dug into and worked the wet clay. In fact, as Patrick Swayze looked on in admiration of this sensual and artistic feat, his hands couldn't resist joining hers at the wheel. Their "touch" was exquisite to behold. The climax came when both pairs of hands moved simultaneously, creating a phenomenon of seductive art. Suffice it to say, seductive art is what you will be creating with your objet d'art—your man!

REAL ROLES

To love deeply takes a lot of courage and guts—a lot of patience, nurturing, and reassuring, but the rewards are great. Are you game? If so, you can gain access to his cache by choosing a sensitive moment to communicate the following: that you will not think him unmanly or weak if he lets you take sexual control sometimes; that he needs to forget all of his preconceived ideas about who's supposed to be dominant and who's supposed to be submissive; that he does not have to perform on any level; that lovemaking is not tit for tat; and that it's not about one person controlling every sexual session. It is about *give-and-take control and surrender*—for both parties.

Your soldier may be prone to hide his submissive side. That leaves it up to you to change his thinking with your skillful processing orientation. To surrender, a man might fear losing his erection and the humiliation that follows. Reassure him that it's not a contest—keeping his erection is not vital. You're simply cohorts sharing responsibility; advancing the art of lovemaking in a collaborative process. In fact, at times it's more provocative when he allows *you* to become his fantasy femme fatale.

Women have tremendous power to be life giving

or life threatening. Lea, a twenty-six-year-old beautiful blonde from Youngstown, Ohio, gets upset when her man is not erect. She said it makes her feel undesirable. Not only is she expecting the impossible, she's also putting unimagined pressure on herself and her fella. It's foolish and insecure to think such thoughts. A man is a human being, not an automaton. He can't be expected to rise on command. In this case, as in many others, the best lubrication and stimulation is still . . . communication!

Take a chance on being the innovator who dares to take your man on the voyage of his lifetime. To be able to get what you want out of lovemaking—kissing, foreplay, orgasm, romance coupled with hot interludes, you need to make love to his body the way you would like him to make love to your body. Show him slowly while expressing, "Does this feel good? I love it when you do this to me . . ." A man will not be able to give you what you need and want if you don't know what you need and want. After you have learned to satisfy your own body, kindly show him by example. No matter how much you wish it to be so, he's not a mind reader, and maybe not as quick as you. Just cut him a little slack. If he's a good one, he's certainly worth it.

Please don't get frustrated if it doesn't happen in one night. It generally takes a few sessions before he finds the right rhythm to draw pleasure from your treasure. Eventually, he *will* get the whole movie and voilà—your phantom lover in the flesh. So tell Tarzan to move over and let Sheena swing on the vines for a while.

Once aware that surrendering is truly sexy, he will give you his weaponry any time, any place. If you doubt me, rent the movie *Desirée* and pay particular attention to the last scene when Marlon Brando, playing Napoléon, surrenders his sword to Jean Simmons, who plays

Desirée—his first love. It is a magic moment. The amazing thing is that both characters emerge from that scene stronger than they were when it began. There are no losers in love. The experience itself is pleasing to a woman.

The main benefit of initiating and leading sex play is you get what you want. Being in control allows you to choose the place, set the pace, tempo, and most important . . . create the right mood to discover and draw out hidden passions. With his body in your hands and at your command, you can make foreplay more sensual and last as long as you desire. Of course, this can only work if you have already earned and *deserved*, not merely *demanded*, his trust.

Go slowly and take your time; feel his anatomy. Let your fingers act as sensors exploring the uncharted territory of his pleasure. Investigate the mysterious regions of his response—what areas and what kind of pressure make him shiver or sigh or moan?

When you've found his bliss, weave in and out, circle around. *Tease* until he's breathless—intoxicated. Then delicately and purposefully use those educated fingers to guide him safely into the quiet glades of Eden, where delirium and emancipation grow with the most incredible foreplay and orgasm he has ever had!

Keep remembering the nonpareil lover who appears to you when you're "petting the pony." He walks through your door or stands at the foot of your bed, drawing you to him like the magnet he is. Unquestioningly, you surrender your whole being to a current of engaging orgasms. After he's drained every last droplet of dew from your orchid, your heart and soul, branch and root belong to him as you lie in his arms perfectly spent.

You see, you do to your man exactly as your ideal sex mate does to you—more or less. Need I say more?

Carry on: treat his entire body as the erogenous zone it is. This kind of communicative lovemaking is more feeling and exploratory than vocal. He might be vocal in expressing his release, but your seductive voice will come later during intercourse. For now, go very, very slowly. Titillate, tantalize, and thrill.

KISSES

We discussed kissing earlier, but now that we're discussing a more intense relationship, here are a few more reminders about kissing. First, as I've stated before, relax your jaw. Since the muscles of the lips are connected to the jaw, when you relax your jaw, the lips relax. Your kiss must be tender, delicate, and with controlled passion, but passion nonetheless. Always kiss gently at first. Cushion your lips against your teeth, so as not to jar or take him out of the moment. He needn't feel your teeth, just your soft, gentle, hungry lips. (A man hates to feel teeth either when you're kissing his lips or his penis.) Also, if you kiss him with tension in your lips, he can't properly relax. He takes his cue from you, remember. And relaxation is the key to enjoyment.

Don't stick your tongue into his mouth before he can taste your lips. After he feels comfortable and wants more, you can gently but firmly rub the tip of your tongue over the front and back of both rows of his teeth. Then delicately suck on his lips. Keep it sensual. No quick movements. (Some men like this, others don't. You be the judge.)

If he gives you his tongue, that means he has accepted you, and his sexual temperature is on the rise, if not risen. But don't let his encouragement rush you. Stay with sensual, tender, and exploring kisses. While you're exploring his lips and mouth with your tongue, keep it pointed, rather than broad and flat. And don't suffocate him by keeping your tongue deep in his throat. You don't have to try to be sensual . . . *you are sensual*—you're a woman!

When his mouth opens more—and I'm certain it will—slip your tongue in a little further. Focus is everything in great sex. Men generally stay focused on one intention. It works! So don't lose yourself in *his* intention and become swept away with *his* focus. Wait . . . Tease . . . Withdraw slowly. If he likes what you're doing and you feel his body rise, carry on with rhythmically bolder strokes, as though you were in the middle of passionate intercourse. When you know for sure that he's following your lead, move on to kiss other areas of his face—his eyes, his nose, his ears. Nibble on his earlobes, his neck, and whatever exposed skin you find.

MASSAGE AND MORE

After all this scrumptious tasting and drawing on his soul, I think now's the time to use his body as a picturesque temple for the high art of massage foreplay. Nothing is more stimulating for your man when done beyond his expectations save fellatio, or hot, heavenly intercourse in his natural position—from behind.

Next, take your time to remove most of your clothing in his full vision. You may want to do a scanty striptease, removing only a few items. Then excuse yourself to don a silky robe with only your sublime nakedness underneath. You will need all of your bodily accoutrements free from any restriction to produce your magnum opus. Beforehand warm the room and the massage oil. It's more thoughtful. And you don't want him to catch a cold as you open much more than his pores.

Exploring your lover's physical being—skin, hair, muscles, lips, and penis—is essential for his pleasure. When done properly it is an undeniable aphrodisiac—

an incredible prelude to lovemaking. It can break the touching barrier while relaxing the body and mind. In minutes, you can soothe, energize, or arouse. You can warm his muscles, loosen tissue, dissolve knots, cramps, and tension. It is the quickest and easiest way to inspire him to open his soul. But he must have trust in you as well as your touch. And the more comfortable you can make him feel, the more he will trust you. When he starts to trust you, his real self will surface. *Trust* is key, especially in successful body massage.

The *first touch* of your fingertips on his skin is the *most important* of all. So take your time—feel him—savor the magic moment when your bodies first connect in massage foreplay. Moreover, this union of skin draws out a man's masculinity and a woman's femininity. If you can imagine that just two and a half square yards of his skin contain five million nerve endings that send sensory signals to his brain with unfathomable speed, you'll better understand why the right touch can feel exquisite.

When you relax a man's brain, he is more apt to open up to you. If you've never done so, it's a good idea to take a look at a skeletal chart. It will help if you visually sketch his outline in your mind before you begin. You will have a better idea of what you're touching. And that helps, believe me.

His skeleton provides the internal framework that supports the rest of his body. He has about 206 bones. His skull encloses and protects his think tank and other important organs, in particular the eyes and inner ears. Gauge the amount of pressure you apply by paying attention to his body language, sighs, moans, and groans. Stay focused and let your sensorial fingers articulate your thoughts—good, positive, generous thoughts that serve to connect your souls.

Give special TLC to the major erogenous zones: the

lips, nipples, and genitals. Tantalize with the musical feel of your fingertips and your tongue. This is only a prelude to the pleasures awaiting him.

Begin your work of art in a heated room with warm oil, unscented or slightly aromatic. Most men are averse to strong smells and greasy liniments. I massage with an oil or lotion of natural ingredients that I include in my romantic kit. I find the subtle, organic scents more palatable to the male taste. Now place a bedsheet or towel over a mat or anything moderately soft. The bed is usually too soft and bare floors are too hard. Your man must feel coddled . . . loved. Relaxing music should be playing in the background, preferably non-vocal. Words might distract.

Ask him to lie down on his stomach. (Most professionals begin with the person on his stomach and I think it works well that way.) Also ask him if he has any injuries before you begin. For example, if he has tendonitis and you unknowingly press and pull, that can hurt him and he will not relax enough to surrender. A lack of surrender will stifle your creativity.

During massage, think of yourself as a sculptor and his body as your clay. Your hands and imagination will mold his clay into a beautiful and fitting tribute to your genius. Use all of his subtle tones and textures to create a golden bronze that would give Michelangelo pause.

Begin: straddle his body so you can have the proper balance and support. Empty some oil into the palm of your left hand and put the bottle down beside you, always within reach. Having access to your lubricant is part of maintaining the massage rhythm. Place both hands on the back of his neck and shoulders, since this is the prominent area where tension is held. Start a rotating motion with your thumbs and fingertips. Gently knead the muscles around, across, and up the neck, into the back of the head, where nerve endings connect, and all around the skull. Spend a lot of time on his head (don't you enjoy a good massage and wash at the beauty shop?), massaging firmly with your fingertips. Then use your nails to gently scratch the scalp. It also feels good to him when you take semilarge sections of his hair and gently tug. As you tug, think of it as pulling out his tension, slowly. Do make sure you tug all the hairs in sections on his entire scalp. It's both healthy and invigorating.

Okay, let's continue back up his spine, rhythmically pumping the muscle with firmer pressure. A good rule is never to let your fingers lose contact with any part of his skin. When a part of you is always touching a part of him, he feels more secure and loved. With the same rhythm, return to the top of the spine and slide both thumbs down the sides of his spinal column. You can feel if he's enjoying your talents. Reverse the movement. Then with the heel of your hands, use a zigzag movement down his spine while blowing air on and kissing each vertebra.

For arms, wrists, and hands, use a squeeze-and-release motion. Squeeze and release—rather firmly—in a pumping kind of motion all the way up to his shoulders, then back down again. Now, spend a lot of time on his hands, those complex organs made up of many small bones. (They're the things he uses the most, other than the obvious thing!) Clasp the sides of one of his hands with both of yours. Use a rotating motion with your thumbs to work in between the palm bones (metacarpals) and finger bones (phalanges). Just feel all portions of his hands.

After you have worked over his torso, gently part his legs and wander on down to the lower half. (No, not that . . . yet!) His buttock muscles will need a much stronger pressure. If your thumbs are tired, alternate with the palms of your hands. Add droplets of oil gen-

erously onto his glorious mounds. Push both cheeks together in a rotating rhythm. Lift them and squeeze
them. Shape his buttocks with your hands and fingers
—lift, separate, and smooth them. Watching and feeling
them as you mold your clay is certainly a turn-on, if
you know what I mean.

With his legs still parted, rub more oil into his inner thighs. Feel the heat. The craving between his legs
will be tormenting, but I'm sure he will let your engaging fingers commence to work the rest of his flesh. His
hamstrings in the back of his thighs are likely to be taut;
therefore, they need a deeper pressure. As you continue,
extend your downward stroke to include the calf muscles and carry on with his Achilles tendons and feet.

You are clearing away all of his thoughts with your
seamless changes and variations. That was your intention! Take his foot in your hands and hold it for a few
seconds while the nerve endings feel the warmth and
energy emanating from your hands. Feel the structure
and massage the five long bones of the foot (metatar-
sals) and toes (phalanges). When you concentrate on his
toes, make sure you give each one a gentle tug. From
the toes, follow with the instep, ankle, knee, thigh, and
up his body once again, but this time using a squeeze-
release motion. When you have finished, ask him to
turn over on his back or, better still, silently guide him
with your hands.

If you happen to get this far, you can continue the
massage up and down the front of his entire body, finishing with his head positioned in your lap, gently
smoothing the oil into his throat, chest, and shoulders.
Then the muscles of his face, temples, brow, eyes, nostrils, and once again . . . his head—which, after all, is
a lovely crown for the finale of body massage. He will
feel so good lying there in your hands—a passionflower
in bloom, readied for your pleasure.

You can enjoy a laid-back, sexy kind of energy in his response. However, in the event your energy is waning, allow for revitalization with tender caresses and sips of chilled champagne. But always have a part of your body touching his. After you feel invigorated, pretend he's the last chocolate éclair you will ever eat. Savoring every nuance, begin to smell, taste, lick, and suck out the creme as if it would be the last time or the first, if you will. While caressing and kissing his neck, shoulders, lips, and face, murmur honest compliments that you sincerely feel from your heart like, "I love the way you taste!" or "I like the feel of your skin!" or "I could drown myself in your manliness."

When you speak with sincerity, he will bathe in the essence. And when you focus on his pleasure, you become liberated. Remember, the only dialogue at this time is flattering and sexy talk, nothing else.

Everything in life is rhythm and timing, as I'm sure you know. Keep in mind the timing of your action and rhythm of the moment. Now for the tongue bath: with silent words of "I love you, I adore you, I worship you" rolling off the tip of your tongue and your soft lips, slowly trace the whole of his anatomy with no stone unturned, and no crevice unattended. To add to his ever growing sensations, you can blow warm air on each spot you lick. Enjoy his delectable manly flavors and smells.

Starting with his fingers, kiss his fingertips, fingers, and the palm of his hand, and hold his hand to your face. Gently put each finger individually into your mouth. Suck and swirl your tongue up and down and around, concentrating on the middle ones as you look deep into his eyes. Let your tongue proceed up his forearm, upper arm, and neck to his hungry mouth. Kiss and gently bite his earlobe while whispering endearing thoughts into his ear like, "Do you like what I'm doing?

Is it okay if I touch you in other places?" Say whatever pure thought your heart is feeling at that moment.

With the tip of your tongue, gently trace the outline of his ear, slightly inserting your tongue at intervals. Don't drown his hearing with a lot of tongue and saliva. That's a sure way to ruin the mood you've been creating.

Whisper sensual and flattering secrets that you've discovered about him while you insert your pointed tongue in the rhythm that you would like your vagina to be penetrated by his penis.

Hmmmmm . . . you certainly know what he's thinking now, right? He has to wait, though, until you are ready. It's not time . . . just yet. Be patient.

You've had a few appetizers, some mouthwatering champagne—now you want to tickle his fancy with yet another delicacy. As you're holding his head in your secure hands, trace your tongue down his neck, planting little kisses as you go. Again, run your fingers through his hair and inhale its aroma. It lets him know that you appreciate all of him as you move down his neck to his pectorals and then his nipples.

A lot of men really enjoy having their pecs massaged (as you did his buttocks—lifting and squeezing), and their nipples sucked, licked, and played with. Others are ultrasensitive and find it rather tickling. If you have a ticklish man, move on. If your man enjoys this procedure (goose bumps on his body are a giveaway), and you'll be able to judge by his reaction as your tongue is sliding in the general vicinity of "the territory"—continue to make love to that area the same way you would like his moist mouth to kiss, suck, and flutter on your sexy breasts and nipples. If he likes it, ever so gently tease the tips of his nipples with the tips of your teeth. Don't bite; rather, gently feel.

For heightened stimulation, you can grasp one of

his nipples between your thumb and index finger, gently rolling it around as you would a grape, without breaking its skin, as your mouth and tongue travel to other areas. Don't forget to alternate from one nipple to the other with the same fervor. Give every part equal attention. You know how you hate it when your guy just sucks one breast all night, while the other is entirely neglected. Don't make the same mistake with him. See, you're showing him in subtle ways how you want it.

At this point, you'll sense how important the right music fits into the layout of your lovemaking. Your body parts dance to the sounds of seduction on his male figure. It only adds to the atmosphere. Without losing tempo, continue with the impression of your soft, moist lips down the sides of his pectorals, rib cage, and belly. Then work your mouth and tongue around his navel area as your hands stroke his thighs, skipping over his genitalia. Remember to tease! At this point, I'd bet my car that your Michelangelo is on the ceiling. Enjoying his response and watching his body come alive in your hands is a definite, if not definitive, reward.

Let your hair and breasts fall and glide around his abdomen, thighs, and accidentally over his groin while your hands stroke and delicately massage his inner thighs. Without touching his penis, kiss all around the area. You're engaging in teasing foreplay before penis play.

Make him hold back while you drive him crazy. He loves it and he hates it. Some men have enormous control. It's challenging to see just how cool they can stay. But others are a bit more expressive. And without warning, the creme in his éclair might suddenly slip out in the middle of your extravaganza. That's actually a compliment to your artistic skill. Nevertheless, it's more exciting when he can last until the last act. But, as the Boy Scouts advise, be prepared!

You've guessed by now what comes next and he's certainly ready, waiting, and deserving. He is absolutely prepared! You have gardened his landscape, made his soul blossom. The time has come to ply your skills in that very special brand of foreplay called fellatio.

FELLATIO

Is that a gun in your pocket or are you just happy to see me?

—MAE WEST

Is fellatio important to men? I can only tell you that almost all the men to whom I spoke told me that fellatio has a place of honor on their wish list. It ties with making love to two women simultaneously as their favorite fantasy. Make it your business to do fellatio so well that he'll forget his ménage à trois. When you really love your man, it's easy to be great!

The other day, as I walked out of a popular chicken diner on Sunset Strip in L.A., I witnessed a pretty "lady of the night" (in this case day) approach two young nice-looking gents in a new white truck. They talked for a few minutes, laughed—when, suddenly, the girl slipped inside the front seat between the boys. The truck pulled to the back of the restaurant in broad daylight, and the girl's head started bopping up and down in a beat, with Snoop Doggy Dogg loudly playing, on both penises. It was amazing. I must confess, I stood there as though I were riveted to the spot . . . watching! Men are visual? Please . . . give me a break!

Some women think "goin' down south" is difficult to do. Actually, you do more difficult things every day. Compared to parallel parking, it's downright easy.

However, you need to know the basics of how his anatomy works. Then, with a little concentration, a lot of practice and self-confidence—*voilà*—good things! Think of it as your favorite food, candy, or ice cream to lick, savor, and play with its flavor. That's a positive step down the bulbous, bronzed path.

For extra fun and play—prime his penis. Do what the geisha do. Get a towel, soap, and warm water, and tenderly wash his sapphire and diamonds. But do it seductively and with great sensitivity. Wash slowly and thoroughly, and talk to it as you tend it.

Now, you're going to play a symphony on his swollen manhood with the orchestra of fellatio. Imagine that you're the great Leopold Stokowski conducting a Stravinsky opus. Your instruments will be his sexual organs in the sensitive rhythms of a violin for handling, a flute for kissing, a clarinet for licking, and timpani for sucking—all orchestrating and conducting a symphony of fellatio.

Usually a symphony is composed in four movements, while the orchestra is divided into different sections (strings, woodwinds, brass, and percussion) to present the creative work.

Fellatio, in a sense, is similar to the colors and harmonies of an orchestrated piece. It usually starts slowly and quietly and builds to a crescendo—an increase in volume. Through the piece, there are highs, lows, ups, and downs—different mood changes, speeds, and rhythms. One minute it flirts, teases, and plays. The next it's passionate, insatiable, and daring. Then it's sensitive, tender, and loving. Feel him. Feel what he wants and give him what he needs.

No matter how sensational a certain action feels, nobody enjoys the same motion on the same spot indefinitely. Variation is the key—spontaneous and rhythmic variation. Whatever music you hear in your mind (whether it be jazz, R and B, soul, rock, Latin, country, or the latest craze), compose with it. Play with your own sense of rhythm and his. Take your time, let things develop instinctively, do not force anything, and be confident. Your sterling skills will tantalize his life force in any rhythmic variation.

HANDLING

Have you ever had a sibling or neighbor take a violin lesson? I have, and believe me, the squawks, squeals, and groans of such a fine instrument in unskilled hands were not only excruciating to my ears, but what about the poor instrument? When a student sticks to the lessons and practices faithfully, what a difference!

A violin, viola, or cello skillfully handled produces mesmerizing music, but only as a result of the right touch. Each musical note is located on a particular string at a specific location. Touching the wrong string will draw the wrong note. Touching the correct string but miscalculating by even a few centimeters spawns a note that is erroneous, sharp or flat, and painful to the ear. And if you happen to touch the right spot on the correct string, too little or too much pressure can cause a dreadful noise. These details are to let you know that when handling your man's instrument the same principles apply.

Handle your lover's penis with the reverence, love, and skill Heifetz bestowed on his violin, Casals his cello, and Segovia his guitar. Their touch came from arduous practice, love of their art, a finely tuned ear, a knowing touch, and the ability to express passion from their heart and soul. The playwright Clifford Odets said, "If you want to be a true artist, you have to see and feel what other people don't." Wise words.

So how *do* you handle a penis? You handle it as if you were holding a Stradivarius. Who will teach you how to play it? Your best "violin teacher" is your man. Ask him to stroke it while you watch. (He may be too shy. If so, let him know that to give him maximum pleasure you need to watch a pro . . . him.)

After watching him stroke, caress, squeeze, admire, and massage his penis, you will be able to mimic the exact grip, area, pressure, and rhythm that he enjoys the most. Pay close attention to every detail, ask questions; educate yourself while mastering his desires.

First, begin by playing scales, slowly graduating to simple melodies, then confidently moving into arpeggios. Only when your lips, mouth, tongue, hands, and fingers make harmonies on his violin will you become the quintessential seductress.

KISSING

Woodwinds are mouthpiece instruments that are more delicate-sounding in character. They can be ethereal and also have a sense of humor.

Create your own sweet sound on his oboe or magic flute with soft, tender kisses from your lips while breathing warm wind across his reed. This is sure to leave him lingering in exotic mystery.

Your lips have tons of nerve endings in them. Use them as sensors. Be a connoisseur who savors that first moment of magnetic contact when your lips first touch his soft flesh. Bathe in the wondrous feeling of intimacy. Taste his juicy desire flowing from the rain-spouting slit in his heavenly helmet. Roll your tongue around the opening as you would roll fine wine on and around your palate.

Since kissing his genitalia is the bosom of familiarity, you want to start slowly by flirting with your lips. Take his breath away and entice him to hold you high in his esteem before you explore the rest of his poetic justice. Allow him to luxuriate in your teasing adventure. Invite him to play, tempt him with artful endeavors.

When your lips meet his crown and glory, kiss it as though you were kissing his parted, hungry lips. Without a doubt, the head and shaft of his penis are the softest part of his body—fine and delicate. It's his treasure chest—the place he stores his gold and lust. When you first cup it in your hands, kiss it lovingly. Appreciate its essence. You may want to close your eyes and yield to his sensuality spreading throughout your body.

Or you may prefer to leave your eyes open and watch his elusive shade formations. Watching is extremely sexy, don't we know? This would be an opportune time to compliment the shape, texture, smell, and feel of his Trojan sword. Admire its intricate design and elegant ridges.

LICKING

The sound of brass instruments will stir the fire in your soul. Their intense, hypnotic notes are notorious for captivating the mind and heart, leaving you spellbound. Why not leave him spellbound the moment you place your mouth and mobile tongue on his trumpet and begin to play? You will feel and see his instrument soar. What glory! What strength! What obedience!

Before you position your mouth to blow, look closely at his member. Imagine a mushroom. After all, a man's penis resembles a mushroom's shape and delicacy. The top of the mushroom is akin to the hood of his penis, the stem of the mushroom is akin to his soft, velvety shaft. The whole of his ne plus ultra, down to his testicles, is extremely sensitive.

Like you, a man must have lubrication. Your wet mouth will always be his first choice. Most men produce their own lubricant, but during fellatio you need an abundance of juicy substance to slide, glide, and tantalize. You want to encourage a flood of artistic expression!

Now imagine that his penis is your favorite aphrodisiac: chocolate truffles, chocolate mousse, tiramisu, butter mints, dark chocolate mints, fruit sorbet, French vanilla ice cream with red, ripe strawberries, loaded with fresh whipped cream, Godiva chocolates, parfaits. Aside from drawing sufficient lubrication from his well, licking his love joy will make him stand firmly at attention, if he's not already.

With the tip of your tongue, circle the mushroom top (called the glans), and then up and down the shaft. The glans is filled with spongy tissue that feels like a woman's inner thigh. The urinary opening (urethral meatus) is the little slit at the top of the head. And the place where the head meets the shaft is called the coronal ridge. (It encircles the base of the glans and is the area where circumcision is performed, if it has been performed.)

The most sensitive part of the whole penile area and the most erotic is the skin within the inverted V, called the frenulum. It's located at the intersection where the head and shaft connect, and it faces away from his body. That's his penile G-spot. (Others are his prostate and perineal areas, but we're concerned with the penis at present.)

Another important area to concentrate on is the tube that runs through the entire length of his penis from the inverted V. It resembles the shaft of an arrow and is known as the urethra; it carries either urine or semen, but don't worry, you won't get a golden shower on top of whipped cream. (Fortunately for you, he's unable to do both simultaneously!) A lot of men are thrilled with a gentle long stroke of your tongue starting at the base of his tube and rolling up to the inverted V, but then an assortment of favorable flutters to focus more on his G-spot.

For variation, play a tune with your tongue by licking around his testicles, then roll your tongue up and down his protrusion while intermittently changing your pattern to a rapid fluttering all around his crown. Alternate with kisses and exploring licks. But remember to keep most of your focus on his G-spot. That will always produce a melody he won't forget.

SUCKING

The percussion section of the orchestra provides the beat—the pulse. A throbbing begins at your female center and spreads throughout your entire womanhood. You'll feel the birth of your body's rhythm from Miami to Zimbabwe. You'll long to move to a certain beat—to dance, to express.

Have you ever passed a concert hall or church where the music has measure and your head starts bopping, or your foot begins to tap to the beat? Just yesterday while I was driving in my car, a big black Bronco pulled up beside me at a red light. The music blaring from the driver's stereo was so infectious that, without realizing, I found my fingers strumming his beat on my steering wheel. The driver obviously sensed that I was enjoying his bass, because when I looked up, he was smiling. Finding your man's rhythm is easy. Just listen to his preferred music and latch onto the beat. Then give him what he likes.

A reminder: in a great piece of music or work of art, start slowly and build. Feel the emotion, ride his wave of desire. You're not going for speed. You're going for gold. Don't go all the way down on his shaft too soon. Don't use harsh, rapid stroking, with vacuum cleaner suction. Don't use quick, jerky movements, sharp teeth, or fingernails . . . *please*. It's not a ham sandwich! And also remember that he needs a wealth of lubrication, especially as you increase the tempo, adapting to the intensity of his fervor.

We know his right brain is visual. Let him look, feel, and hear the seduction. Give him the pleasure of watching his timbales being played. Let him revel in the hedonistic joy of your gifts. When Mr. Vesuvius decides to erupt, it will be a generous flow of warm, orgasmic lava.

After you have kissed and licked his penis sufficiently, hold the base of it with one hand while your other hand gently strokes the swollen member (recall the handling section above), and place your mouth on the head and delicately suck. Continue to tease him by going very slowly, gracefully sliding your mouth up and down, up and down. He needs to anticipate your charms. Use your most valued agents—teasing, flirtation, and mystery. Together with true love, these components are the basis of seductive lovemaking—an intrinsic and vital part of your symphony.

At this point in your sucking, you can begin to use your throat as a receptacle for the tip of his penis. Whether the complete penis can be taken into the whole of the throat depends entirely on your gag reflex, whether it's hyperactive, mild, or absent. Most women I interviewed said that when they relaxed, became uninhibited and totally involved, they were able to take the penis into the deepest parts of their throat.

Vary your techniques during the course of fellatio. Suck and lick a while; then suck and simultaneously stroke the shaft with one hand, while your opposite hand caresses his testicles. The point is be inventive, mix it up, and most of all *have fun*!

If you're having fun, it's almost a given that your man is going to be having fun, too. Several men that I interviewed talked about what it was like to be on the receiving end. Harry, for example, a forty-six-year old successful screenwriter, gives his view of why he likes "deep throat" and what he feels are the electrical connections: "It's like acupressure. You touch a spot, it has a response; you touch two spots, it has another response; you touch three spots, it gives you a totally different response. When my penis goes all the way down into my woman's throat, I feel a suction and an envelopment around the head. I also feel a suction and pressure at the base of my penis where it joins at the balls. That's why it's such a total turn-on, both of these things are happening simultaneously. Talk about all-encompassing. Man!!!"

It's possible to create a facsimile by taking your hand and making a ring out of the first finger and thumb. Place that at the base of the cock and, for support, apply gentle but firm pressure while working on the head of the penis with your mouth.

"Deep throat" is not such a no-no anymore. In this day and age it's often par for the course. No matter what size a man's penis (of course within reason), it can be done, but it must be learned. Compare it to swallowing a big chunk of food. You really don't think about it, do you? Well, it's the same with a man; he's just flesh. Begin by loosening the muscles of your throat.

Learning "how to" and practicing is the key, just as your fella has to learn to be your "little raspberry" by practicing the coordination of his tongue muscles. He wants to be the best at satisfying you during cunnilingus. So when he sent you to nirvana with his expertise and technique, you didn't think his van Goghlike strokes of the tongue were from a novice. Oral lovemaking is definitely not something that comes naturally to every guy or gal. So practice, practice, practice.

RHYTHM

After you become familiar with the various aspects of pleasing his penis, you need to find the right rhythm for him. Rhythm is like a heartbeat or the underlying pace in music. It's smooth, flowing, sensual, and romantic— we're not talking 78 rpm on the turntable here!

With rhythm in mind, cup his testicles with one hand, hold his shaft with the other hand, and put your mouth around his head. Now one hand gently massages his testicles while your head and other hand are going up and down in the same direction with the same tempo.

For rhythmic variation, you can move your hand up and down on his shaft, independently of your mouth, which is licking and sucking his head, while your other hand gently massages his testicles and central perineum (another erogenous area between the scrotum and anus). This latter requires more skill and, at first, sounds uncoordinated, but is really analogous to a poly-rhythmic African dance that synthesizes several seemingly different body movements into a unified whole. It can only be done if you and your lover are really in tune with each other—emotionally, mentally, physically, and spiritually. At such a point the common rhythm in your souls coalesce. This rarity is reserved for the fortunate and is the kind of sexual chemistry that transcends eroticism.

You've probably never milked a cow or even had the pleasure of seeing one being milked. But if you haven't, make an effort to do so. It's invigorating. You sit on a little stool in front of the cow's udder and put both of your hands on her teats. (Using a special ointment helps.) Start from the top of the teat and, in a controlled manner, actively work all five of your fingers, drawing the milk out in a form of massage. Pull in a rhythmic sequence—left, right, left, right. Latching on to a perfect rhythm is an unforgettable experience for you and the cow.

Animals understand a natural rhythm—men understand a natural rhythm. It's really that simple. An animal will not object to a confident pull, nor will your man object if you are confident. He gets nervous when you appear self-conscious and insensitive while doing the act, or pull too harshly with one hand, or fumble with your fingernails or teeth on his sensitive skin. If you did that to a cow, she would kick you in the mouth with her hoof; fortunately, a man is more kind. He just squirms, grits his teeth, and holds his breath, hoping you'll stop hurting him and find a more conducive stride.

Pace yourself and don't forget to breathe. Begin with soothing, gentle strokes, then as he responds, you can be a little more firm and aggressive. If you feel his penis becoming engorged and you taste or feel fluid flowing from the opening in the tip, it could be a sign that he's close to ejaculation . . . sometimes. You need to look at the expression on his face from time to time and pay close attention to his moans and groans. He will definitely let you know how fast, how slow, how pleasurable the experience. His body and verbal language are your guiding lights to the end of his tunnel.

In addition, you may want to observe how he's caressing your head, hair, face, mouth. Unconsciously, most men start to move in their own rhythm. Sometimes, they will gently move your head in the rhythm they desire. So if he's pleased with your composition, continue. If you see, feel, or hear that he may be in pain, *stop instantly*! You may be hurting him. And if this is one of your early lovemaking experiences, your man may be too shy, embarrassed, or macho to let you know that he's in pain. Don't be afraid to ask if everything is okay. It will not alienate your man, but, in fact, make you all the more resplendent to him.

SEMEN

A man's semen has the faint taste and texture of clam sauce in a bowl of pasta. Very, very few men have the taste of a persimmon, which is to say sweet. You're a lucky lady if your man has the "drink of the gods," which is similar to the nectar of a honeysuckle.

There are many factors involved; but most probably, the taste of semen is determined by diet or stress. A large intake of amino acids, a lot of salt, herbs, vitamins, garlic, curry, et cetera, can cause strangeness in its flavor; sometimes a large intake of pineapple juice can produce a sweetness. If your fella has a sour or bitter taste all the time and it displeases your senses, don't try to swallow—you'll probably gag. Off the record, when a man's semen has a sour taste, it can mean he's had an orgasm recently, possibly through masturbatory means. If he ejaculates more than twice in one session for a day or two, he may also become a little sour or acidic.

Different men ejaculate different textures of semen. To draw an analogy, the yolk of an egg has more viscosity than the egg white. Right? How about the analogy of icing on a cake? Some cakes have thick frosting, others a thin glaze that dribbles down the side. Your man's semen may be as viscous as thick egg yolk or frosting, whereas other men's semen may be similar to the thinner egg white or glaze. The point is that consistency does not dictate flavor.

SWALLOWING

Swallowing is not an obligatory thing. Don't ever think you have to swallow if you don't want to—end of sentence! Also, don't ingest on a full stomach. You'll be sorry.

If your guy is having a hard time ejaculating and you're starting to get lockjaw because you've lost that "lovin' feeling" . . . stop! Unless, of course, you've become Spartan just to prove the point of orgasm, which is not terribly exciting, but rather mechanistic.

In the event he absolutely cannot ejaculate, don't worry about it. He's only human. Just maybe, he had a hard day at work; he's worried; he had one too many beers. Maybe he masturbated earlier while thinking about your overwhelming beauty. Or maybe he was ready to come and you unknowingly changed rhythms. That'll do it every time! However, once a man starts to ejaculate, his apparatus functions in such a way that he cannot stop, even if he wants to. It's a runaway train!

Swallowing the fluids of the man you love is akin to fulfilling yourself in a matrimonial exchange of soul. It's the closest thing to penile insertion that a woman can do. Whereas a man can insert his penis into his woman's vagina, a woman has nothing to insert into her man; swallowing can substitute. The easiest way to swallow is to keep the head of his penis at the back of your throat and, as he pulsates and spurts out semen, gulp it down using the back of your throat in a rapid rhythm. As he squirts, you swallow quickly. And don't think about anything else but opening the throat to receive.

This unabashed enthusiasm is definitely not shared by all women. Unless great love or lust supersedes, women in general will not suck or swallow a man's semen. Therefore, ingestion is the ultimate sign of acceptance (unless, of course, he's paying for it).

Aside from swallowing semen, women often rub it on their faces and breasts for a few reasons: love; nastiness; pure adult lust; or desire for a natural facial, similar to an egg-white protein mask used for cleansing and rejuvenation. At any rate, handling semen is a sensitive issue all around. The male psyche is more fragile than you might suspect. When he offers a gift of his precious fluids, any form of rejection is a slap to the face of his manhood. Lovers must be sensitive to these particular needs.

If you should decide to swallow, you will be bestowing on your lover the ultimate sign of acceptance. Given that you want to give him this gift, is it safe? In this day and age, I'm obliged to warn you that swallowing is safe if your partner is healthy. According to the most current data available, it's not the semen that transmits disease; it's blood from an open sore or a cut. However, data change every day. Let me remind you that the act of love about which I am writing and which I am supporting applies only to monogamous, trusting relationships.

FELLATIO FOR THE NOVICE

You've probably been programmed to think: "Don't put that thing in your mouth. It's nasty and dirty." Change your programming to: "What a delicious new food! Why, it tastes like a bonbon. I want more! More!! More!!!"

Above all, don't be afraid. His penis will not harm you. Quite the contrary, it will love you if you treat it well. Like his finger, toe, or nose, it's part of his anatomy. Needless to say, the most important part! The most supple part!

The way a penis operates is truly fascinating. It can swell in a matter of seconds—go from very little to very big with just your gaze. In Trinidad they say, "The penis is the lightest thing in the world. Even a thought can make it rise." Don't you think that his "expression of desire" is a wonder of the world? It's so delicate in feel, yet when it's firm and throbbing, it can be tough and hard. Because he loves it, you should grow to love it, too.

I can never talk too much about cleanliness. It should be a given. If not, do as the experienced lovers. Always work showering or bathing separately or together into your dates. Oftentimes, washing one another is a sensual part of lovemaking. For example, if you bring your date home, tell him to relax, then seductively whisper in his ear that you're going to slip into something more comfortable. You know you're going to clean yourself, right? The same idea for your man. When he brings you to his home, he usually offers you a drink while he excuses himself to either wash off or take a quick shower. Providing you know for a fact that you're both clean, you might use the time to undress and slide into bed.

Suffice it to say, you may encounter some residue of urine, sweat secretions, body odors, and so forth. In which case, do as I suggested earlier: fetch a warm, soft rag, warm water, and delicate soap. Seductively wash his entire genitalia. It is a part of foreplay, especially among the famous courtesans. When done expertly, it's deliciously arousing. The gentle washing gives you a chance to introduce your charming self to his miracle of life, and also to investigate the miracle. Lather his lovables with slippery suds and wash with tender strokes. Talk to it, if you feel the incentive. Only when you're ready, tenderly stroke your cheek, nose, and eyes with his tip and shaft. Maybe this caressing contact will dispel any bogus myths about his organ.

Take a few drops of unscented cream and gently massage along the shaft of his penis and sac containing his testicles. Feel what you're touching. Explore with all your senses. It will be a pleasurable experience for him and for you, too.

A few rules to remember: Develop mutual trust and comfort by starting slowly and gradually building. Please don't go from zero to sixty in five seconds with an up-and-down, up-and-down stroke as if it were a race to the finish. Pace the action. The slower you go, the bigger his "trumpet lily" will grow. Be loving. Be patient. It takes time and the right rhythm for a man to have an orgasm. No woman wants a man to go straight for her clitoris and turn on the vacuum. No man wants a woman to dive straight for his whole piano and hammer on his keyboards with frantic strokes. Actually, they hate that. Relax. They want to bathe in the poetic feelings—from the stroking with your hands, lips, and mouth to the rubbing and admiring. All mouth doesn't work. You can't blow his live instrument without using your breath, tongue, lips, fingers, hands, and whole being to siphon beautiful music. Allow him to grow in your hands and mouth while you explore the delicate, tender, smooth flesh of his manhood.

Lubrication is absolutely necessary to avoid chafing his sensitive area with multi-stroking. Best is your own saliva, but for fun you can use honey, jam, jelly, whipped cream, maple syrup, caramel, chocolate syrup, and all flavors of ice-cream toppings for his cone. Pick your flavor.

Sucking requires actual entry of the penis into the deeper parts of your mouth. Just as the penis enters your vagina little by little, so the penis should enter your mouth gradually while you are loving and adoring it—in and out, in and out, gently. I'll keep reminding you, don't forget to tease. To tease is to please.

As time goes by, the penis can be taken in more deeply, but only as you feel comfortable. If your man's penis is extremely large or if your mouth hurts when he enters, use a different approach. Lubricate his penis with your saliva, then circle his hood and V with your tongue. Start licking and nibbling on his hood and down the length of his member while cupping the top and caressing it gently with the inside of your palm. You need to use your hands in this situation. Cup both hands, caress around the top, and nibble around the sides. Maybe his penis is too wide and too curved. Then you need to put both hands gently around the top while licking down its body. Once you work your way down, don't neglect his testicles. Cup them gently with your hands while your open mouth licks the lower part of the shaft. The reason you must have your hands around him is to bridle in his passion if he happens to start bucking out of control. In a millisecond, he could go from a trot into a full gallop. Be warned that your hands should be in command at all times to corral the situation, otherwise your mouth could feel a stampede.

A normal penis can reach into the deepest part of your throat. Use your hand around the base of his shaft to control the depth of penetration. Most men feel good if you use one hand on their shaft and the other hand to gently caress and feel their testicles.

Now, let's not forget that some men ejaculate somewhat quickly, and there will be times you wish he would. Most men manufacture a substance called pre-ejaculatory fluid first. Acquiring a taste for semen is like cultivating a taste for wine or beer. Some people don't particularly care for wine or beer at first, but after several stages of tasting, they acquire a true liking or even a passion. During the evolution of your palate, take small tastes of semen at first. You can use water, wine, Binaca breath drops, or the chaser of your choice to cleanse your mouth. In time you will build toward a more complete consumption.

During your next lovemaking session, experiment

in the same manner. When he comes, taste some of it, but don't swallow. Keep it in your mouth and then use a towel or sheet or whatever you have near you to let him expel the rest of his semen while you're acquiring a taste. Or if there's nothing to wipe with, let it drop out of your mouth onto your chest, if you prefer. The key is don't be afraid to take it out of your mouth. He will certainly understand.

The third time you're together, be adventurous. Take a gulp and you will see it's just like milk gravy. Not bad, really. It's simply a matter of getting accustomed to doing it. And I believe these tips will direct you on a new, fun, and daring journey.

You may ask yourself, "How does it feel in the mouth just before he comes? How do I create a rhythm when swallowing? Or, how long do I continue?" The signal is when his penis becomes extremely tense and inflexible. There are definite lines of engorgement along its sides, the glans pulsates and becomes top-heavy as it contracts. Throbbing is key. Take some advice from the comedians in Las Vegas: "You keep on lickin' till it stops tickin'!"

However, some men have severe sensitivity and find it difficult to ejaculate with any motion. They will usually grab your head and/or your hand to give pause while their sperm flows freely.

It's best not to let the semen sit in your mouth and then swallow. Rather, when the semen shoots, gulp it down as quickly as you can. You create a rhythm by pulling the head of his penis out of your throat into your mouth cavity and pushing it back against your throat—all the while swallowing rapidly. You can feel when a supply of semen is pushing through the urethra, because the glans will pulsate. Continue to swallow in rhythm.

FELLATIO FOR THE ADVANCED

To complete this section, I offer an advanced technique of fellatio. While you take him on your fantastic voyage, let your hair and breasts fall and brush all around his abdomen, thighs, and over his groin, while your hands stroke and delicately massage his inner thighs. Without touching his penis, kiss all around those same areas. Welcome him to penis foreplay!

Now lightly kiss his glans, shaft, and scrotum while your hands fondle the surrounding area. Position yourself over him so you'll have more control of what you're preparing to do. It's sexy for both of your legs to straddle one of his. That way you can massage your own clitoris with his leg as you go through the various stages of loving.

Ever so gently, take his penis in both of your hands and admiringly caress it against your face. Look lovingly at its shape, color, size, aroma, and texture, all blossoming into full maturity from your nurturing. Compliment and talk to it while sliding it against your lips, cheeks, eyes, and throat. You say the things that you feel and mean. Like, "Hmmmm, you smell so good. You feel so big and firm in my hands. I want to taste you. I want to put you in my mouth and rub my tongue all over your head, especially that tender spot. Then I want to take it down my throat. I want to lick your come like melting candy. I want you to rain all over me. You make me wetter than the Mississippi River. I can't wait for you to explode in my mouth!" This is just an example of what you might verbalize, if it's true and comfortable for you.

Now's the time to do all the things you told him you were going to do. Continue teasing. Play and suck and lick around his nipples, stomach, and legs, passing by his penis. Then start to play with his balls. (Again:

some men don't like their balls played with or squeezed, but most men do.)

Begin nibbling and kissing the tip of his penis along the shaft and over the testicles. Give the entire groin area your complete focus and total attention. While holding his property in one hand and gently massaging it, kiss in between the folds or creases where the groin starts.

Okay, enough teasing. Here's where we really begin. As Candy Sample likes to say, "It's serious cock-sucking time!" Lick and kiss the hood and shaft of his penis with your moist lips, making sure everything gets wetter than wet. You can never get it too wet, as I'm sure you know. Even the ooh-ahh sounds of saliva mixed with sucking are hot for him. You are letting your man know that his penis is being worshiped at the altar of a love goddess.

Did I mention that you need to look into his eyes once in a while? You do. It will be your barometer of appreciation. I can't imagine at this point that he would be in pain, but one never knows when the stakes are high. Maybe he's excruciatingly ticklish and everything except sucking tickles him. Don't rule that out. Paying close attention to his body language and checking the expressions on his face regularly help you on your journey. As I said earlier, every man is different, and if your man is ticklish, give him time to learn and trust your loving and sensitive hands. He'll come around eventually. It's all about *trust*.

After your saliva has gotten him wetter than an Amazonian rain forest, sucking will be comfortable and fun. Always start at the top and work your way down, neglecting nothing. Everything should be slow and easy, building to a crescendo. Remember the symphony!

Every move, stroke, lick, and suck must have a melody, a rhythm, a flow all its own. With one hand on his shaft, the other hand on his testicles, and your mouth wrapped around the hood, the rapture expands. Men need reassurance, so continue talking to his animated member with mmmmms, ahhhhs, and ooohhs—inhaling and stroking, kissing and blowing on it. Be honest! If you think it's big, tell him how big and beautiful it is. If not, compliment other things you sincerely like, maybe the shape, color, or smoothness. If you love him, you'll love it. Compliments will make him feel proud. But he needs truthful communication, not just blind sex. Blind sex is like eating bland rice cakes as an aphrodisiac. It doesn't wear well.

With one hand still wrapped around his shaft, the other on his testicles, and your mouth around the hood, slide, slide, slip and slide—up and down, up and down. Your head and hand are moving in the same direction, as your other hand massages his sac to the same rhythm. It's as if your hand and mouth form a tunnel with a soft wet suction at the top, or a sheath filled with a slippery substance in which his penis is inserted and massaged. You start with an hum pa pa, hum pa pa, hum pa pa, hummm. Recall milking the cow. It must be done with confidence and a smooth rhythm. Be confident that you're gentle; that you know what you're touching; that you've discovered his desired pressure; and that you're in sync with his body language. His penis is coming alive and pulsating in your hand.

If he's growing bigger and bigger and a few oohs and ahhs are escaping his lips, or inaudible words are being murmured, then you know you're breathing spring into his happy seasons.

Another great inspiration for this day of reckoning is when you make tiny circles with your lubricated thumb around his inverted V, as your mouth and tongue suck and lick his glans.

After you know that he is slippery wet, circle your

erect nipple around his secretions at the slit in the top of his penis. You can gently hold it open while your nipple peeks further inside. Then do it with the other nipple. Let him look. He loves to look! If you have ample breasts, put his penis in your cleavage; squeeze the breasts together in an up-and-down massage, catching onto his penis's rhythm. Make sure there's plenty of oil or saliva in between your breasts and on his tip and shaft. Keep these playful parts as wet as possible.

Rub his penis on your cheek and circle it around your mouth. Kiss and lick all around his shaft and balls, slightly pulling his testicles into your mouth with a very, very delicate sucking motion. Be extra careful not to hurt this area. Some men prefer it harder, most don't. Sensitively ask and explore to find out what your man likes. He'll tell you, I'm sure.

After you've used all your senses and different pacing, pressures, and strokes with your hands, mouth, and tongue; after you've exhausted your erotic repertoire and are totally satiated; after gratifying yourself and your lover: put one hand at the base of his cock and push down on his sac to show him how long his rock-hard organ is now that it's been thrilled by your aggressive, knowing composition. Keep it pressed down while you take the fingers of your other hand and gently swirl them around his juicy top as you look deep into his eyes with your throaty voice asking, "Darling, where do you want to come? Do you want to come on my breasts, my face, my stomach? Do you want me to drink you? Or do you want a piece of my apple pie?"

If he can even think at this point, I'm sure he will say, *"Anything you want!!!!"*

Now, don't take advantage of his vulnerable condition and ask him for the moon, the stars, and rain every minute. That's not nice or kind. Don't use the intimate gift of surrender to barter or trick. Lovemaking is pure and holy. Plus you'll lose his trust, the asset you took so long to earn.

Angles in all forms of lovemaking are very important. Maybe you want to be positioned at an angle for deeper swallowing. When your lover is ready to come, having his penis all the way at the back of your throat is best for direct shooting. There, his spurting penis will feel like someone is simply shooting water down your throat; the reflex to swallow is all you'll feel. Always keep your hand around the shaft so your firm grip can control the rhythm and penetration of the situation.

He may scream, have body spasms, and let out primitive sounds during his orgasm. It's such a spiritual release for him when you push all his sexual buttons simultaneously. Also, during ejaculation, it's sexy for him if you massage his central perineum, the area between his testicles and anus. A light rubbing or slight massage encourages a more enjoyable orgasm.

I don't want to get into the anus right now because that's such an individual call. But again, some men love the whole idea of your inserting a lubricated finger to slightly massage their prostate just before they begin to achieve orgasm. When done professionally, it will blow him away. However, other men are just too embarrassed to participate in that particular activity. Ask him seductively whether he so desires.

When all is said and entirely done, you may want to delicately kiss the top of his penis and tell him how much you love him. As I'm sure you know, the above experience is best when there is passion between kindred spirits, great love, chemistry, and enthusiasm for one another. Never be uptight and repressed about loving your man. Savor, relish, wallow in your passions without shame. You have just evoked a delicious sensation of arousal—yours and his. Be proud of your talents and communication skills.

Fellatio is a large part of loving your man completely. It's truly an art when done to his desired and erotic expectations. When you become his magnificent seductress, he will forget his ménage à trois fantasy.

Love is a total release of all the senses; and like beauty, it is in the body of the beholder. Two people in love have the right to do anything that pleases both of them. Love is never judgmental. Everything I've discussed only applies to *real love*. That's the only time you can create heavenly music.

Men generally love receiving fellatio, partly because the act itself is pure pleasure and partly because they don't feel the performance pressures they often feel during intercourse. You are his "lady of the night," his dream come true. So do allow your man his pleasure. He deserves it! And in return, he will kiss and lick you from head to toe, devouring every moist and succulent inch of you in an unabashed orgy of lust, love, and gratitude that will leave you in a limp, sweaty, smiling state of bliss.

INTERCOURSE

When you engage in intercourse, you enter into a mystery as deep as the ocean; as old as time; as new as the birth of the present moment; as vast as the universe; and as near as the heart of your lover lying beside you. It's been experienced by human beings since before they even understood that they were human beings. It's an eternal dance in which all things in nature take part, and it's been going on since before the beginning of what we understand to be time.

I marvel at the lyricism of butterflies. Only minutes ago, I looked outside my window and was enchanted to witness the duet of a male and female butterfly mating in the warm wind. It seemed as if the male was riding on the wings of the female. They were so tightly connected that, at first glance, they appeared to be one—floating in the same rhythm as would a rose petal if it were dropped from the Eiffel Tower.

With this thought in mind, let us move on to the composition and choreography of intercourse. Foreplay was the rehearsal—now you dance . . . Feel your bodies vibrate to the sensuous rhythms of your minds—music created by the two of you together that no one else can hear. That's the miracle of your duet. So listen carefully to the music that weaves your dance of lovemaking. It will make the difference between a satisfying orgasm and no orgasm at all!

Each person has an individual style of dance. Some dances are as carefully choreographed as the Ballet Russe, while others are as primal and abandoned as a pagan fertility rite. You want to have both of those styles and everything in between too in your sexual repertoire.

Watch how people move on a dance floor. Some couples are as smooth as silk, others look like wild mustangs, shaking their heads, arms, and feet to God knows what music. Oftentimes, I wonder exactly what sound those individuals are hearing. But give them credit. They do hear something. They've surrendered to "it" and are expressing themselves with a vitality and courage that promise extraordinary delights in the evening ahead.

Since there is an array of personal styles, techniques, and accoutrements in lovemaking, you must follow your own instincts as did Martha Graham and other trailblazers of dance. Your instincts will never let you down. If you and your lover prefer drifting in an easy, relaxing, mesmerizing tide, move to that sensation; if you enjoy jazz, find that tempo; if you fancy blues, rap, rock and roll, or country, find that cadence. Follow the natural rhythms that belong exclusively to you and your lover. No one can teach you that. It's innate. Explore and experiment with one another's whims, desires, and fantasies. You bring your interpretation, he brings his, and then when your sex organs finally meet and merge, your emotional centers unite and spin into a soaring spiral that spills into the night.

Sometimes, Prince Charming will take you in his arms and lead your glass-slippered Cinderella around the ballroom floor while you gaze lovingly into his spellbinding eyes during a Strauss waltz. Did you know that during the Regency period the waltz was considered too risqué for young maidens? Although we smile at the thought, the guardians of virtue of that period were not fools. Just think of it. All that twirling and spinning around, having a lady's breath taken away while being firmly held in the arms of a beautiful man was very exciting. Isn't it still?

A visual pantomime of seduction can be seen by Fred Astaire and Ginger Rogers in the film *Gay Divorcée* as they dance to "Night and Day." He tries to draw her close. She withdraws. He tries again. She becomes interested and allows him nearer. They touch and begin to move. By the end of the dance they're spinning together over the shining surface of the floor —her skirt billowing and floating all around them in celebration.

Watch Torville and Dean dancing on ice to their gold-medal interpretation of *Bolero*. Who could miss the eroticism of that build in intensity and the ending that might be "death" or merely the state of being "spent" that follows climax?

Check out the film *Romeo and Juliet* starring the premier danseur Rudolf Nureyev with Margot Fonteyn. Everything that can be expressed about romantic and erotic love can be seen in their interpretation of that ballet. The power of their genius enables you to see the joining of not only their bodies but also their spirits and souls. They show to the public what you and your lover will do to each other in private.

As a dancer of love, you need to prepare. Do you think Nijinsky could make his breathtaking leaps on legs that weren't superbly conditioned by exercise? Well, your vagina is a muscular organ; hence, the more you exercise it properly, the better conditioned it will be to pleasure both you and your man.

Your pleasure muscle—pubococcygeus or PC—extends from front to back across your pelvic walls. It supports your bladder and surrounds the urinary, vaginal, and anal passages.

Let's get those muscles into condition by exercising them! They're the same ones you use to start and stop urination. Contract—hold—release. Do sets of fifteen to thirty, three to five times a day, any time, any place —in the car, at a board meeting, or in line at the grocery store.

After a few weeks, you will be able to latch onto his penis like a loving boa constrictor. You, in turn, will more easily feel his thickness growing inside. Also during orgasm the involuntary muscular contractions of your uterus will be stronger. That's good! The strength, dexterity, and mobility with which you use your PC muscles can either take him to a Paphian paradise or a horizontal ride around the block. It's your trip.

There are sex shops that have tiny balls or a lightweight bar bell designed for exercising your PCs. However, it might be a lot more fun to let your lover participate in your "exercise program." He inserts his finger slowly into your vagina and you practice gripping and releasing around his finger. He can begin to feel how proficient you become after a few sessions. You want to duplicate this exact motion when he's inside. The idea is to grip his penis with your vaginal muscles as he slides out, then relax as he reenters. Once you catch on to the rhythm, you can't beat it. But most of all, he will think a thousand fingers are massaging him to orgasm.

Now that you've thoroughly prepared your vagina to make love to his penis, there's something that he needs to do to prepare his penis to enter your vagina. That is, of course, if you're not in a monogamous relationship, which I hope you are.

Scenario: You think it's love, because it's definitely hot and heavy. You're ready for the big moment. He didn't bring a condom. *Stop!!* Lovingly and firmly explain that you both may think you're disease-free, but people can be "positive" and not know it. You also need a condom to protect you against pregnancy and other transmittables. Be safe and keep a supply on hand. Or if you prefer, use a female condom until both of you are tested. Simply tell him that the precaution protects you both, since you care so much about one another. Enough.

Now you're both ready to make love. Hold him in your arms, caress him, kiss him, and treat him as the totally special and unique discovery that he is. Before he glimpses heaven's gate, respond to him as if it were the first time. Every way you touch his body or move your pelvis with "him" inside should be a new experience—every time you love him. You can't lose with this attitude!

Ignore all rules that make men active and women passive. After you come together, each partner will usually take a turn at the lead before returning back to a central unified rhythm. You create and choreograph as you go along, mutually inspiring one another with equal parts imagination, flair, energy, reverence, and passion—ending in total fulfillment.

The beauty of intercourse is in the magical flow of positions—the endless gliding of two units in one synchronized rhythm. Think of your vagina as Ginger's arms wrapped around and holding on to Fred's confident and secure penis while he glides you around the floor in different rhythms, tunes, and dance steps. You never miss a beat. You feel nurtured in his gentle yet firm embrace.

At the most basic level, there are really two positions of intercourse: horizontal and vertical—up and down. However, there are many variations on these two themes that you and your lover can discover when your bodies are attuned. Positions should be comfortable and satisfying for both of you at all times.

Most of the women with whom I've spoken say that there are three basic positions in which they can achieve orgasm: missionary, woman on top, or doggy. Men are slightly more adaptable, preferring doggy style or woman on top, followed by any and all positions in which they can achieve ejaculation comfortably. It's individual.

Permit me to offer a few more suggestions in the event you have only experienced one or two positions. And please don't hesitate to guide your lover through a few of the movements listed below. It will be an artistic endeavor. Learning positions is comparable to doing pliés at a ballet barre. After you warm up properly, if he's willing and you're able, you will make toe tap-

pin', power packin', soul possessin', mind messin' love
. . . until you catch your breath for more!

The choreography of the first few positions before
doggy style (where he will need to pull out) offers
choices of movement while staying solidly connected.
When you shift, move slowly and keep the rhythm. This
fluid connection will sweep you both toward the sweet
madness of overwhelming gladness.

THE MISSIONARY POSITION

I feel the most important position to experience orgasm
at the same time is the missionary. With his manly body
atop your feminine self, you can look into each other's
eyes and gradually create a gentle, soft pulse that builds
and builds, until you both explode into the high-voltage
concurrent orgasm—the stuff dreams are made of.

In the missionary, you're lying flat on your back
with your legs apart. Your man is over you with his
knees bent or stretched, appearing to be doing a push-
up between your open legs. Resting his body weight on
his elbows and knees, he can touch your breasts with
his free hands and suck on your nipples as his penis
penetrates your vagina.

The key is flow. Some bodies fit and flow perfectly
together. Other bodies need to experiment with positions several times before shouting hallelujah! But while
dancing to the music, take care not to overextend your
anatomy with too much enthusiasm. It could cause
injury.

So, you're on your back, right? There's little variation on this theme except for his flexibility and the
mobility of your legs and, of course, the possibility of
jackknifing your spine. For example, your knees can be
bent with your feet on the bed; your legs can be
wrapped around his waist, pulling up your lower torso
for better control; in the same wraparound leg position,

let the heels of your feet encircle his buttocks, pressing him into you rhythmically; tuck your toes under his calves for firmer support.

Your hands can gently guide his torso back, preparing him for your legs to go over his shoulders. One leg can be over his shoulder while the other hangs loose; your straight legs can be opened outward almost into a side split; your knees can be pulled in close to your chest or to the sides of your upper torso.

THE SCISSORS POSITION

This adaptation actually looks like two pairs of open scissors meeting at the center. Without him pulling out, gently coax his torso back over your body in the stretched-out missionary once again. This readies him for another modification—the scissors.

Straighten out your left leg as your left hand gently guides his right knee over that leg and in between your armpit close to your left breast. After he's positioned, pull your knees up. This will encourage his buttocks to rise giving him more support as he shifts onto his knees. Now . . . he can more easily pump your pelvis to the rhythm he desires. You too can enjoy the shakin' and bakin' of a sexy ride.

When you've exhausted the scissors position, return to the flat missionary by stretching out your left leg and sliding it underneath his right leg. Circle your legs around his waist and with both hands gently push his chest back so that his buttocks are sitting on his heels.

LEGS OVER SHOULDER

Lift your legs high in the air over his shoulders and point your toes. Your free fingers can circle around the base of his penis in lubricated massage while alternately stimulating his balls.

SITTING POSITION

With his knees bent and him seated back on his heels, clasp your hands around the back of his neck and slide onto his lap. Your legs can either fall over his legs freely or circle his torso with your feet clasped together. This will give you tremendous security for the ride.

While you're still facing each other, he can lift you up with his body weight, simultaneously straightening his upper torso. With his strong hands hoisting your buttocks higher and closer into his penis, his mouth can suck on your breasts and nipples as he continues to pump in his rhythmic flow. This position is still his ball game. You're a loving participant enjoying his lead.

You may want to reverse the love flow. Same position, but you hang onto his torso while he straightens out his legs. Go very slowly and be careful he doesn't slip out. He can lean back onto his arms, supporting himself as you bring your torso down with your weight on your knees. Then you can ride him, encircling his neck with your right arm and holding onto his right knee with your left arm concurrently. It puts you in the driver's seat.

WOMAN ON TOP

Sitting on top of him, reach your arms back, holding onto his ankles for support as he massages your breasts. Now release his legs. Then smoothly straighten the entire length of your body over his. Your body weight can be completely on top of his. In this position you can feel the thickness and length of his penis sliding in and out. This is an excellent time to squeeze and release your buttock muscles as he slips in and out. You can also control the exact amount of his penis you want to take inside. Your elbows can support your body weight as you lean forward and kiss his lips and slide your pubic bone over his for maximum sensation. Oftentimes, this motion massages your clitoris and stimulates you to a quickened orgasm or two.

This would be a good time to lift yourself up while he is completely stretched out. Squat over him with your knees in the air and feet planted firmly on the sides of his torso. In this arrangement, you have complete control of the depth of penetration. You can take as little or as much as you desire.

At this stage, he can slide his body around and let his feet fall on the floor while you once again wrap your legs around his torso. Now, provided he's strong enough, he can stand up with you fully attached, encircling his torso with your arms wrapped around his neck and your legs around his waist. His arms and hands can hold your buttocks as he massages them and rhythmically pulls you on and off his protrusion.

At this time, he can walk over to a chair and sit down in it with you still fastened to his body. For a terrific feeling, you can use the base of the chair to balance and control your movements. Sitting on him, sitting in a chair is a very pleasurable and erotic sensation for both of you. A good orgasm can come from this technique.

DOGGY STYLE

In the film *Clan of the Cave Bear*, Daryl Hannah was endlessly on all fours servicing her husband. Hopefully her character was being fulfilled, too! The eroticism of penetrating from behind can be an enormous turn-on for both lovers. It's a virile thing and exceedingly primal, and some women can only achieve orgasm in this position. It blows their mind every time.

This preferred position gives your man better access to your G-spot (which is about the size of a quarter and located two or three inches inside the vagina di-

rectly behind the pubic bone and clitoris at once, plus
he can control your body with graceful aplomb. By the
same token, you can reach your hand through your legs
and massage his scrotum. Also in the doggy position,
inhibitions seem to fade for both partners, which is key
to orgasm.

You can alter this position by both of you lifting
your torsos together. Okay, both of you are on your
knees—upright—with your back to his torso. His advantage is that he can kiss your turned face, massage
your breasts and clitoris while sliding in and out at a
desired angle. At this point, he can sit back on his heels
while you sit back, resting on him.

With a little more energy and still connected, he
can lie back on his elbows while you sit on his erection
with your legs over his knees and possibly wrapped
around his torso. From this very sexy position, he sits
up as you bend over, placing your elbows on the floor
for support and resting your head on your forearms. Of
course your legs are wrapped around his waist back-
wards, right? Your genitalia is facing his face. His penetration is seriously erotic and visual. He can see, play,
and satisfy as he takes over the floor.

Next! Still connected, but with the same flowing
rhythm, he's lying down again as you stretch your left
leg out and over his left shoulder. His left leg is bent
and to the side of your left torso. His right leg is curved
over your right extended leg. In this position, you are
almost completely on your stomach and he is completely on his back. He has better control of penetration, but your wild tigress can still roar.

This would be a good time to disconnect for a
while and in the same position, slide your genitals back
gently into his mouth as you position your mouth on
his fields of Bali.

POSTERIOR SLIDE-IN

You can lie on your stomach while your man approaches your vagina from behind, laying his chest on your back. You can enjoy the weight of his pelvis hitting your buttocks and the length of his penis traveling between your legs, arriving at your vagina. For more rhythmic waves, he can put a pillow under your buttocks and satisfy that G-spot a bit more.

CUDDLE POSITION

This is nice for waking up in the morning. You're both on your sides facing in the same direction (often called "making spoons"). He slips his penis into your vagina from the back. He can also hold your slightly bent leg up as he slides his penis and his legs in between yours. The advantage is the snug, cozy, comfortable fit as well as the ability to massage your breasts and clitoris and hug you from behind. It's a very loving position.

WORKERS' POSITION

It's a variation of the cuddle. You roll onto your back while he stays on his side. You lift your leg closest to him and place it over his pelvis to give his penis access to your vagina. For the sake of comfort, he inserts his top leg between your legs. From this position he can easily suck on the breast closest to his mouth. This position is for lovers who are a bit tired from long hours of work.

Any position is great, as long as it's comfortable for both lovers. The way your bodies fit together will determine the best sequence for any given position. It's amazing how creative lovers become after experimenting a few times. Invent. Use your instincts. Go with the flow. Flash and dash with maximum confidence.

A few tips: Work with his penis to find what rhythms and pressures he enjoys the most. Also experiment with angles that will give you good hip mobility. In this way, you can control the rhythm and tempo of the complete sex act. Use your hips and pelvic area to pump and slide—up and down, around and around, side to side, as your vaginal muscles squeeze and release, squeeze and release.

As you maintain a graceful rhythmic flow, your tempo will vary in degrees. The spiral growth of your vine tendrils should start to wrap around his penis and pull him in slowly while you gently open wider—inch by delicious inch—feeling his firm tenderness inside your warm, wet enticement.

After a great while, when you sense the time is right, accelerate from a slow leisurely walk of holding hands, smelling the flowers, and getting to know him, to a moderate trot. Only when you feel absolutely primed, harmoniously ride into a quickened pace—fast, faster, fastest. At which point, he is probably beginning to end. Ahhh, such immense vibrations to his penis!

Also, know that when your lover first penetrates, he will automatically begin to gauge the depth of your vagina. It's his natural instinct. His penis is measuring how much depth he has to play with—whether you have a shallow or deep vaginal vault. This lets him know what action to take, how to react to your enthusiastic aggressions, and when to go forward. That's essential for a duet. Allow him to survey the exact width and circumference of your vault. In case it's shallow, he may accidentally push too hard, too soon, and bang up against your cervix, sending you screaming in pain. It's a good idea always to take him in slowly before playtime.

In a luscious and loving moment, take him in completely and let him rest inside your walls while the only movement between the two of you is your vaginal muscles squeezing and releasing, hugging, gripping, massaging, and playing with his organ. It's a great sensation for a fella to just hang out while your muscles make magic around his wand. But please understand that your progressive movements may feel too good and he may ask you to stop moving for fear of losing his cool. A perfect example is the intimate lovemaking scene between Robert Redford and Meryl Streep in the film *Out of Africa*. Redford whispers to Streep, "Don't move!" She says, "But I want to move!" He repeats with complete conviction, "Don't move!!" The translation is: "You feel so good, I'm ready to explode. If you move a muscle, I'll come right now." The choice is yours. If you want the lovemaking to end . . . move. If you want it to continue . . . do as he asks.

Now, when you hear those beautiful words from the breath of your lover, your heart will silently smile. I admit, it is tempting to feel the meat of the matter at that sexy, vulnerable moment, but providing you want more, I suggest you allow him a few seconds to compose himself before you restart your engine. The words *don't move* are his way of saying, "Honey, you're incredible, I'm losing control!" N-I-C-E . . .

Take this opportunity to compliment his sexiness —his manliness. Seductive sounds can be highly effective. Keep your words truthful and simple: "Your hair smells so good, your hands are so strong, your skin is beautiful, you make me so wet, I want your tongue everywhere. I want to feel all of you." Then when you're ready for him to ejaculate you can say, "Come inside of me. Come deep inside of me. Deeper, deeper, harder. Yes, Oohh, yes. Yes, yes, *yessss*!!" My feeling is that you will probably both orgasm together. But let's enhance his pleasure a bit longer before you do. Remember, *you* are driving the car! Go where you wanna go.

Anyway, I know I refer to the sac that holds his two perfectly cut diamonds quite a lot, but try not to forget them. While holding his jewels securely in your hand, think of being in Tiffany's and having the gems between your fingers, feeling all the facets—the brilliance, the fascination. With the same sentiment, gently work his testes in a circular motion. Feel them rolling in their sac. It's a kind of loving sensation for both of you.

Again, pay attention to his every nuance. He will quietly or silently let you know what pressure he prefers—gentle, more firm, or none at all. Follow his lead and give him what he wants. As he penetrates in and out, find a rhythm of massaging his testicles that coincides with the rhythm of his motion. Also, gently slide your finger up and down his perineum—the area between his anus and scrotum. Your fingers will intoxicate him. It's also extremely sexy to circle your thumb and forefinger around the base of his shaft as he's sliding in and out of your vagina. A little pressure can be enjoyable; however, too much of a good thing can cause the cake to bake prematurely! And we don't want that to happen just yet, do we, ladies?

Licking, sucking, and touching his neck, shoulders, mouth, nipples, ears, and fingers are erotic during intercourse. Don't stop your heavenly touches because "foreplay" has ended and "intercourse" has begun. All of your parts should continue to be giving him pleasure. And don't use the same tactile stimulation pattern for too long. It gets boring. Stimulation should be exhilarating.

I talked about the frenulum of his penis being one of his G-spots. Well, his other G-spot is his prostate. You may want to explore this sensation; you may not. If you decide to touch upon it, clean, clean, clean is key.

Some men will invite your explorations, while others may feel embarrassed, awkward, and violated. I'm sure he'll let you know immediately exactly what his feelings are on the subject, either verbally or with silent and very tight body contractions. Like, "*No! Not there! Don't touch that!*"

Unfortunately, to touch his prostate you must go through the rectum. That's the rub. To make matters more difficult, the anal area does not produce its own lubricant. There is also an element of "total recall." Many men associate this sort of probing to the extreme discomfort of a similar procedure given during their physical examinations at the doctor's office. It happens to be a crucial part of his physique. No wonder a man gets nervous. Wouldn't you?

Yet there are many uninhibited men who may encourage your gentle rummaging. If so, make sure you have plenty of lubrication at your disposal. Make sure your nails are short and smooth and that you enter gently and slowly with great sensitivity, as though it were your own private part.

His prostate is located a few inches inside the rectum on the anterior (front) wall. It's about the size and shape of a walnut. Proper massage of the area is usually a healthy deterrent to future prostate problems. I'm not recommending that you do this, but when he's ready to orgasm, a little prostate massage will detonate the dynamite.

Did you know that a lot of people around the world engage in touching and probing of the anus but refuse to talk about it? Some men insert finger size vibrators for added stimulation. The anus is all part of your anatomy, like your mouth. In fact, it's the bottom of your throat, isn't it? It's important to always keep it clean with thorough washing and proper diet.

After you've discovered the opulent and naughty treasures at the bottom of his emerald sea with your inviting glance, touch, movements, enhance his pleasure by expressing your true erotic needs and feelings. For example: "Wait, slower, yes, that's it, faster, harder, no, not yet, hmmmmmmm . . . hold it, yes, ohhh, that feels so good, yes, stay—just stay there. Oh, I like that . . . it feels so good. Ohh, don't move, let me grab onto you, let me feel you. I love your thickness. Yes, that's right, slow and easy. Give me more. I want to feel more of you—deeper, deeper, yes . . . give me more, more, more. Oh yes, that's it. Faster, faster, deeper. I feel you growing inside me. It's so big and hard!" Express all of your emotions. Verbalize. It will only serve to heighten his ecstasy.

When you have arrived at this final destination and you know that he's throbbing to release, if you're also ready to experience the highest form of orgasm—that sacred ground of the universe where you melt and mold into one being, catch his rhythm, and ride his wave into the vibrant orange, yellow, red, and amber hues of the sunset—tell him, "Come with me, come now, please come. I want you to fill my body with your hot come. Yes, yes, *yes, yessssssss*!!!"

As you feel his semen flooding your insides, suck gently on his tongue in the same rhythm as his penis is pulsating inside your womb. Talk about otherworldly? Hmm, ummm! Your vaginal muscles will organically pulsate around his penis as you both contract in orgasmic delirium.

During this dizzying orgasm, you will not know where he ends and you begin. It's the ultimate symbolism of sexuality and true love. Your mind leaves you. Your twitching, quivering body and soul belong to him; and his blushing heap of muscle, sinew, and significance belongs to you. The two of you truly become god and goddess in the empyreal land of Zeus. You don't exist anymore. He doesn't exist. Your wet, sublime molecular structures are swimming in the ocean of embryonic fluids united in poetic motion.

For variety, he may want to be nasty and come on your breasts, your stomach, your back, your face, or in your mouth. If that's his choice and yours, let him pull out and enjoy. It can be very exciting for him to watch while his semen expresses itself all over your body or inside whatever orifice he chooses to implement. You have no idea how exciting love play can be for the two of you until you let go—explore, experiment, and invent.

Before we leave this section, I want to inject a warning. If you're on top of your gent and you accidentally bend yourself backward, it's extremely possible to hurt the spongelike tissue inside his organ. Also, torsion, which is a twisting of the testicles, can obstruct the penis's blood supply and kill off the testicles. Please be careful. His organs are much more delicate than you can imagine.

If you use a reasonable amount of care combined with a little skill, a little practice, a lot of imagination and love, you can make intercourse a glorious experience each and every time.

A WOMAN'S PLEASURE

One half of the world cannot understand the pleasures of the other.

—JANE AUSTEN

I've given you some techniques for pleasing men. These techniques are, after all, essential elements of a seductress's tool kit. But never underestimate the importance of finding your own pleasure—not only for your sake, but also for his. A woman who is responsive and enjoys the act of making love is a much more exciting partner than one who is diligently working away, practicing her technique, but deriving no pleasure or joy from the act herself. I promise you, men can tell the difference. If you don't naturally explode in pleasure, you can learn how. And after you've learned it, you can show your man when you're in bed together.

Imagine that you're the legendary Sacagawea guiding your Lewis or Clark on the expedition of his life. Lewis and Clark might have received the credit, but it was Sacagawea's instinct, knowledge, bravery, and guidance that paved the way. However, if Sacagawea had not known the territory, the expedition would have been a tragic failure. You can't travel up that mountain unless you know exactly what your body and spirit needs for the ultimate journey. So first become a connoisseur of your own body. Explore it to discover what areas give you pleasure when touched and what kind of touching or stroking is most effective. When you know what touch, pressure, and stimulation genuinely feel good to you, you can communicate that information to your man. Show him by touching him in the ways you would like to be touched and say the words out loud. Men like to hear them.

It's a biological fact of life that men don't have to spend a lot of time positioning themselves, being in the "right mood," or feeling sexy to enjoy a good release —ejaculation feels good whenever it happens. We women do need to be in the right mood and feel sexy. But don't make the mistake of thinking you are at the mercy of your mood as if it were some kind of weather over which you have no control. You can make choices to adjust and manipulate your mood.

One way to get into a sexy mood is the use of

imagery. Think: I am beautiful, I am wonderful, I am special, I love my hands, my breasts, my legs, my hair, my womanhood. Another way is to treat your physical senses. Turn off the world and turn on your favorite music. Run a warm, soothing, bubbly tub; light a few candles; use gels, oils, or slippery soaps to spread all over your entire body. Now you're stimulating the senses of hearing, sight, smell, and touch. This is a good time to explore your body. Feel your softness and cherish your lotus blossom. Before you leave the tub, use a handheld shower or open your legs and let the faucet water run over your clitoris, but make sure the water is comfortable for your delicate parts. You may orgasm, but if not, continue to rub oils or lotions on your soft clean skin, paying more attention to your nipples and clitoris. Is this helping to put you in a sexy mood? If it isn't, try something else.

Some women get into a sexy mood by wearing certain kinds of clothing. But it's different kinds of clothing for different women. For some, it's silky lingerie. For others it's beautifully cut classic clothes in wonderful fabrics. Other women feel very sexy when they're wearing tight jeans, leather, latex, or Lycra, and others feel beautiful in gowns of billowing silk, chiffon, or lace. Find out which outfits make you feel like the "It" Girl. No one but you has to know why you're wearing them. But the sexy mood you're feeling will give off positive vibrations.

Put on an erotic video, read sexy passages from a book or magazine, and look at erotic pictures of other women, men, or couples. Buy erotic toys—whatever excites your libido. Just do it! Do whatever you deem necessary to promote pleasure.

Drink wine or champagne if it helps you feel more free. Guide your lover's hands up and down the length of your body, exploring all erotic portals. Learn which

parts are hungry for attention. When you find them
. . . experiment. What touch turns you on? What type
of stroke do you prefer—long or short? What kind of
pressure do you enjoy—light or firm? What type of
rhythm feels best—fast or slow?

Let's move on . . . Teaching your man to give you
the proper stimulation to orgasm during cunnilingus is
extremely difficult. Either he has a mobile tongue and
loves a woman's juicy vagina or he doesn't. Learning
fellatio is much easier for you than it is for him to learn
how to properly give you cunnilingus. He needs to have
an aptitude and a strong desire with no hang-ups.

You must be exceedingly clean for him to draw
pleasure from the experience. The only way to really
show him is to literally let him put his face between
your legs as you massage and titillate your own femininity. Now let him watch as you pleasure your love
bud. Then encourage his fingers to mimic your previous
motions by either placing your fingers over his and
guiding him or slowly whispering your needs. Men
learn very fast when they're given specific instruction.
They understand clarity.

So as he licks, don't be shy in letting him know
what strokes, pressures, tongue rhythms, fingers or no
fingers, you prefer. Again, relaxation and rhythm are
everything. Without the proper rhythm you won't orgasm during intercourse or cunnilingus. This, of course,
takes practice and plenty of patience.

Remember the old joke where the stranger in New
York asks a passerby how to get to Carnegie Hall? The
answer was "Practice, practice, practice." That's what's
needed here. But in this instance, the practice itself can
be a lot of fun. And when the desired level of expertise
is achieved, each of you will be playing in a throbbing,
pulsing duet.

HOW TO MASTURBATE

One of the most effective ways to learn how to pleasure your own body is to masturbate. Does the subject embarrass you? It shouldn't. "Hey, don't knock masturbation! It's sex with someone I love" (from the film *Annie Hall*).

To be a goddess, a magnificent seductress, you need to feel, understand, and express all of your womanhood. You must experience orgasm. God gave you all the tools, all the parts. Work with them, use them for your pleasure, and the pleasure of your lover, your main man.

Alan Jay Lerner reminds us that "Pleasure without joy is as hollow as passion without tenderness." The word *pleasure* comes from the Old French *plaisir*, which means "to please." Before you can please anyone, you must first rid yourself of that block in your brain that tells you pleasure is not good. Pleasure *is* good!!! Pleasure is what every female needs to feel and express to be complete. You deserve all the joy and sensual gratification in life—simply because you're you.

Relax. Open your mind, and feel your sensuality. Give yourself a present wrapped in joy with a card attached that reads: To Yourself . . . From Yourself.

No one can awaken your sensuality as well as you. Only you hold the key that unlocks the door to Wonderland. Your brain is the lock, your fingers are the key. You are on your own. Are you ready, Alice?

Prepare to love yourself for at least thirty minutes or more in total seclusion. Find a part of the house— basement, attic, garage, or separate room—where you can lie down in a soft comfortable spot. Make certain that you will not be disturbed, and if possible, put on slow, sensual music, turn the lights low or light a candle, burn incense or spray the room with your perfume, drink a few sips of wine or champagne, and wrap your body in a silky piece of lingerie. Actually, a warm room is preferable, but if you don't have immediate access to these accoutrements, work with what you've got at hand—you and your imagination. That's all you need anyway.

Now lie down. Take your time to explore. Go very slowly—very, very slowly. Start touching the fabric of your gown over your skin. Touch your hair, your ears, your nose, your lips, your throat. Slide your fingers up and down your arms and shoulders, pass over your breasts, touching your stomach, your navel, your hips, and down your thighs. Feel the warmth of your silky skin emanating through the fabric. Stroke your thighs on the outside, then slightly part your legs and run your fingers along their inner flesh. Feel the texture, the smoothness of your skin. Feel the warmth of your hands traveling back up your body, reaching the softness of your breasts. Circle your hand all around the plumpness of your breasts, brushing over your nipples. Gently slide the fabric over their erectness. Observe their color and shape. Pinch them, make them harder. Lick your index finger and circle it around the protrusion of the nipple. Roll it slightly between your thumb and index finger. Squeeze it. Play with it for a while. Enjoy the sensation. Now use both hands to massage your breasts. Feel your sensitive nipples as you massage. As you gently squeeze and pull them, you can also feel throbbing sensations arising from your clitoris. You are experiencing their direct line of communication.

Now take a few deep breaths and let your hands drift down your navel and over your thighs again. Ever so gently, lift the cloth up as you feel that triangle of curly hair between your thighs. Look at the beauty of your erect nipples as you caress the outside of your nether lips. With your fingertips, tug slightly on your curly hairs. Feel how they are connected to your ripening vulva. Run your finger up and down the smoothness of your silky inner lips. Open your legs wider. Slide your index finger down the hot, moist crevice, feeling the desire of your beautiful and natural secretions. See how your body is responding to your touch? It's moaning in silence.

Put the same moist finger up to your parted lips. Lick it with your tongue. Taste and smell your own sweet nectar. Now liberally wet your fingers and put them back on your aroused clitoris (the highly sensitive knob that protrudes slightly just underneath the pubic bone). With your probing fingers, very gently move the hood up and down to stimulate arousal. Try to focus more on your left side. Because there are more nerve endings on that side, sensations tend to be greater. Experiment with different rhythms, different pressures, until you find the desired touch for your particular pleasures.

As you play, always be gentle. Since your rosebud is the most sensitive part of your genitalia, it does not like direct stimulation. So take care not to hurt it. With a little tenderness, it will reward you greatly. (And beware of too much intense stimulation. This could result in numbness of the area, thereby ruining your orgasm.) With the proper stimulation, your entire feminine area will become more and more sensitive with its increasing engorgement. You are on your way to the joy of complete pleasure.

Gently reduce the pressure, but continue the natural rhythm you have found. Continue to relax, to breathe, to enjoy this delicious moment. Your face will be flush, your nipples will be hard, your heart will be racing. At this point, you have found the right plateau. (If you haven't, a little troubleshooting may be in order. Try adjusting pressure and rhythm until you find the right balance.) Your body will easily remember these sensations; they are like a guidepost for future sessions. Do not try to orgasm just yet, continue to ride the wave.

Orgasm at this stage is not important. What is important is that you find a comfortable and stimulating rhythm and pressure. When you hit the right plateau, the force of life will take over. Orgasm generally follows when you let your body take over your mind. However, don't make the mistake of stopping once you feel it coming on. This is not the end. The end occurs when you feel several contractions in a row. In a word, keep stimulating until you can stimulate no more—until it becomes too sensitive to touch. Then you know you've done it. Alice has been to Wonderland.

P.S. Don't forget to breathe and do not masturbate to excess. Once or twice a day is okay—from time to time, but too much will desensitize you, rub the hairs of your pubis away, and diminish the possibility of intense orgasm with your man.

Masturbation is not only the most useful and widely used substitute for loving sex with a partner, but it is also the way to taking your lovemaking to new heights by increasing your awareness of your own body.

FOR THE EXPERIENCED

For you ladies who are experienced at masturbation, you may want to try something new and fun. Since you already know your body, maybe this creation will offer a little more satisfaction, titillation, or extended lustiness.

Always make sure that you are undisturbed for at least an hour. Lie down on your bed, couch, or floor in front of a mirror, if you will. Bring yourself to that euphoric feeling by massaging the hood of your clitoris with your wet fingers. As the erotic sensations increase, slip several fingers of the other hand into your vagina, hook them upward and massage your G-spot (urethral sponge) at your heartbeat rate. As your vagina expands, add more fingers, keeping it half full. When you feel the need to orgasm, resist the sensation. Stay relaxed and keep that lovin' feeling. The sensation will increase, and by resisting orgasm at this point, you will feel simultaneous pleasure/pain.

Now your right hand is pushing against the clitoral hood while the fingers of your left hand are feeling the spongy tissue inside while pushing against your G-spot (which is really the back of the clitoris). Now you are performing a "bimanual palpation" of the clitoris. This heartbeat rhythm actually pinches the clitoris, urging on a swell of jubilation. You can feel your walls twitching at your heartbeat rate. But don't be fooled. It's not an orgasmic contraction . . . just a twitch!

P.P.S. Some women use vibrators to enhance this method. If you become too attached to your vibrator, you might become impatient with your main man. And that would be a shame.

At this time, you will arrive at the spiritual level . . . When orgasm starts, stop all stimulation! More stimulation at this point will probably be painful. Your vagina should powerfully contract about six times, then pause for one contraction. Squeeze your PC muscles and stroke your love bud a few more times. The orgasm should increase and your vagina will go another six contractions. Your entire body will feel like one big clitoral head in a whole-body orgasm.

During this whole-body orgasm, you are already self-excited, so do not apply any hand stimulation. Nevertheless, leave your hands in place. Especially, leave your fingers in your vagina. It needs something to squeeze and push against to continue orgasm; otherwise it stops. Oftentimes, by applying a steady pressure on the hood of your clitoris with your outer hand, it can increase your orgasmic sensations.

At contraction twelve, there will be another pause. Squeeze your PC muscles, give your clitoris a few more strokes, and you will fly out of your body. Time and place and space will escape reality. Your feminine senses will be swimming in the high seas of erotic sexuality. You may hear the romantic voice of Luis Miguel accompanied by the classical guitar of Segovia serenading your orgasms in the distance.

Utopia will be reached, ideally, when you teach your man to take you to this place. After this experience, he will never leave you and you will never leave him. Not after crossing over into the divine milieu—the realm of spiritual eroticism—together!

MASTURBATION

Love is like cigarette smoking. If you smoke four or five a day you enjoy the smoke to the fullest. If you smoke two packs, you get nothing out of it but hardening of the arteries.

—HENRY MILLER

"It's pink. It's hard like an engorged weeping animal— a live piece of flesh—a succulent plant growing out of the moss of pubic hair engorged with fluid. The open slit which looks like a little mouth is waiting to kiss or be kissed. Then the mouth gets full and ejaculates," says Graham, a thirty-nine-year-old journalist in Washington, D.C.

From a man's point of view, this definitely explains why masturbation makes a fella feel alive and well. It's a way of loving himself, so to speak. We all know that love is blind, so a man needs to feel his way around!

Of course, there are many other reasons a man engages in this visual heaven: he enjoys watching his symphony grow and feeling its thin, sensitive skin; reveling in the nerve sensations while it fills with blood and stiffens; experiencing lewd fantasies during its awakening; and hearing Ludwig van Beethoven's "Ode to Joy" from his Ninth Symphony, while seeing bright lights and angels at the finale.

His penis is naturally on the outside of his body, so he can watch fluids flow from the little slit at its head while he's massaging it, then spreading the slippery secretion around the shaft.

The delicious sensation of masturbation also allows a man to forget his worldly woes for a few stolen moments. He wanders into his testosterone head where only warriors can see the other side. Because no matter how strong a woman's orgasm or how rejuvenated, enthusiastic, and relaxed she feels, it will never produce the same effect that a man experiences when he ejaculates. It is magic to him. When he's done, he can even go outside and give a thirsty branch or tree a golden shower from several feet before it lands. It's a lot of fun for a man to put his hands on all that miraculous equipment and watch its workings. When it's working and giving him pleasure, it makes him feel proud and thankful that he is a man.

Men who especially love the missionary position have been known to use pillows (the soft, downy kind) for masturbation. For example, when men masturbate, not only is it common practice to use their hand with a bit of lubrication spread over the penis, but certain men have discovered a way to actually duplicate the feeling of the woman they fantasize. For example, while in the missionary position the man puts on a condom, faces downward on the bed, places a pillow underneath his stomach with his testicles free-falling, and another pillow underneath his chest. He circles his arms around the latter as if he were hugging the woman, then proceeds into a copulating motion. I'm told it's a great facsimile. You would be surprised to learn just how many men continue to masturbate after marriage. A lot! Mary Louise, twenty-six, has been married to Glen, thirty-four, for eight months. One morning, she returned home after forgetting her briefcase to find Glen still in bed holding a pornographic magazine in one hand while the other hand was massaging his member. She was taken aback at the sight.

Mary Louise could not believe her eyes. She and Glen had a great sex life. So why, she asked herself? Before Mary Louise married Glen, she knew that he was prone to compulsive masturbation, but she believed that marriage would change him. Wrong! Marriage doesn't change anyone. Instead, the comfort of marriage brings out the real person. If a man derives joy in self-stimulation, oftentimes he will continue. Married men *do* masturbate! It's not bad or abnormal. Wouldn't you rather he masturbate than have coitus with another woman? Think about it!

When a man masturbates, there's a lot more going on than just the physical activity; his *imagination* is creating sexual fantasies in glorious living Technicolor and stereophonic sound that is akin to virtual reality. Try to get your man to share his fantasies with you. Knowing exactly what arouses his imagination is advantageous to your lovemaking.

During my interviews, a lot of men were embarrassed to reveal that intimate part of themselves for fear of being judged improperly. However, a few strangers did express themselves rather enthusiastically. They all came from a different background of fantasies. For instance: Ross, thirty-two, a paralegal in Saint Louis, Missouri, and married, said: "I was obsessed with these three girls in my office. They all looked different—different color hair, faces, bodies, but all tens. For weeks I couldn't talk to them without seeing them naked in my imagination. Driving home I would fantasize all three of them in my cubicle at work. They would all be completely naked except for wearing CFMs (come-fuck-me four-inch spike heels). One would be sitting on my desk with her legs spread-eagle, playing with herself. The second girl would be sitting in my chair, sucking on her nipples and bouncing her tits, and the third would be standing in the conference room door, waiting to undress me when I arrived. They were there to give me pleasure.

"The girl standing in the door unzipped my pants and sucked my cock. The girl sitting in my chair walked over and while putting her tits in my mouth said, 'Suck on these, big boy!' The girl sitting on my desk turned around and got on all fours with her pussy facing me while she masturbated herself to orgasm. They were all down and talkin' dirty. I loved it! I know it was unrealistic, but it's that unrealistic quality that turns me on."

Does Ross's wife have anything to worry about regarding these three co-workers? Probably not. But she might feel a little intimidated, to say the least. This is a situation where Ross's discriminating good judgment should take over. Certain fantasies might be harmful to the relationship if vocalized unless a woman is completely self-confident and not the jealous type. Do you know any?

The dominating power of a woman can inspire many a male fantasy. Darrin, thirty-seven, a stamp collector living in Sioux City, Iowa, relates an ongoing fantasy that most men have about attractive lady doctors. "I was on my way to a dental appointment. I hate going to the dentist. I usually put off my appointment until the pain is so excruciating, I have no choice. One day, it was an emergency. My appointment was the last one of the day. To my surprise, my usual dentist had taken ill and a stunning woman, Dr. Taylor, filled in.

"I sat down in the chair. Dr. Taylor started probing around in my mouth, trying to find the root of the problem. She found it, shot me with Novocain, and it started: As she cradled my head in her arms, her breast softly brushed against my face. She said, 'Open wide! Yeah, that's right. Stay just like that. Move your tongue over to the side. Now, keep it there. Open a little more. Good, good, don't move, stay where you are. Yeah, that's it!'

"She dabbed the side of my mouth with a napkin. All of a sudden, my fears diminished. All I could think about was having her. I shut my eyes and felt her fingers slowly unzipping my trousers. She rubbed and massaged my penis before she slid her hand inside. Her hand knew exactly what I wanted. I felt like exploding. Before I realized it, she was straddling the chair and me. She unbuttoned her blouse and opened her bra, exposing pink nipples. She decisively leaned over, unhooked the nitrous oxide and placed it over my face. Then she inhaled a bit herself as she sat on my erection. She put my hands on her breast and held onto them as she massaged them back and forth. Her hips were gyrating. Her pussy was sucking me to orgasmic spasms.

"You wanted to know my fantasy? Now you know. That was an ongoing picture reeling around in my mind every time I saw my lady dentist. Unfortunately, Dr. Taylor moved. Now I have a male dentist. Nope, I've got nothin' to add to that!"

Some men are into pain-dominance from a mistress figure. Others like Al, twenty-eight, a gofer on a movie set in Madison County, Virginia, enjoy fantasy subservience. Al confides, "When I masturbate, I like to think of my girlfriend wearing a mask, thigh-high black leather boots with spike heels, a black bra with the nipples cut out, and crotchless black panties. She's my mistress and I'm her slave boy. She ties my hands behind my back. She walks over to me with a dominating look in her eyes, slapping a paddle against her leg. She commands me to get down on my knees and lick her boots and then she puts her spike heel into my mouth and says 'Suck.' When I do something that displeases her she thrashes my bottom with the paddle. She orders me to lick and suck her entire body. She makes me stay there until she is completely appeased. When I don't please her, she pushes my mouth away and makes me wait while she does it herself to show me the proper way. Then she makes me do it over and over until I get it right." If Al's girlfriend knew about his fantasy, she might be able to play the role and make it fun for the both of them. I wonder if Al will ever tell her.

A man's fertile mind can turn any co-worker into a sudden siren as Brendan, forty, an actor in Los Angeles, shows. He enjoys a recurring fantasy about his present leading lady. "When I return to my hotel room, usually late at night, I'm too wired to sleep. I often picture Natalie walking into my room dressed in a trench coat and high heels. She takes off the coat and underneath, her shapely, long sinuous legs are sheathed in black nylons with the narrow tabs of a black garter belt, bustier, and tons of white pearls. I watch as she unknots her raven hair, letting it cascade to her waist. She says, 'Don't touch me. Don't even move. I want you to lie still while I grind my luscious juices over your big hard rock and straddle your face!' " I wonder if Natalie knows about Brendan's feelings for her. Should he tell her? Faint heart never won fair lady.

Other men derive even greater pleasure from

slightly pain-giving fantasies where he takes on a more sadistic point of view as Jason, forty-six, an advertising executive in Savannah, Georgia, exhibits. He fantasizes himself a plantation owner giving discipline to one of his gorgeous slave girls. Once a week, he needs to show his authority: "My butler brings Sophie into my study. She grins defiantly as she walks through the door. I tell her that I will not tolerate her disobedience one more time. I pull her by her golden mane over toward the piano, where I bend her over the bench and tie her arms and legs. I go in back of her and slowly lift her skirt, the layers of petticoats exposing her bare white buttocks. I remove my belt, feeling the smooth hard leather across my palm. Then I slide it across her bare flesh and between her alabaster thighs. She squirms against her will. I stand back and lay one across her backside, watching her buttocks redden. The more they redden, the more excited I become. Watching them lift and fall, lift and fall with every swat. Her moans and groans make me delirious. After a few more licks, I stick my boot between her legs and part them even farther. I pinch her pubic lips to feel her moisture. I can see the glistening of sweet nectar flowing down her thighs. I tell her she's a bad girl and she's disappointing. I can feel my rod getting the best of me. Her writhing makes me hotter. She says, 'I'll do as you say, anything, anything, my lord, my master!' With that plea, I kneel down behind her, taking her ripe globes into my hands and opening her wider. I watch her pink folds quiver with desire. I know she's ready. I spank her with my hand once more before running my fingers up and down her lips, parting them farther. I play with her clitoris before inserting my two fingers, then three, pumping them into her pussy as she grabs onto them with her whole sex. The more she begs, the more time I take. My tongue finds her pink bud and flicks around its firmness. Then sucking, pulling, biting until I feel her body jerking from orgasm. My erection is painful. I walk in front of her, unzipping my pants to relieve my throbbing member. I hold it in my hand watching it quiver in front of her flushed and delirious face. She opens her insatiable mouth and drinks from my tumid fountain as I shove it into the depths of her throat!" This is a pretty popular fantasy, although Jason articulates it better than most men.

There are women out there who would love to role play in a bondage/domination fantasy. Maybe Jason should spend a little bit of time seeking someone out. Or, maybe, he could carefully introduce his girlfriend to the idea in easy stages. What do you think?

A lot of men watch porno flicks. It's extremely common. In their minds, they place themselves on the screen. Especially in these days of virtual reality, some men even go so far as to imagine the actress from the film they are viewing walking out of the television set and into their room. One such man is Fisher, a twenty-nine-year-old automobile assembler from Dayton, Ohio. Fisher explained to me one of his favorite fantasies, which revolved around a specific movie.

In the story, a full-figured, succulent blond woman, dressed in a black crotchless cat suit with a patch over one eye, crawls on all fours into a room where two studs are standing at each corner of a mat, stroking their erect penises. She crawls over to one guy, rises up to her knees, and begins kissing his balls and licking the shaft of his penis. She becomes ecstatic as her quivering hands and tongue wrap around his organ. The second man becomes impatient and suddenly walks over, pulls her hair back, positioning her face in front of his hard member and thrusting it in her mouth. She begins to perform the same subservient licking and sucking along his grand erection. While she's enjoying the action, the first man spreads her legs wide apart, and as he lifts her hips high in the air, pierces her from behind. With his entry, she lets out a primal cry of pleasure, and for several minutes she has multiple orgasms. After a while, both men simultaneously ejaculate—one in her mouth and the other in her vagina. They pull out and leave the mat.

Still on all fours, the blond bombshell turns around and looks straight through the TV at Fisher lying on the bed. She slowly stands up, walks through the screen into Fisher's bedroom, and proceeds to plant a wet kiss on his hungry lips, whispering, "You're next, Big Boy." Her tongue slides slowly over his body until she reaches his throbbing erection and wraps her lips around its thickness. She urgently guides his penis into her vagina and begins to gyrate her hips and squeeze her nipples in rhythm. In a frenzy, Fisher throws her on the bed, spreads her legs, lifts her buttocks, and savagely plunges into her from behind, exploding his semen deep into her wanton walls.

The gamut of male fantasies is wide, and what I have presented is a small slice of the pie. Other fantasies include golden showers, cross-dressing, voyeurism, sex with older women, sex with coeds, watching two or more girls.

In most cases, men do not live out their fantasies. But their orgasm may be associated with some kind of fantasy that is either recurrent or changing, depending upon their whim.

Let's be honest, ladies. We all need fantasies at one time or another, and some people need more than most. So if you need a little encouragement, buy a desired porno flick acted out by the people you find sexy and attractive, put on the movie, pull down the shades, and enjoy an exciting adventure with your man.

Chapter 5

•••

*If Things
Go Wrong:
Troubleshooting*

MENOPAUSE—HIS AND YOURS

There is nothing permanent, except change.

—HERACLITUS

HIS

When I first heard of male menopause, it was from my mentor, Henry Miller. I asked him if all men go through a change of life the same as women. He assured me that indeed they do, and the effects can be just as disturbing. It's all part of the aging process—waning sexual desire, losing hair, diminishing eyesight and hearing, coming to terms with his mortality. And most men in our society are just not ready for it. The ones that slide through have great self-worth and high self-esteem. They sincerely like themselves, their jobs, and their families. For them, menopause is not a bowl of cherries either, but neither is it therapy time.

Men don't get hot flashes, genital dryness, mood changes, or other symptoms associated with women, because it's not about fertility or hormones. As men age, their hormones remain steady. There is a gradual decline in testosterone production from eighteen to ninety. Around the age of thirty-five, a man begets fewer sperm and less semen, but men free from disease and illness continue to produce testosterone, sperm, and semen until the day they die.

Their angst is more about libido and mortality. Their midlife crisis is usually between ages thirty-eight and sixty. It begins when a man's body reminds him that he is no longer young. His injuries don't heel as quickly; his sex drive slightly diminishes; and he begins

236 • Brenda Venus

to fear sexual dysfunction. You know exactly what happens when fear sets in—self-doubt, weight gain, insomnia, infidelity, unhappiness at work, increased use of alcohol, low self-worth, and low self-esteem are just a few characteristics. Also, his physique, emotions, and behavior alter. During this midlife crisis of feeling unsettled and bored, men sometimes go into therapy or trade their jobs and families for newer, younger models.

The solution: relax into maturity; gain a better understanding and acceptance of the aging process; keep a sense of humor and deal with problems as they arise; eat nourishing foods, take vitamin and mineral supplements, get plenty of exercise, and change goals. Meet each day with enthusiasm, while not letting ego stand in the way. Embrace new ways of life by being grateful for the little things. They really do mean a lot.

Be supportive of your man and boost his self-esteem. Once a man has the realization of his own self-worth, that he's still sexy and appealing, that he can still enjoy good sex, he'll start to sing again. Most men become better human beings. It's all about acceptance. Accepting a new life, a new way of being, and a new attitude.

Most men realize their true selves after forty, and oftentimes are much happier in a new career. And today, several men are having children at fifty, sixty, and seventy. Look at Clint Eastwood, Sean Connery, Warren Beatty, Norman Mailer, Kirk Douglas, Ted Turner, William Devane, John Forsythe, Leslie Nielsen, Robert Redford, Sidney Poitier, Jake La Motta, Dick Clark, and others who are doing great. In fact, some are actually better, happier, and more content. All are more successful!

YOURS

We live in a generation of women who have very high expectations about looking good well into their forties and beyond. In fact, these women don't even have an age, they have a wonderful style and flair. They're also determined to stay sexually active, lustful, and romantic through it all. Let's give a cheer for those ladies! Bravo! And, there are many men who feel as did the actor Liam Neeson when he professed, "The truth is, I've always just loved women—every shape, color, age . . . and I always gravitate toward their company." Gold stars for them!

Now, for ladies who have not been introduced to menopause, or "the change," let's get familiar. First of all, it's a crying shame that your mother, aunt, or somebody doesn't prepare a woman for the biological and physiological oddities your body will undertake. Many ladies confessed that they thought they were going crazy until they went to a doctor and were told the shocking news, "You are going through menopause—get used to it!"

It happens to every woman. No woman is immune. It isn't a disease. It's just your last menstrual flow. And some women are glad, because they hate their periods —PMS and heavy flows. Your body will go through a hormonal change. Since every woman is different, her clock will vary. Some experience it as early as their thirties, others as late as their late fifties.

Hormones play an active role all through your life. Dramatic changes occur in the brain, sex hormones, and regularity of ovulation when a woman approaches her forties. Estrogen levels can drop off over a period of fifteen years, but for most women it's a brief three- to four-year span. The development of osteoporosis (depletion of calcium stored in the bones) is directly related to estrogen loss. That's the reason women can look so much older than their years. Heart disease is another common consequence.

Ovarian exhaustion is the culprit that underlies menopause—decreased vaginal lubrication, thinning of the vaginal walls, and changes in the entire genital area encompassing the urinary tract. Lack of estrogen causes tissues, nerves, muscles, veins, and organs of the pelvic area to alter. Without hormone-replacement therapy, the likelihood of vaginal and urinary infections increases, and hernias of the uterus, bladder, or bowel may occur. Hernias can protrude or totally collapse into the vaginal walls. These are just a few of the symptoms making intercourse painful.

Several women complain of numbness in the genital area, but these changes do not necessarily alter a woman's ability to have orgasms or diminish her desire, and aging by itself does not reduce a lady's libido or her ability to enjoy good sex. In fact, some women enjoy it more. Actually, the hormone associated with desire is testosterone! The adrenal glands continue to produce testosterone, and oftentimes a woman becomes "very sexy" after menopause.

At the onset of menopause, other symptoms, such as hot flashes or night sweats, insomnia, mood changes, vaginal dryness, and loss of pubic hair as well as head hair, increase when the production of estrogen and progesterone in the ovaries tapers off.

Since all women experience this change differently, and some may need more progesterone than others, it's best to see a doctor you trust to find the right combination for your particular body. What works on one woman does not necessarily work on another.

To prevent negative changes in the genitals and urinary tract, there are other alternatives available. Estrogen and progesterone creams are widely used. The sources of these creams are the barbasco plant and soybeans. (The barbasco plant is a giant yam grown in the jungles of Mexico.) Also the use of evening primrose is recommended, and 1,500 mg of calcium a day and 1,200 mg of powdered vitamin E are beneficial. If you decide to go the natural way, consult a homeopathic physician. There's no reason for any woman to suffer. You can always find a way to better health, if you investigate and keep a positive attitude.

To really understand what it must be like for a lot of women, watch the movie *Fried Green Tomatoes*. Kathy Bates gives a wonderful comical and realistic impression of what it's like to go through a change and not have a clue about what to do. Also, if you ever feel depressed, let the following women be an inspiration to you. They have either gone through it, are going through it, or will soon: Lindsay Wagner, Sandy Duncan, Sophia Loren, Candice Bergen, Ali McGraw, Angela Lansbury, Jane Fonda, Jane Seymour, Lynda Carter, Jaclyn Smith, Lauren Hutton, Victoria Principal, Cicely Tyson. These women look great and carry on full, exciting lives no matter what their age. Most of them have families, a demanding career, and celebrity to balance. A lot can be learned from these and many more admirable ladies.

HOW TO KEEP HIM ERECT

Husbands are like fires. They go out if unattended.
—ZSA ZSA GABOR

If you have ever been the recipient of a loose noodle, I don't need to tell you how awkward it is to recover from this embarrassing moment, especially for him. Women need to have a much greater understanding of this phenomenon, because there's probably not a man alive who hasn't had that curse fall upon his "friend" at some point in his life. As in: "What are you doin', buddy? This is not the time to let me down!!!"

Women are mighty lucky that they don't have to contend with such delicate matters. And delicate is an understatement. Men go through hell on earth worrying about Hoppin' Harry's health. Keeping Harry happy is a big responsibility. No matter how much a man wishes it were in his control, it's not. I've heard so many women complain about how their men get an erection every time the wind blows or with any passing beauty. Yet when his apparatus doesn't rise, those same women become undone, responding as if it were a personal affront, and often criticizing their men irreparably. You don't ever want to do that. It's just not fair.

Often a man's momentary inabilities have nothing to do with his emotions for a woman. There could be a number of reasons for his temporary impotence: insensitivity on the woman's part, fear of rejection, self-consciousness, distraction, substance abuse, stress, illness, response to medication, a death in the family, a desperate desire to please, a muscle relaxant, or a simple headache or backache. Perhaps he just doesn't feel sexy, or maybe he's worried that you may find his penis unattractive. Men are extremely sensitive about their penises.

If you subscribe to the theory that an impotent man may be the consequence of an unknowing woman, you can help dramatically. So . . . what are you going to do if this happens to you? The secret is not to bring attention to the fact that his erection is napping. For heaven's sake, don't do that!

For most men, loss of erection is mental. If and when it happens to your man . . . *empathize*. Realize that it may be hard for him to discuss the situation with you, but that it's better for your relationship if you are able to talk about it lovingly. Reassure him by letting him know that you understand his fears, worries, and anxieties . . . that his stalled engine is not important, because you love him, not his car. Don't put pressure on him. Don't start kissing, fondling, sucking, or trying to get him excited for your own ego. That's counter-productive. He must feel that you love him, no matter what.

My friend Darla had a similar situation with her boyfriend Ted. She confided, "I met this wonderful man. Everything was too good to be true. We clicked on every level. Every time we made love it was magic. Then we decided to move in together before we got married. From that moment on, he couldn't get it up. I thought it was me. But he assured me that it was just a temporary setback.

"Weeks passed and still nothing. I became really worried about our sexual relations. Then I decided to keep him busy around the house and try to keep his mind off his deflation. I suggested he build another room. He took a course in home improvement and began hammering away. I also suggested that we sleep in separate beds for a while. We hugged and snuggled and kissed from time to time, but I never let it get past a certain point.

"Months passed. The added room was almost finished. Ted was so proud of his accomplishment. Then one night during a rainstorm, he brought some wood in for the fireplace while I cooked a spaghetti dinner. The smell of good food, of kindling and pine; the sound of sultry jazz; and a bottle of red wine were so relaxing. I started massaging his shoulders and neck. He gave me the most delicious kiss of my life, and ka-boom, before I knew it, I was naked on the couch and Ted's detonator was about to blast off. I was in wet heaven!"

The bottom line is don't make him feel any pressure. Eventually, when he believes in his heart that you don't expect him to jump through hoops or give you umpteen orgasms with a twenty-four-hour-a-day erection, he *will* produce.

Of course, problems with male sexual performance run the gamut and may be deeply rooted in physical and/or psychological origins that require professional medical aid; when a problem has become progressive and long-standing, such may be the only alternative.

But, perhaps, before deciding to bring in the white coats, you and your man may want to experiment with a few physical aids to facilitate his erection. Although surgery is definitely necessary for penile implantation, there are other varieties on the market today such as: cock rings, vacuum pumps, injections, et cetera. Injections of phentolamine, papaverine, and prostaglandin as smooth-muscle relaxants at the base of the penis are commonly used.

Rings and pumps are favored by many. After erection results from arterial blood flow into the penis, these aids prevent outflow of venous blood, temporarily enlarging the penis.

Several women mimic the process during lovemaking to a milder degree. They tightly cup their hand around the man's shaft base and testicular base. He becomes thicker as he continues pumping inside her vagina. It's a turn-on for these ladies to feel his building grow bigger and harder in structure.

The more organic devices are sparking a revival of the classical styles of the nineteenth century, which grew out of the old "bow tie theory." Building on the past, as it were, men have been using this trick for thousands of years; partly because it was simple, and partly because it was plain common sense. Take the infamous Beau Brummel, for example. He allegedly claimed that he could enlarge his organ and enhance orgasm during lovemaking by untying his perfectly formed cravat and wrapping it to strangle the base of his penis. You see, there is beauty in tradition and inspiration in history.

A well-known scientist from Los Angeles, California, has discussed with me the idea of venous engorgement temporarily enlarging the penis at great length. He explained: "I advocate what I playfully refer to as Dan's Bands." Two rubber bands can make a man a king. However, it's essential that the rubber bands fit the man's penis. Rubber band sizes 82 and 83 are most commonly used by the average penis. (They are about half an inch wide with a five- and six-inch circumference.) A man can experiment by putting a number 83 rubber band behind his testicles, encasing both penis and testicles, then placing a number 82 rubber band in front of his penis at its root. The bands should fit like a glove. If they're too tight, they will shut off the circulation and that's very bad. If they're too loose, they won't work at all.

"The rubber bands restrict outflow of blood through the penile veins. The male spongy tissue (corpus cavernosum), which is erectile tissue, fills with blood and becomes more swollen. The more blood that is retained by the spongy tissue, the more will be the swelling, and hopefully the greater the penile rigidity and orgasm.

"Now, you may think this is balderdash, but you must view the penis as a balloon that can be pumped up by the man's own blood instead of hot air."

These methods are not completely fail-safe, but they can enhance penile engorgement and sexual performance. However, I do want to stress that when a problem has grown beyond a reasonable level, couples will need professional help—therapy and/or surgery.

Even within this realm, the same basic fundamentals still apply: treat your man with empathy, consideration, patience, and lots and lots of love. It's a most delicate item indeed.

HOW TO COPE WITH PREMATURE EJACULATION

Love him, love him, love him.

—BV

"It was so exciting! He pulled up to my bumper in his long black limousine. He entered eagerly! He was slow at first because of his large size! His moves were legendary, almost magical! And then . . . it was gone," recounts Maureen, a thirty-two-year-old receptionist at Kaiser Permanente. It had promised to be an unforgettable night. It was unforgettable, all right, but not the way she had hoped.

The big question is when should ejaculation be called "premature"? Most men reach orgasm within two minutes of starting coitus. Technically, the average guy goes from penetration to ejaculation anywhere from ten seconds to three minutes. The average woman takes about eight minutes providing she's hot, thoroughly aroused, and knows how. But who cares about technical when the mood is not set and she's just beginning to spread her legs?

Bravo for the man who thinks that he's coming too quickly when he only lasts five minutes. And super bravo for the man who can wait until his woman has her mystic moment. Time is irrelevant. It all depends on how long it takes an individual woman to become completely relaxed, thoroughly stimulated, really wet, and ready to blast off. Making "great" love has nothing to do with how long. How long is a question reserved for little children who can't wait to go out to play.

Certain men just detonate too fast period, no matter whom they're making love to. Their premature ejaculation is probably due to our evolutionary past. If a man were to have lingered around in a delectable sugar wall thinking of nothing except the end of his penis, being at his most vulnerable while sexually aroused, he would probably have been eaten by a lion or other voracious carnivore.

Anthropologists say that our physical natures have not changed much in the last one hundred thousand years or so. Fortunately, today men are adaptable. A lot of men have become so goal-oriented that the result has detrimental effects. They begin to feel anxious about either having an orgasm or giving their partner one. This, however, interferes with a man's ability to relax into a pleasurable experience. Inadvertently, men who have a problem delaying detonation are considered "quick shooters."

Several of these "quick shooters" have tried all manner of things to last longer, such as numbing their penis with topical anesthetics, taking herbs, chanting, pinching themselves during intercourse, thinking about sports, a work deadline, et cetera. But premature ejaculation is not caused by an overly sensitive penis; it's simply lack of emotional control. With your considerate and loving help, he can learn how to control his orgasm.

Luckily, there are three or more methods of postponing inevitable ejaculation. One is the stop-start method, developed by James Seman, M.D. A man can either (a) masturbate during this exercise or (b) use it during intercourse. However, I feel that masturbation will yield better results, simply because a man can practice more often with no distraction, whereas inside his partner he will definitely be distracted. How does it work? When a man feels close to the point of orgasm, he should stop and rest from five to twenty seconds or when he judges it okay to continue, then begin again. This requires repetition and practice until a man can last longer than his usual or until he feels he, not "Waldo," is controlling the show. The other method is to squeeze the head or the base of his penis momentarily to slow the onset of ejaculation.

Dr. John Whipple, a psychiatrist in Topeka, Kansas, agrees that either technique can be effective.

William Masters and Virginia Johnson developed the Penile Squeeze. It works thus: when a man feels he's ready to come, he stops and pulls out. Then reenters after he and his "friend" are composed.

Another highly effective method is controlling his orgasms by contracting the same pelvic muscles that stop his urethra from expelling its golden stream. Your fella can practice this exercise while driving in his car. All it entails is the ability to contract his penis in his pants. He can do several sets of twenty repetitions.

Many doctors that I interviewed in all fields of practice recommended the simple and more pleasurable technique of pulling down the testicles. Here's how it works: when your man is ready to explode, his testicles contract, harden, and pull close to his body. It's kinda cute to watch. Pay careful attention to this moment. When his balls rise and become firm, you know that he's getting close. Take your thumb and finger and circle it at the top of his scrotum or base of his shaft and give it a gentle jerk downward. Not too hard, because you don't want to hurt him and ruin the erotic mood. It's actually fun and exciting for you to do it, but he may want to explore the feeling himself. No matter.

Whoever does it will contribute to a longer-lasting, loving, stimulating session.

Thinking about anything other than your ravishing beauty during lovemaking may be an effective way to postpone ejaculation, but it's no way to achieve harmony and togetherness. In the event a man tries everything, but nothing seems to work, there is a pleasure enhancer called "Long Joy," developed in China, based on an ancient herbal formula, and available for purchase in the United States. It's said to increase a man's endurance possibly long enough for you to reach orgasm.

But never subscribe to Murphy's Law of whatever can go wrong will. Participating in your man's glorious "point of no return" when his pelvic muscles contract in orchestration with his Cowper's gland, seminal vesicles, and prostate to spill his spectacular seed is a breathtaking occasion. The longer you can help him last, the better the sensation. Be gentle. Be patient on a continuous basis and you are sure to be rewarded by "Murphy's" new attitude.

Another positive way to view his premature ejaculations is to consider his first ejaculation as advance troops, or "sperm cadets," with the real army following soon. The night is young—talk, play, eat, drink, smoke, massage. Enjoy each other, and I assure you his army shall return! Your calla lily will blossom again, and you can get down to the real business of spending the night together, which is more than the sum total of strict sex. This is the whole experience of love.

IMPOTENCE—REAL AND IMAGINED

A man in the house is worth two in the street.
—MAE WEST

There are exceptions to every rule, but impotence is often self-induced. It can be caused by a negative mental attitude, arising from childhood humiliation or abuse, or from the feeling of inadequacy—a smaller-than-small situation. Some men seem to be born with an inferior attitude and they can't get over it.

It's not easy for certain males to keep their priorities straight. At some point in a man's life, he will suffer from temporary impotence. This occurs in about ten percent of the adult male population. Some older men suffer from recurring impotence, which can be treated either with an injection of the drug papaverine or with an apparatus such as a penile splint or implant, or even an artificial penis.

Men who have active sex lives are the lucky ones, because they are more likely to avoid the curse of impotence during old age. For most men the saying is true, "If you don't use it you might lose it!" You see, there is a muscle at the base of the penis and muscles need exercise, just as his prostate needs to be massaged. It's not advantageous for a man to fall into an asexual mode from a lengthy abstinence.

Before you throw in the towel and visit a doctor or a clinic that specializes in this type of trauma, ask him what he feels the problem is. Communication and positive, knowing action with the right woman can often be a cure. However, there are a few age-old common explanations: anxiety about his performance, fear of intimacy, possibly the wrong woman, guilt owing to religion or self-imposed ethics, depression or stress, or the influence of alcohol and drugs. But whatever the cause, don't kid yourself. Impotency, either real or self-induced, is a problem. We are what we think, remember? So if he truly thinks he has a problem, he does have a problem. Maybe he needs a change—a change of venue—a change in his sleeping patterns, eating patterns, lovemaking patterns. Sometimes all a man needs is a familiar and responsive partner and the opportunity for lively sex. Maybe he needs to know that you really want him. Try conveying a genuine interest in his pleasure. You have nothing to lose!

Epilogue

To love someone is to invite them to grow. Being happy in a relationship means communicating your needs—in bed and out of bed. Love and great sex demand everything—courtship, surprise, playfulness, humor, thoughtfulness, forgiveness, passionate moments, exercise, massage, music, good food, aphrodisiacs, and . . . a happy face!

Start today. Be positive and adventurous. Be your fantasy—the woman you admire and revere—but stay true to yourself. The secrets of seduction? Giving and receiving, controlling and surrendering, putting your whole heart and soul into pleasuring your lover, using the magic of music, candlelight, imagination, and the feel of something silky against your naked body—with complete confidence in your seductive skills. Only then will you succeed in being the greatest lover he's ever had.

On the subject of love, the actor Gerard Depardieu said, "On a movie set, when I'm working with a beautiful woman, I may enjoy a little seductive teasing. I don't go beyond that, however; I value fidelity over flirtation. Conquest is not heroic—what's heroic is to make love last!"

I'll leave you with these two thoughts: truth comes from the heart, not the tongue. And a life lived in fear is a life half lived. Happy trails . . .

Bibliography

Abelman, Paul. *The Sensuous Mouth*. New York: Ace, 1969.

Archer, W. G., ed. *The Kama Sutra of Vatsyayana*. New York: G. P. Putnam's Sons, 1963.

Balch, James F. and Phyliss A. *Prescription for Nutritional Healing*. New York: Avery Publishing Group, 1990.

Barr, Tony. *Acting for the Camera*. Boston: Allyn and Bacon, Inc., 1982.

Bechtel, Stefan. *The Practical Encyclopedia of Sex and Health*. Emmaus, PA: Rodale Press, 1993.

Burns, Minique. "Sex Drive: A User's Guide." *Essence*, vol. 21, no. 4 (Aug. 1990), 29.

Camphausen, Rufus C. *The Encyclopedia of Erotic Wisdom*. Rochester, VT: Inner Traditions International, 1991.

Chang, Stephen T. *The Tao of Sexology: The Book of Infinite Wisdom*. San Francisco: Tao Publishing, 1986.

Chia, Mantak, and Michael Winn. *Taoist Secrets of Love: Cultivating Male Sexual Energy*. Santa Fe: Aurora Press, 1984.

Cowan, Connell, and Melvyn Kinder. *Smart Women, Foolish Choices*. New York: Clarkson N. Potter, 1985.

Davis, Ben. *Rapid Healing Foods*. West Nyack, New York: Parker Publishing Company, Inc., 1980.

Dextreit, Raymond, translated and edited by Abehsera, Michel. *Our Earth Our Cure*. Brooklyn, New York: Swan House Publishing Company, 1974.

Dunne, Lavon J. *Nutrition Almanac*. 3rd ed. New York: McGraw-Hill, 1990.

Elisofon, Eliot, and Alan Watts. *Erotic Spirituality*. New York: The Macmillan Co., 1971.

Ellis, Havelock. *Psychology of Sex*. New York: Emerson Books, Inc., 1944.

Federation of Feminist Women's Health Centers. *A New View*

of a Woman's Body. Santa Monica, CA: Feminist Health Press, 1991.

Fensterheim, Herbert, and Jean Baer. *Don't Say Yes When You Want to Say No*. New York: Dell Publishing Co., 1975.

Gawain, Shakti. *Creative Visualization*. Mill Valley, Calif.: Whatever Publishing, Inc., 1978.

Grof, Stanislav. *Beyond the Brain*. Albany: State University of New York Press, 1985.

Hartman, W., and M. Firthian. *Any Man Can*. New York: St. Martin's Press, 1984.

Hopkins, Andrea. *The Book of Courtly Love*. Harper San Francisco: Labyrinth Publishing, 1994.

Jacobsen, Karl. *Dynamic Intercourse*. New York: Cybertype Corp., 1967.

Keen, Sam. *Fire in the Belly*. New York: Bantam Books, 1991.

Kendall, Henry O., Kendall, Florence P., and Wadsworth, Gladys E. *Muscles: Testing and Function*. 2d ed. Baltimore: The Williams and Wilkins Co., 1971.

Ladas, Alice K., Whipple, Beverly, and Perry, John D. *The G-Spot*. New York: Holt, Rinehart, and Winston, 1982.

Lloyd, Joan E. *Nice Couples Do*. New York: Signet, 1959.

Ludwig, Emil. *Cleopatra—The Story of a Queen*. New York: Garden City Publishing Co., Inc., 1939.

Ludwig, Emil. *Napoleon*. New York: Garden City Publishing Co., Inc., 1926.

M. *The Sensuous Man*. New York: Dell Publishing Co., 1971.

Masters, William H., Johnson, Virginia E., and Kolodny, Robert C. *Masters and Johnson on Sex and Human Loving*. Boston: Little, Brown, 1982.

McKenna, Terence. *Food of the Gods*. New York: Bantam Books, 1992.

Milonas, Rolf. *Fantasex*. New York: Grosset & Dunlap Publishers, 1975.

Moore, George. *Héloïse and Abélard*. New York: Liveright Publishing Corporation, 1921.

Nin, Anaïs. *Aphrodisiac*. New York: Crown Publishers, 1976.

Parsons, Alexandra. *Facts & Phalluses*. New York: St. Martin's Press, 1989.

Reich, Wilhelm. *The Function of the Orgasm.* New York: Simon & Schuster, 1973.

Rector-Page, Lynda G., N.D., Ph.D. *Healthy Healing: An Alternative Healing Reference.* 9th ed. Healthy Healing Publications, 1992 and 1994.

Reinisch, June M. *The Kinsey Institute New Report on Sex.* New York: St. Martin's Press, 1990.

Rohen, Johannes W., Yokochi, Chihiro, and Romrell, Lynn. *Color Atlas of Anatomy.* New York: Igaku-Shoin Medical Publishers, 1993.

Rutgers, J. *How to Attain and Practice the Ideal Sex Life.* New York: Cadillac Publishing Co., 1940.

Shepard, Martin. *Ecstasy.* New York: Moneysworth, 1977.

Taberner, P. V. *Aphrodisiacs: The Science and the Myth.* London and Sydney: Croom Helm, 1985.

BLUE CHRISTMAS

BLUE CHRISTMAS

Mary Kay Andrews

An *Imprint of* HarperCollins*Publishers*

This is a work of fiction. The characters, incidents, and dialogues are drawn from the author's imagination and are not to be construed as real. Any resemblance to actual persons, living or dead, is entirely coincidental.

HarperCollins books may be purchased for educational, business, or sales promotional use. For information, please write: Special Markets Department, HarperCollins Publishers Inc., 10 East 53rd Street, New York, NY 10022.

Originally published in 2006 by HarperCollins Publishers. This revised edition, with added material, published in 2007.

FIRST EDITION — 2006

REVISED EDITION — 2007

Designed by Joy O'Meara

Ornaments by Kara Strubel

Library of Congress Cataloging-in-Publication Data is available upon request.

ISBN: 978-0-06-137048-9

ISBN-10: 0-06-137048-7

07 08 09 10 11   ID/RRD   10 9 8 7 6 5 4 3 2 1

*For my Savannah posse: Polly Powers Stramm and
Jacky Blatner Yglesias, with love and thanks
for all the years of friendship and fun*

acknowledgments

First and foremost, thanks go to Carolyn Marino, my amazing editor at HarperCollins, for the idea to set a Christmas novella in Savannah, and to Stuart Krichevsky, the best agent in the world, who convinced me I actually *could* write a story in less than four hundred pages. Thanks and hugs also go to Polly Powers Stramm and Jacky Blatner Yglesias, for their unfailing help and friendship, and to food writer and cookbook author extraordinaire Martha Giddens Nesbit, for her encyclopedic knowledge of Savannah foodways—and the inspiration for our family's favorite crab cakes. Ed Herring at Seaboard Wine Warehouse in Raleigh helped with wine research, and Liz Demos, owner of my favorite antiques shop in Savannah, @Home Vintage General, showed me how Weezie's shop should be run. David K. Secrest helped with sports info, and friends like Virginia Reeve and Ron and Leuveda Garner gave me shelter on Tybee Island. And as always, thanks and love to my family, Hogans and Trochecks, and now Abels, whose love remains the best Christmas gift of all.

BLUE CHRISTMAS

CHAPTER 1

I was just hot-gluing the last popcorn-and-cranberry strand to the second of two five-foot-high topiary Christmas trees when my best friend came breezing into Maisie's Daisy.

BeBe Loudermilk stopped dead in her tracks and gazed around the first floor of my antiques shop, wrinkling her nose in distaste.

She gestured toward the half-empty crates of apples, oranges, and kumquats scattered around my worktable, at the halved pineapples and the pomegranates spilling out of grocery sacks, and at the freshly fallen drifts of popcorn littering the floor.

"What the hell?" she said dramatically. There are very few statements BeBe makes that are not laden with drama.

"Are you now turning to fruit vending as a sideline?" She shook her head sadly. "And I thought you were doing so well with the antiques."

"Christmas decorations," I said, pressing the popcorn strings onto the surface of the topiary tree, which I'd already covered with what seemed like a whole orchard full of tiny green crab apples and kumquats. "For the historic district decorating contest."

"Ohhh," she said, drawing it out.

With one tentative fingertip, she tapped the tree I'd completed, knocking off a kumquat, which rolled onto the floor, joining half a dozen other pieces of fallen fruit.

"Cute," she said dismissively.

"Cute? Is that all you can say? Cute? I've spent three whole days with this project. I've blown a good three hundred dollars on fresh fruit and nuts and Styrofoam forms, and strung what feels like ten miles of popcorn and cranberries. And just look at my hands!"

I held them out for her to see. There were needle pricks on my fingertips, hot-glue burns on my palms, and multiple bandages from self-inflicted skewerings.

"Criminal," BeBe said. "But why?"

"Because," I said, "I am, by God, going to win the commercial division decorating contest this year, even if I have to cover the entire surface of this building with every piece of fresh fruit in Savannah."

"Again . . . why would you bother? I mean, what's in it for you?"

"Pride," I said. "Last year I really thought I had it sewn up. Remember, I did that whole deal with the gilded palmetto fronds and magnolia leaf swags? And I had all the dried okra pods and pinecones? And I didn't even make honorable

mention? They gave first place to that stupid boutique on Whitaker. Can you believe they won with those lame-o kudzu vines and hokey bird's nests and stuffed cardinals? I mean, stuffed birds! It was absolutely Hitchcockian!"

"A tragic oversight, I'm sure," BeBe said, looking around the shop. "Remind me again why it was so crucial that I come over here today?"

"You promised to watch the shop," I said. "There's an auction at Trader Bob's, over in Hardeeville, that starts at noon. This close to Christmas, I can't afford to close up while I go on a buying trip. I was also hoping you might help me put up all the decorations before I leave in an hour."

She sighed. "All right. What are we doing?"

I gestured toward the pair of topiary trees. "Help me drag these outside. They're going in those big cast-iron urns by the front doors. Then we've got to tack up the over-door plaque with the pineapples and lemons and limes, and swag the grapevines around the show windows. I've got two kinds of grapes—green and red, and we'll hot-glue those once the vines are in place. Then the only thing left is the window display. But I'll set that up once I get back from Hardeeville."

With a maximum amount of huffing and puffing, and some very un-Christmas-like swearing when BeBe broke an acrylic nail, we managed to get the decorations in place.

"There," I said, standing out on the sidewalk, gazing at our masterpiece. "Take that, Babalu!"

"Babalu who?"

"Babalu them," I said, pointing across Troup Square.

"My nearest and queerest competition."

"That's not very nice," she said. "I thought you loved gay men."

"You don't know Manny and Cookie," I told her.

Manny Alvarez and Cookie Parker had opened their shop on Harris Street the previous spring. Manny was a retired landscape designer from Delray Beach, Florida, and Cookie? Well, Cookie *claimed* he'd been a Broadway chorus boy in the road show of *Les Misérables*, but he was fifty if he was a day, going bald, and weighed close to three hundred pounds.

"I tried to be nice and welcoming. I took flowers over there on their opening day, invited them to dinner, but since the minute they opened, they've been trying to put me out of business," I told BeBe. "They've tried to snake some of my best pickers. They called up the city and complained about my customers parking in loading zones; they even went to the gift mart and came back with the exact same line of aromatherapy candles and bath salts I carry, and now they sell them for two bucks cheaper."

"The nerve!" BeBe said. She craned her neck to look across the square at their shop. "Looks like they're working on their Christmas decorations too. Must be half a dozen men swarming around over there. Wow, look. They've got like a phone company truck with one of those cherry-picker buckets hanging lights along the front of the building."

"I'm sure whatever they do will be gaudy as hell," I said, flouncing back into the shop with BeBe following close behind. "Remember what they did for Halloween? The whole façade of the building was a red devil, with the shop's windows lit up with yellow lights as the devil's eyes."

"Hmm," BeBe said noncommittally.

"They blinked off and on all night. I thought I was having a seizure the first time I looked over there and saw it. It damn near drove me nuts," I said. "And it was *so* over the top."

"Not Savannah at all," BeBe agreed. "But flashy. You gotta give 'em that."

"Anybody could do what they've done," I said. "If money was no object. And those two are apparently rolling in it. I heard Manny personally donated twenty thousand dollars for the downtown business district's new Christmas lights. Of course, it's nothing but a thinly veiled attempt to buy the decorating contest."

"That is a lot of cash though," BeBe said. "Where do they get their money?"

"The old-fashioned way," I said. "Inherited. I heard Manny had a much older lover down in Florida who died two years ago. He had a start-up telecommunications company, and when he died, Manny got everything."

"Except good taste," BeBe said. I shot her a grateful look. She really is the world's best best friend.

"All righty then," I said, wiping my hands on the seat of my jeans. "I'm gonna head over to Hardeeville. I should be back by about four. There's plenty of change in the cash register. Prices are marked on everything. Anything brown or orange should be considered Thanksgiving merchandise, and you can mark it down fifty percent. And if you see Manny or Cookie lurking around outside, trying to steal my decorating ideas, just sic Jethro on 'em."

"Jethro?" She sighed heavily.

At the sound of his name, Jethro the shop dog poked his nose out from under the worktable where he'd been hiding, hoping I'd perhaps drop a sausage biscuit along with all that runaway fruit.

"He adores you," I told BeBe. "And he's great company."

"He sheds," BeBe said. "He drools. He farts."

"At least he's consistent," I said, heading out the back door to my pickup truck.

CHAPTER 2

It was one of those winter mornings that remind you why you live in the south. Sunny, with a hint of coolness in the air. Despite the fact that we were less than two weeks away from Christmas, the thick grass in Troup Square was still emerald green, and Spanish moss dripped like old lace from the oaks surrounding the iron armillary in the middle of the square. And on this beautiful winter morning, I was just as thankful for what wasn't as I was for what was: no gnats, no blistering heat, no suffocating humidity.

I should have been headed in the opposite direction, but instead I turned my beat-up old turquoise truck around the square. Just a quick drive by Babalu, I promised myself. Just to reassure myself of how superior my decorations were. But my heart sank as I slowed my roll.

The three-story shrimp pink exterior of Babalu had been transformed. Twining vines magically covered the façade. A

pair of towering palm trees in rococo concrete urns flanked the shop's front door, which itself was wreathed in a fabulously elaborate swag of moss, boxwood, smilax, and cedar. Everything, including the palm trees, had been painted flat white, then sprinkled with glitter. Hundreds of cut-glass chandelier prisms dangled from the white vines, and sent crystal refractions of light onto the sidewalk. It was a winter wonderland.

And standing right there on the sidewalk, directing the man in the bucket of the cherry picker, was the Snow Queen himself, Manny Alvarez.

"No, darling," he called, cupping his hands to be heard. "You've got the lights all bunched up there on the right side."

The bucket-truck had traffic blocked in front of the shop, and I had no choice but to stop behind it. My truck's brakes made a grinding noise, and Manny whirled around to see where the noise was coming from. A smile lit his face when he spotted me.

"Eloise?" he said, one eyebrow lifted. "Checking on the competition, are we?"

I gritted my teeth. "Hello, Manny. Looks like your side of the square has had some unusual weather for Savannah."

"You know me," he said airily. "Fantasy is my life. And really, that whole nuts and fruits and berries thing all the locals down here seem to be clinging to is so five minutes ago. Don't you agree?"

"The historic commission's guidelines specifically call for using natural, vernacular design elements," I pointed out. "I guess that's why the 'locals' as you call them tend to follow the guidelines."

"Oh, guidelines," he said, shaking his head. "Boring! Cookie and I believe in following our muse, in order to allow the full range of creative expression in our work."

"How nice," I said. "It'll be interesting to see what the judges think of stylized white palm trees in the context of an eighteenth-century historic district."

"Won't it though," he said.

CHAPTER 3

Trader Bob's Treasure Trove Auction House is a grandiose name for what is, in reality, a converted chicken house on a dead-end street on the outskirts of the tiny town of Hardeeville, South Carolina, just across the Talmadge Memorial Bridge from Savannah.

Because Trader Bob, aka Bob Gross, doesn't usually believe in wasting time or money on a catalog or advance flyer, a Trader Bob auction is always an adventure. Some days he'll have a container load of fine English or Dutch antiques, mixed in with odd lots of tube socks and bootleg videos bought from distressed merchandise brokers. More than once I've arrived at Trader Bob's to find him hammering down cases of half-thawed frozen pizzas and slightly dented cans of off-brand pineapple.

But on this December morning, the parking lot, nothing more than a mowed cornfield, was only half full of the usual

assortment of dealers' vans and trucks, which was fine by me. Fewer dealers should mean lower bids and better deals.

I was greeted at the door by Leuveda Garner, Bob's sister and business partner, with a friendly nod and a proffered cardboard bid paddle.

"Hey, Weezie," she said. "Long time, no see."

"Merry Christmas, Leuveda," I said. "Got anything good today?"

"Are you in the market for refrigerated dairy cases? Bob bought out a Piggly Wiggly grocery store over in Easley. We've got a bunch of old fixtures and display racks. There's a couple good cash registers you might be interested in."

"I was thinking more of antiques. Is everything going to be store stuff?"

"Not all of it," she said quickly. "We got everything from the owner's estate, too. Some furniture, dishes, linens, all the junk from the attic and basement, and from a couple of barns on the property too." She wrinkled her nose. "Old crap like you like, Weezie. Better go find a chair. Bob's starting early today because he's driving to Hendersonville tonight to pick up a load of furniture, and we heard there's rough weather in the mountains."

Sure enough, as my eyes got accustomed to the dim light of the chicken house, I saw Bob standing at his podium, microphone clipped to his shirtfront, holding aloft a life-size cardboard cutout of the Birds Eye Jolly Green Giant.

"All right now," Bob chanted. "I need a giant bid to start us off. Folks, this is vintage advertising art. Whadya give now? Whadya give? Gimme a hundred. Let's go, ho, ho, ho. Get it?"

The audience groaned, but they got it, all right.

With no time to stroll the merchandise, I picked a folding metal chair down close to the front and did my best to eyeball the offerings from there. Some auctioneers don't mind if you shop while they talk, but Bob Gross runs a tight ship, and he doesn't like any distractions once he starts working.

As Leuveda had promised, there was an entire small grocery store's worth of fixtures and display racks lined up on both sides of the chicken house walls. My eyes locked tight on a battered red-wire three-shelf bread display rack with a tin Sunbeam bread sign affixed to the top. The Sunbeam girl's topknot of golden curls still shone bright as she bit into a slice of white bread. It would be just the thing for a display fixture at Maisie's Daisy. I could already envision it piled with stacks of old quilts, tablecloths, and bed linens.

Right beside the Sunbeam girl leaned an old turquoise painted wooden screen door, with a bright yellow Nehi orange soft-drink metal-door-push advertisement.

"Mine," I whispered to myself. Again I lusted after the screen door for myself. I could already see it as a kitchen door for my own town house on Charlton Street.

I looked nervously around at the other auction-goers to size up the competition, and was elated to see that most of them seemed genuinely interested only in the more modern fixtures Bob was rapidly auctioning off.

When the Sunbeam bread rack came up half an hour later, Bob started the bidding at two hundred dollars. I kept my paddle down. Way too high, I thought. Today, with this

thinned-out crowd, he'd be lucky to get fifty bucks, the price I had already budgeted spending on it.

"Two hundred?" Bob implored, searching the room for a bidder. "How 'bout one seventy-five?" He held his arms wide in disbelief. "Folks, this is Americana. You can't put a price on Americana."

"One hundred eighty." The voice came from the back of the room, and I'd heard it recently. Only this morning, to be exact. I whirled around in my chair to see Manny Alvarez, frantically waving his bid paddle.

"That's more like it," Bob said approvingly. "A man who knows values."

Manny Alvarez! What was he doing slumming over here in Hardeeville? I'd been buying from Trader Bob's for years and I'd never seen any other Savannah antiques dealers make the trek over to my secret source before. Had Manny followed my truck over the bridge?

"We've got one eighty," Bob said jovially, looking around the room. "Anybody else?"

My fingers turned white as I gripped the paddle. A hundred and eighty was actually a fair price for the bread rack, cheap even. But I hadn't budgeted spending that kind of money for something I had no intention of selling.

"One eighty going once," Bob droned, staring directly at me. "Weezie Foley, I can't believe you're not bidding on this thing. I thought of you as soon as I saw that little Sunbeam gal."

"One eighty-five," I said through gritted teeth.

"One ninety," Manny fired back.

My heart sped up. "One ninety-two?"

Bob rolled his eyes but nodded, accepting my chintzy raised bid.

"Oh for God's sake," Manny said. "Two hundred."

Bob cut his eyes in my direction. My paddle stayed where it was. Christmas was coming. I had gifts to buy. Bills to pay. The commode in the shop was making weird gurgling noises that foretold a high-priced plumbing problem.

Bob looked at Manny. I looked at Manny. He had his checkbook out, and a smug nonny-nonny-boo-boo expression on his face. I hate smug. But I hate broke worse.

"I'm out," I said, shaking my head.

"You sure?" Bob asked, his gavel poised midair.

I nodded.

"Sold for two hundred dollars," Bob said. "You got yourself a great buy, mister."

"I know," Manny said. He gave me a broad wink and went over to Leuveda to cash out.

I turned around and tried to concentrate on the rest of the auction, consoling myself that I would probably have no competition for the screen door with the Nehi advertisement.

The screen door was a twelve-dollar steal, for which I gave myself a pat on the back, but my paddle stayed in my lap after that, as Bob auctioned off the rest of the Piggly Wiggly people's earthly belongings, which included an astonishing amount of Tupperware containers, Beta format videotapes, and case after case of empty canning jars.

Finally Bob paused to take a swig of coffee from his Sty-

rofoam cup. He glanced down at his watch, and at the greatly diminished crowd of bidders.

"Folks, it's getting late, and I gotta head for the hills. Tell you what. I got three mixed box lots here. We don't have time to drag the stuff out of 'em. Leuveda," he called toward the back of the room. "Hon, tell 'em what all's in these boxes."

Leuveda stood up and ran her hand through her sandy blond curls. "Bob, there's good stuff in there. Some nice old glass Christmas ornaments, some vintage linens. I think there was at least one Christmas tablecloth, and some old aprons and things. Miscellaneous pieces of china, and a jewelry box full of odds and ends. The family took all the really good stuff. But there's probably some good old costume jewelry left."

Bob nodded approvingly and Leuveda took her seat again and resumed cashing out the dealers who were preparing to leave.

"Gimme twenty—one money for all three boxes," Bob urged.

Two men in the front row got up, stretched, and started toward the door.

"Twenty," Bob repeated. "Leuveda, didn't you say those ornaments were Shiny-Brites? Still in the original boxes?"

"Four, maybe five Shiny-Brite boxes," Leuveda agreed, not looking up from her adding machine. "There's a strand of bubble lights too."

My pulse blipped upward. I've collected old glass ornaments for years, and Shiny-Brites—especially in their original boxes—were at the head of my want list.

But before I could say anything, a skinny redheaded woman in front of me cocked her head to one side. "Give you five bucks, Bob."

"Five," he howled. "You can't buy a single Shiny-Brite for that."

"Five," she repeated, standing up.

"Weezie?" he said, noticing my fidgeting.

He had me and he knew it. "Seven," I said, mentally crossing my fingers while trying to keep a poker face.

"Estelle?" He went back to the redhead. "You gonna let her get away with that?"

She shook her head resolutely.

Bob sighed. "You're killing me. Seven once, twice, sold for seven dollars."

I smiled and waved my paddle number at him, which he called out to Leuveda, who'd already added it to my total.

"I gotta get out of this business," Bob said, shaking his head in disgust.

It was nearly four by the time I got the truck loaded. BeBe, I knew, would be champing at the bit to be relieved at the shop. Still I couldn't resist peeking inside the heaviest of the cardboard boxes as I loaded them in the bed of the pickup alongside the screen door.

The bitter loss of the Sunbeam bread rack to Manny Alvarez was quickly forgotten as I lifted out four yellowed cardboard boxes of Shiny-Brite glass ornaments in their original cartons.

"Yes!" I exclaimed, peering inside the brittle cellophane box-top window at the glittering colored glass orbs. The

boxes contained not just unadorned round balls, but rarer, and more desirable, glass figural ornaments in the shapes of angels, snowmen, and Santas. Some had flocked swirls or stripes, and a few were kugel and teardrop shaped. Each box held a dozen ornaments, and all were in fifties colors like turquoise, pink, pale blue, and mint green.

I never bother to read price guides for the things I collect, because these days I buy only when the price is cheap, and I'm never looking to resell, but still, even I knew my seven-dollar purchase was a winner.

Beneath the boxes of ornaments, I unwrapped a neatly folded, if slightly stained, fifties Christmas bridge cloth, with decorative borders of red and green holly leaves interspersed with playing card motifs. There were eight kitchen aprons, all with Christmas themes, ranging from practical red-and-white gingham and rickrack numbers to a flirty red ruffled chiffon number to a starched white organza one with hand-crocheted lace edging and an appliquéd snowflake pocket.

"Adorable," I said, happily patting the pile of aprons. Beneath them I found a cardboard box filled with dozens of delicate vintage lady's handkerchiefs, and beneath the aprons, I found the jewelry box Leuveda had promised.

The box itself was nothing special. I'd seen dozens of embossed leather boxes like this one at yard sales and thrift stores over the years. Inside I found the expected jumble of old glass beads, discolored strands of cheap pearls, orphaned clip-on earrings, and inexpensive dime-store bracelets and brooches.

I rifled the jewelry jumble in the bottom of the box with my forefinger, like a painter stirring paint, until something sharp jabbed me, drawing blood.

"Oww!" I exclaimed, sucking my wounded finger. With my left hand I picked up the piece that had stuck me.

It was a brooch. A big, gaudy blue-jeweled brooch, maybe two inches high, in the shape of a Christmas tree. A blue Christmas tree.

My cell phone rang. I looked at the caller ID panel and winced. BeBe. Time was up. She was tired of playing store, I knew. Anyway, I had to get back and finish decorating the shop before getting ready to go hit the holiday party circuit tonight.

"Hi," I said, cradling the phone between my ear and shoulder as I pinned the brooch to my blouse. "How's business?"

"Great," BeBe said unenthusiastically. "Your dog drooled on my shoe. Your toilet sounds like it's going to explode. But all is not lost. I sold that ugly brown stick-looking table by the door for two hundred fifty dollars."

"You what?" I exclaimed.

"Yeah, I couldn't believe it either," she said, laughing. "And I got cash, so don't worry about the check bouncing."

"Two hundred and fifty," I repeated dumbly.

"Great, huh?"

"Not so much," I told her. "That was a signed, handmade Jimmy Beeson hickory-stick table from the 1920s. It came out of one of those old lake lodges up at Lake Rabun in North Georgia. I paid almost a thousand for it myself."

"Oh," BeBe said. "So marking it two hundred fifty dollars was kind of a loss leader thing?"

"No," I said sadly. "The price tag was twenty-five hundred dollars. Two zeroes."

"Whoopsie," BeBe said. "Look, I'll make it right with you when I see you. But I've got to lock up and go get ready for your uncle's party tonight. Is it all right to leave Jethro alone until you get here?"

"Go ahead on," I said. "He used to like to chew on the leg of that table. But that's not a problem anymore."

CHAPTER 4

When I got back to Maisie's Daisy, I parked the truck and walked across the street to get a better perspective of the shop's decorations. The fruit garlands and topiaries were tasteful and by the book. And yes, I thought ruefully, Manny was right. BOR-RING!

But rules were rules. And if I wanted to win the historic district decorating contest, I'd just have to be a by-the-book kind of girl.

As I ferried my auction finds from the truck to the shop, an idea came to me. The outside of my shop might have to look like Williamsburg proper, but the inside of the shop could be anything I liked. And that box of vintage Christmas stuff had put me in a funky kind of mood.

I switched on the shop lights, and Jethro ran to my side, planting his big black-and-white paws on my chest. "Not now, sport," I said, giving him a quick scratch behind the

ears. I went over to the pine armoire that hid the shop's sound system and flipped through my collection of Christmas CDs, passing on the tasteful instrumentals, the Harry Connick, Nat King Cole, and Johnny Mathis selections.

"Here," I said aloud, sliding a CD into the player. "Here's what I'm in the mood for."

It was my all-time favorite Christmas compilation, *A Christmas Gift for You from Phil Spector*, featuring all the legendary (and nutty) sixties producer's acts: the Crystals, the Ronettes, Darlene Love, even the inimitable Bob B. Soxx and the Blue Jeans.

A moment later, Darlene Love's powerful voice swung into "White Christmas," done in Phil Spector's trademark "wall of sound" style, sounding nothing like Bing Crosby, but just right in her own way.

I picked up the boxes of Shiny-Brites and headed for the display window. For the past few years, I'd been buying every aluminum Christmas tree I could find at yard sales and flea markets, but the rest of the world had gotten hip to fifties, or midcentury modern as it was now called, and the trees had become expensive and scarce. This year I'd managed to scrounge only three trees, and I'd had to turn down dozens of customers who wanted to buy them out of my window. Now I flitted from tree to tree, placing the Shiny-Brites on the window side of the trees, where they could be seen by passersby. I interspersed the vintage balls with newer, reproduction ornaments I'd ordered at the Atlanta gift mart in September. With the tiny white flicker lights, they were glittery and wonderful.

But the window was still too stiff, too formal. I'd created a living room vignette, with a pair of red tartan–slipcovered armchairs, a primitive fireplace mantel and surround with peeling green paint, and a red-and-green hand-hooked rug. A twig table held a stack of old leather-bound books, including an opened copy of Clement Clarke Moore's *'Twas the Night Before Christmas* with illustrations by N. C. Wyeth.

I'd thought the window perfect only a few hours ago, but now it seemed way too safe and predictable.

I crossed my arms over my chest and gave it some thought. Suddenly the Ronettes swung into "Frosty the Snowman," and I got inspired.

I moved the twig table and replaced it with a just-purchased could-be Stickley library table. An improvement, I decided. Reluctantly, I brought out my stack of dime-store Christmas gift boxes. I'd have to fight my customers to keep them to myself, but really, they were too wonderful not to put on display. I arranged them under the tree and took another critical look. It needed more. Much more.

Glancing at my watch, I realized I'd lost track of time. The party started at seven, and Daniel was supposed to pick me up in fifteen minutes!

Later, I promised myself. Genius can't be rushed. I whistled for Jethro, picked up the box of costume jewelry from the auction, and hurried over to my house.

As always, when I stepped inside my front door, I said a silent prayer of thanks. Mine was not the grandest, oldest house in the historic district, or even on Charlton Street. It was built in 1858 and had austere lines. But it was made of

coveted Savannah gray brick, had beautiful lacy wrought-iron trim, a wonderful courtyard garden, and a fantastic gourmet kitchen of my own design. And it was mine. All mine. I'd found the house when Tal and I were still newlyweds. The $200,000 price tag was more money than we could afford, but I wrote the down payment check without a second thought, and plunged into remodeling it, doing much of the work myself.

This house was my anchor. My dream. It had outlasted the marriage to Tal. He'd been awarded the town house in our divorce settlement, and I'd only gotten the carriage house. But through a strange turn of events, Tal's fortunes had taken a dive, and he'd needed to sell the town house. I was overjoyed to buy him out. And when my antiques business started to take off, I'd been able to buy the twin to my town house next door. I moved Maisie's Daisy out of the carriage house and into the ground floor of that house and rented out the top two floors to a young couple who both taught at the art school.

After bribing Jethro with a dog biscuit, I bolted upstairs to dress for the party. Earlier in the day I'd laid out a simple pair of black capris and a black lace top to wear. But the blue Christmas tree pin had made me rethink my outfit.

Only vintage would match my mood tonight. Once I was out of the shower, I rifled through my closet, looking for the right combination.

Aha! But could I still get in it?

The black fifties cocktail dress was one I'd found at a great vintage shop in Atlanta called Frock of Ages. It usually killed

me to pay retail for old stuff, but when I'd spotted this dress in the shop window one Saturday while cruising down McLendon Avenue, I knew I had to have it. Even at forty bucks.

The bodice was beaded black brocade, with a deeply scooped neck and cap sleeves, and the full, ankle-length bouffant skirt was black chiffon over two layers of black tulle crinoline. I spritzed my neck and breasts with my favorite perfume, then struggled into a black waist-cinching Merry Widow, stepped into the dress, sucked in my breath, and struggled with the zipper. When the dress was still at half-mast, I heard the doorbell ringing downstairs and Jethro barking.

Damn. True, it was ten after seven, but Daniel was never on time these days. His restaurant, Guale, was always swamped at the holidays, and since he'd bought out BeBe's interest in it, he seemed to work longer and longer hours. I hadn't even put on makeup or fixed my hair properly, but it wouldn't do to keep Daniel waiting.

Not this time of year. Christmas seemed to make him grumpy. I knew it was because he was overworked, but it still made me a little sad that he couldn't enjoy what should have been a happy holiday.

Especially this year. My business was doing well, and after all those years of working as a chef in other people's kitchens, Daniel had finally realized his dream of owning his own restaurant. After three years of dating, I had secretly halfway convinced myself that this Christmas could be the one. . . .

I ran downstairs to answer the door. He stood on the doorstep, key out, with a funny look on his face.

"What's wrong?" I gave him a quick kiss.

"Nothing," he said, glancing around at the street behind. "I was going to let myself in, but I had the eeriest feeling just now. Like I was being watched."

I poked my head out the door and looked up and down the street. I saw a flash of red disappearing through the square.

"Maybe you *were* being watched," I said, drawing him inside. "I bet it was those creeps Manny and Cookie."

"Who?" Daniel asked, kissing my neck. "Mmm. You smell good." He held me at arm's length and smiled. "Looking good too. I don't suppose that's a new dress?"

"New in 1958, I think," I said, twirling so he could get the full effect.

"Could you zip me, please?" I asked, holding my hair off my neck. "Manny and Cookie own Babalu, that new shop across the square, over on Harris. They're trying to put me out of business. I think they were probably over here spying, checking on my decorations for the business district Christmas decoration contest."

He zipped me up without any funny business. So I knew he was distracted.

"What makes you think they're trying to put you out of business?" he asked.

"Everything. But don't get me started. I just have to run upstairs and slap on some makeup, and I'll be ready to go."

"You look fine to me," Daniel said. "Anyway, we really need to get a move on here, Weezie. I've got to go back to the restaurant in a couple hours. We've got two law firm

Christmas parties tonight, and the partners all expect the owner to put in an appearance."

"Daniel!" I protested. "It's James and Jonathan 's first party. You can't cut out early. And I don't want to."

"You can stay," he said. "But there's no way I can. Now, can we get going?"

"One minute," I promised.

Upstairs, I dabbed on some eyeliner, mascara, and lipstick, and slipped into a pair of black velvet high-heeled pumps. I grabbed my black velvet shawl, wrapped it around my shoulders, and fastened the blue Christmas tree pin to it.

"Ready," I said, still breathless on the bottom stair.

Daniel picked up my house keys and handed them to me. He looked at me and frowned.

"What?" I asked, tugging the neckline of the dress. "Are my boobs falling out again?"

"No," he said slowly. He reached out and touched my shawl.

"This pin. Where did you get it?"

"At Trader Bob's auction today," I said, surprised. Even though he's a chef, and more arty than most, Daniel is all man. He rarely notices things like jewelry or shoes. "Why? Don't you like it?"

"Yeah. It's fine," he said, still staring at the pin.

"What? You're still staring."

"My mother had a pin just like that," he said, looking away. "My brothers and I pooled our lawn-mowing money and bought it for her the year my dad left. She used to wear it, every Christmas. She said it was appropriate. You know,

because my dad left, we were all having a blue Christmas that year. Like the Elvis Presley song."

"Oh," I said softly. Daniel never talked about his mother. Or his father, for that matter. I knew that his dad abandoned his mom and their three sons when Daniel was just a kid. I also knew that Daniel's mom, Paula, had wound up in a scandal involving her married boss at the sugar refinery here in Savannah, where she worked. When the dust settled, the executive had been sent to a federal prison in Florida, but not before he divorced his wife and married Paula. Not long after that, Paula Stipanek Gambrell had followed her new husband to Florida. Daniel and his two older brothers had been raised by his aunt Lucy. It was not a happy story.

I tucked my arm into his. "If you guys bought a pin like this, it just proves you had great taste. These pins were quite the craze from the forties through the sixties, although not so much in the war years, because metal was hard to get for jewelry. I've seen hundreds of variations of Christmas tree pins. Every costume jewelry company made them. Coro, Carolee, Trifari, you name it. And some of the more expensive ones that were sold in jewelry or department stores, signed pieces made by Weiss or Eisenberg or Miriam Haskell, sell for hundreds of dollars now."

Daniel gave a short, humorless laugh. "Yeah, well, I can guarantee you that one ain't worth hundreds. We bought my mom's pin at the Kress five-and-dime on Broughton Street. Between us, we scraped up maybe five bucks to pay for it."

As we walked to Daniel's truck, I heard Jethro give a plaintive howl from inside the house.

"Poor guy. He hates staying home alone."

Daniel tugged at his tie, a rare concession on his part. "Yeah, well, I'd gladly trade places with him tonight."

"Thanks!" I said sharply.

"Sorry," he said, giving me a conciliatory peck on the cheek. "I just really don't get into Christmas parties. Never have. But what I should have said was, I wish you and I were staying home tonight. Just the two of us. I'd love to help you get out of that new dress of yours."

"Hmmph," I said, unconvinced.

CHAPTER 5

Shortly after celebrating his silver jubilee in the priesthood, my uncle James hung up his clerical collar and came home to Savannah to practice law and live a quiet life in the modest house he inherited from his mother. Not long after that, he timidly snuck out of the closet, and not long after that, met his current partner, Jonathan McDowell.

My conservative uncle had waited three long years before finally giving in to Jonathan's request that they live together openly. In September, Jonathan, a charming, forty-five-year-old assistant district attorney, and his adorable mother, Miss Sudie, had moved in to James's house on Washington Avenue.

Tonight would be their first party. For weeks, James had been as nervous as a cat in a room full of rocking chairs. "What if nobody comes?" he'd fretted as we'd gone over the menu for the open house "drop-in."

"People will come," I'd promised. "You and Jonathan have

lots of friends. And everybody loves Miss Sudie. And besides," I'd said, "people are dying to see what Jonathan has done with your house."

James shook his head and ran his fingers through his thinning hair. "He's painted the living room brown, you know. Brown! My mother would be rolling in her grave if she knew. She always kept the downstairs rooms pink."

I shuddered. "Pepto-Bismol pink. Old lady colors. Anyway, it's not really brown now. It's a dark mocha. And it's wonderful. Jonathan has divine taste. And I'm so glad he talked you into getting rid of that horrible old stuff of grandmother's."

"I thought you liked antiques," James said.

"Not all antiques were created equal," I informed him. "That horrid pink velvet sofa was butt ugly, and you know it. And those baby-blue tufted armchairs . . .yeecchh."

"The new sofa is really comfortable," James admitted. "And Jonathan's leather armchairs are great for reading. And he did let me keep the stuff in my bedroom."

So tonight was my uncle's coming-out party. In more ways than one. As we approached his house, I happily noted that the old house was aglow with Chistmas lights, with a big evergreen wreath on the front door and half a dozen people standing on the front porch sipping wine and chatting. And both sides of the street were lined with cars.

"James was afraid nobody would show up," I told Daniel, directing him to pull into the driveway behind my father's dark gray Buick. "Mama and Daddy never stay out past eight," I reminded him.

Daniel glanced over at me. "So your mother's okay with them living together? She wasn't shocked?"

"I wouldn't say she actually approved," I said. "But you know what a snob Mama is. The McDowells are old Savannah money. She's thrilled that James is seeing somebody of quality. And she adores Miss Sudie."

James met us at the front door, resplendent in a snappy hunter-green plaid sport coat and a rust-colored turtleneck sweater.

"Wow!" I said, kissing him. "You're right out of a Ralph Lauren magazine ad."

He frowned. "Is that good?"

"Very good," I said with a laugh. "And you didn't even have to put on a tie."

"Not even for Jonathan," James said. "Not even for Christmas."

Jonathan walked up and slung an arm around my shoulder and Daniel's. "Is he complaining about the damned brown paint again?"

"No," I said. "He's congratulating himself on not having to wear a necktie."

"Well, come on in and get something to eat and drink," Jonathan said. "Daniel did an amazing job with the food. Those baby lamb chops are to die for."

"Thanks," Daniel said.

"Just don't mention the cost to James," Jonathan said. "He still thinks cocktail wienies and Cheez Whiz are perfectly acceptable party food."

"It's the Foley family curse," I told Jonathan. "We're all so tight we squeak when we walk."

While Daniel went into the kitchen to check on the food, I circulated around, chatting with friends and family.

I found Mama and Daddy seated in the living room, Daddy, looking uncomfortable in his good suit, and Mama wearing her traditional Christmas party outfit, which consisted of a green wool skirt and one of those awful seasonal sweaters she adores—this one featured giant knitted Christmas trees adorned with tiny ornaments that actually lit up and blinked. Unfortunately, two of the blinking red lights were located directly in the middle of her chest, so that from across the room it appeared that her nipples were winking.

"Weezie," Mama said, reaching out to pull me down beside her on the sofa. "Don't you look nice tonight!"

I glanced down at my dress and tugged at the neckline. Old habits die hard. "Really? You like this dress?" Mama usually hates my vintage clothes. She can't understand how I could stand to wear what she calls "dead people's cast-offs."

"The pin," Mama said, reaching out and touching the Christmas tree fastened to my stole. "I had a pin like this when you were little. Do you remember?"

I looked down at the pin. "Just like this one?"

She frowned. "Well, no. Mine was sort of gold, with branches, and there were all different colors of pearls on it."

"Pins like this were really popular years ago," I told her. "Daniel says his mother had a pin exactly like this one. It was blue and everything."

"Ohhh," Mama said. She had a long memory for scandal and remembered everything about the Hoyt Gambrell trial. "Does he ever hear from his mother?"

"No," I said briefly, already regretting I'd brought up the subject.

"Where is Daniel?" Daddy asked. "Working at the restaurant, is he?"

"He's here," I said. "Guale's catering the food tonight, you know."

"Nice," Mama said vaguely. "What do you call that mushy rice stuff they're serving with the lamb chops?"

"Risotto?"

"Interesting," Mama said, and then brightening, added, "I brought James one of my famous fruitcakes to serve for dessert. Don't forget to try a slice."

"I won't," I said, secretly vowing to avoid the cake like the plague. My mother had been a closet alcoholic for most of my life, but after she'd gone through rehab, she'd turned her newfound energy to cooking. Unfortunately, sobriety did nothing to improve her culinary skills.

"I've added something new to my fruitcake this year," Mama confided. Lowering her voice and covering her mouth with her hand, lest someone try to steal her secret ingredient, she whispered it.

"Maple syrup!"

"Really?"

Daddy nodded sadly. "She like to run the IGA out of Aunt Jemima's."

"Two dozen cakes," Mama reported. "It's a new record. I've got yours out in the car, if you want to follow us out when we get ready to leave."

"I'll do that," I promised, getting up. "Well, I better check

in with Daniel. He's got to leave early and get back to the restaurant. They've got a couple of big private parties tonight, and he has to put in an appearance."

"Don't forget about the cake, now," Mama chirped. "I've only got a dozen left. They're a big hit this year."

What, I wondered as I drifted through the rooms, alive with light and laughter, could people be doing with maple-syrup-flavored fruitcakes?

Doorstops. Boat anchors. Bookends.

I found Daniel in the dining room, sprinkling chopped parsley on a chafing dish full of shrimp gumbo.

"Looking good," I said, giving him a quick kiss.

"You too," he said absentmindedly.

"Something wrong?" I asked, knowing already that something was.

"There should be a bowl of trifle on the sideboard over there," he said, pointing at my grandmother's massive mahogany server. "It was in the kitchen when I first got here, but it's gone now."

"Everybody loves your trifle," I said. "Maybe people just scarfed it all up."

He shook his head. "No. There were two whole bowls of it in the kitchen. We made enough to serve a hundred. Should have been plenty. And the bowls are gone too."

"Really?" I went over to the sideboard to investigate. Beside a cut crystal bowl of punch I spotted a silver tray layered with slice after slice of fruitcake. Maple scented.

"Case closed," I said, reporting back to Daniel. "Marian Foley strikes again."

"Your mother ate a whole bowl of trifle?"

"I doubt it," I said. "Yours is afloat in sherry. Mama's terrified of falling off the wagon. She won't even take cough syrup anymore. No, I suspect Mama did away with your trifle because it was competing with her fruitcake."

"No!" Daniel said. "So that's where that cake came from? I thought it was a gift from one of James's clients."

"Afraid not. She told me herself that she'd brought one for the party. That fruitcake is her pride and joy."

Daniel went over to the aforementioned tray, bent down and sniffed, and grimaced.

"What the hell?"

"Family secret," I said, crossing my heart. "I've been sworn to silence."

"Dueling desserts," Daniel said. "Only the Foleys."

"I'm sorry," I told him. "Do you want me to see if I can figure out what she did with the trifle?"

"No," he said. "Let James deal with it. Listen, sweetie, I hate to mention it, but I've really got to get over to Guale."

"Already?" I checked my watch. "It's only a little after eight."

"You could stay," he suggested. "Get your parents to take you home."

"Never mind. Let's find James and Jon and say good night."

He headed toward the living room, but I pulled him back. "Not there. I've got to sneak out without Mama seeing me. There's a fruitcake with my name on it out in Daddy's car."

"Ow," he said. "I hope he left the windows rolled down."

Daniel was quiet as we rode home.

"You okay?" I asked, scooting over and rubbing his neck.

"Just tired," he said.

"That's all?"

"It's a busy time of year," Daniel said. "There's a lot more involved in owning a restaurant than there is in just cooking."

"I know. But there's something else going on too, isn't there?"

He sighed. "I hate Christmas."

"Daniel!"

"It's no big deal. In two weeks, it'll all be over. Life can get back to normal."

"This should be a happy time of year. I'm busy too, but I love Christmas. I love everything about it. . . ."

"That's you," he said abruptly. "Not me."

I sighed. "Anything I can do to help? Do you want to talk about it?"

He shot me a look of disbelief.

When we got to the house, he parked the truck and left the motor running. "You can't come in, even for a minute?" I asked.

He shook his head and walked me to my front stoop. He took his keys out and unlocked the door. "I'll call you later," he said, opening the door wide.

Before I could say anything, Jethro came bounding out. He was gone in a flash.

"Jethro!" I screamed. "Jethro, come back!"

"Damned dog," Daniel muttered. He stepped out onto the sidewalk. "Here, boy," he called. "Here, Jethro."

His voice echoed on the deserted street. A skinny yellow cat slinked across the square, and I heard an owl hooting from the limb of a nearby tree. But no goofy barking.

I stood in the middle of Charlton Street and yelled his name.

"Jethro!"

"Now what?" Daniel asked, annoyed.

"Just go on and leave," I snapped. "I'll take care of finding the damned dog."

"Get in the truck," Daniel said. "We'll look together."

"No," I said stubbornly. "He's my dog. I'll take my own truck and look for him. Go on to Guale. You're late already."

"All right," Daniel said. He gave me a quick peck on the cheek. "I'll call you, okay? And don't worry. He can't have gone far."

I locked the front door and got in my truck, pitching my high heels onto the floor, and the shawl, which was hard to drive in, on the front seat. I cruised the streets of the district for more than an hour, stopping every block or so, calling his name.

Every person I saw along the way, I stopped and asked if they'd seen a black-and-white dog. But nobody had. I went back to my house and checked the courtyard garden, in hope that my own Lassie had come home. But the gate was locked, and there was no dog.

I got back in my truck and retraced my earlier route, calling for my lost Jethro, trying to reassure myself that he would be safe. He's a city dog, I told myself. I'd found him when he was just a stray puppy, literally in a heap of trash in

front of a decaying house in the Victorian district. He could take care of himself. And he was wearing his collar and tag. Somebody would find him and call me.

It was close to midnight when I gave up the hunt and went home. Dejected, I got a blanket and pillow and decided to sleep on the sofa—just in case Jethro came back, and I heard him scratching at the door.

The message light was blinking on my answering machine. I pressed the button and prayed. Maybe Jethro had already been found.

But the caller was Daniel.

"Hey," he said, his voice sounding tired. "Don't be mad at me. We'll find Jethro. Everything will be all right. Call me as soon as you get home."

Fat chance, I thought, tears welling up in my eyes. I pounded my pillow, pulled my quilt over my head, and fell into an uneasy sleep.

CHAPTER 6

Three times during the night, I got up, opened the front door, and looked up and down the street, willing Jethro to materialize there, ears pricked up, tail wagging, tongue lolling from the side of his mouth, big brown eyes begging for a treat. Each time, I dragged myself back to the sofa and tried to sleep.

At seven o'clock, I gave up. I trudged into the kitchen and poured myself a Diet Coke, followed by an ibuprofen chaser. I had no appetite, so I picked at a granola bar before discarding it in the trash.

Flyers, I decided, would be a good idea. I could print them up on my computer and post them around the neighborhood. And at nine, when I figured the county animal shelter probably opened, I would call and see if Jethro had been picked up.

I was in the living room, folding the quilt, when I heard

the faint sound of whining coming from outside. I ran to the front door, opened it, and peered out.

The morning paper was on my front stoop. I looked up and down the street again, but saw nothing. Where was that whining coming from?

Dressed only in my flannel pajama bottoms and a camisole top, I stepped out onto the sidewalk. My truck!

A familiar black-and-white face bobbed up and down in the front seat of my truck, whining and pawing at the window.

"Jethro!" I cried, running over to the curb. I opened the door and he leaped into my arms, licking my face, tail wagging a mile a minute. I laughed until I cried. And two tattooed and body-pierced art students, who happened to be walking by, stopped to enjoy the spectacle of my reunion with my dog.

"Excellent," said the androgynous kid with the purple spiked hair.

"Radical," agreed his/her counterpart, who had a skateboard tucked under his arm.

"How in the world?" I asked, when I was able to speak again. "How did you get in that truck?"

Jethro licked my face in answer. I noticed for the first time that a frayed piece of yellow nylon cord was tied to his collar. Tucking my squirming dog under my arm, I looked inside the truck. A large, damp bone rested on the driver's seat, beside my black velvet shawl, which, judging by the amount of dog hair clinging to it, had been used as a bed during his stay there.

I grabbed the shawl and carried both it and the dog inside.

As soon as we were in the house, he jumped out of my arms and ran into the kitchen. I followed him there and watched with relief as he scarfed down an entire bowl of chow. When he was done, I sat down on the floor and gave him a thorough examination. But he was fine. No scratches, cuts, not a mark on him.

He rolled onto his back and allowed me to give him a welcome-home belly scratch.

"You had me worried sick," I scolded. "How did you get in that truck? Who found you and brought you home?"

Instead of an explanation, he went to the back door and scratched, letting me know it was time for a bathroom break. But before I let him out, I went into the garden first, making sure the gate was securely locked.

Satisfied that Jethro was safely fenced in, I ran upstairs and got dressed in blue jeans and a flannel shirt. I was dying to know where Jethro had spent the night, but my investigation would have to be put on hold. I had a full day ahead of me, finishing my redo of Maisie's Daisy window and getting ready for the open house tonight.

I was hanging up the cocktail dress I'd left in a heap on the bedroom floor when it occurred to me that I'd need to take the velvet shawl to the cleaners. I love my dog, but not his scent. I picked it up to see if there were any visible stains, and to remove the blue Christmas tree pin.

There were no stains, but there was also no pin.

I turned the shawl inside out, to see if it had come unattached, but it was definitely not on the shawl.

I went outside to the truck and ran my hands under the

seats. I searched the floorboards. I even looked in the bed of the truck, which was uncharacteristically empty. Still no pin. But I noticed that the driver's-side window had been cranked down about an inch. I knew with a certainty that I'd had the windows rolled up last night and the heater on, because it had gotten downright chilly once the sun went down. Had I locked the truck?

Usually I did keep the truck locked. An unfortunate side effect of living downtown was that crime was a nagging constant. Over the years, I'd had batteries stolen out of my car, potted plants stolen from my porch, and once somebody had even stolen the gas lamps outside my front door. But I'd been in such a state last night, I couldn't say with a certainty whether or not I had locked the truck.

What was unquestionable was that somebody, sometime during the night, had tethered my dog to that makeshift leash, placed him in the truck, given him a bone for solace, and cracked the window so that he wouldn't suffocate. That same guardian angel had also, apparently, decided to reward himself with my Christmas tree pin.

Fine, I thought. I'd have paid a real, and handsome, cash reward to anybody who'd brought Jethro back home. And I'd have gladly thrown the pin in as a bonus.

Before going back to lock up the house, I walked across the street to take another look at the Christmas decorations on Maisie's Daisy.

What the hell? My daisy had been plucked! The topiary trees were virtually denuded of fruit. Apples, oranges, lemons, limes, even the cunning little kumquats I'd paid an indecent

price for, were all gone. The garland around the front door was similarly picked clean. Pieces of popcorn littered the sidewalk, and I felt cranberries squashing under my sneakers. The only fruit left was the pineapple I'd nailed to the plaque above the door, and a couple of random pomegranates.

Without the fruit, the storefront looked naked and pathetic. Had the same thief who'd taken my pin also made off with my fruit? Some crime spree.

"Son of a bitch!" I muttered. Now I'd have to start all over again. With the open house tonight, and the decoration contest judges due at six, there was no time to waste.

Still I wondered if other businesses had also been victimized during the night.

I took a quick hike across Troup Square. Babalu was even more resplendent than it had been yesterday. It was a winter wonderland on steroids. New to the scene was a pair of eight-foot-high snowmen. I had to touch them to make sure they weren't real. Although they glittered like fresh snow, they were actually made of some kind of cotton batting sprayed with iridescent sparkles. The snowmen held aloft shiny black snow shovels crossed over the shop's doorway. Standing outside the shop, I could hear Chrismas music being piped out onto the sidewalk. And yes, as I sniffed hungrily, I realized these men would stop at nothing in their quest for world domination. That was undeniably the scent of fresh-baked gingerbread wafting into the chilly morning air.

The bastards! Manny and Cookie's decorations were breathtakingly intact.

The shop door opened with a merry tinkle, and a small black powder puff with legs emerged. It trotted over to the fire hydrant at the curb, and daintily took a morning pee.

"Good Ruthie!"

Cookie Parker poked his head out the door and looked at me quizzically. "Yes?"

He was wearing a black satin bathrobe, and his chunky white legs ended in a pair of black velvet monogrammed slippers. His dyed blond hair stood up in wisps, and a black satin sleep mask had been pushed up over his forehead.

"I'm Weezie Foley. I own Maisie's Daisy, across the square," I said.

"I'm aware of who you are and what you do," he said coldly. "But what do you want here?"

"Somebody vandalized my decorations last night," I said. "Most of the fruit is gone. And my truck was broken into. I was just checking . . . to see."

"If we'd been hit?" Cookie smiled. "Your concern is touching. But as you can see, nothing here has been touched."

He clapped his hands smartly. "Come, Ruthie." The little dog trotted down the sidewalk a few yards and looked back at Cookie, as if taunting him.

"Naughty girl," Cookie said, shaking his finger at the dog. "Come along now. It's cold out here. You need your sweater if we're going to take a walk. And I need some pants."

"You didn't happen to see anybody suspicious last night, did you?" I asked.

"No more so than usual. Just the usual avant-garde types who wander the streets at night," he said. "Ruthie!" He

clapped his hands again, rapidly. "Come right here, right this minute, miss."

"Odd that my decorations were trashed, and yet yours weren't touched," I commented.

"Maybe it was the birds. Damned pigeons!" Cookie suggested.

"Pigeons that carry off oranges and apples? I doubt it."

The dog trotted farther down the sidewalk, and I did the same.

"Pricks," I muttered to myself. It was way too much of a coincidence that my decorations had been pilfered, while Babalu remained untouched.

But I had no proof that Cookie and Manny were the culprits, and no time to look for any other suspects.

Instead I went home, got Jethro, and went to work at Maisie's Daisy.

First thing, I stripped off the grapevines and what was left of the popcorn strings. I took down the pineapple plaque too. Now that I had a clean slate, I could think again. But it was nearly ten o'clock. Where was I going to come up with natural, vernacular Christmas decorations—prizewinning decorations, this late in the game?"

I sat down in one of the plaid armchairs in the window and closed my eyes. A minute later, I jumped up and loaded the CD player with Christmas albums. I put on all the good stuff: the Phil Spector compilation, Elvis, another compilation I'd gotten at Old Navy, and a couple of CDs from a Rhino Records promotion I'd ordered off the Internet. I hit shuffle and sat down and waited for inspiration.

As luck would have it, the first song was the Ronettes version of "I Saw Mommy Kissing Santa Claus."

For some reason, I thought instantly of Daniel's mom, Paula Gambrell. Had Daniel ever, I wondered, crept downstairs like the kid in the song, and thought he'd seen his mother kissing Santa Claus? Did he have any good memories at all of his parents? I'd probably never know. Family just wasn't something Daniel liked to discuss.

When the next song started, I laughed out loud. Eartha Kitt singing "Santa Baby." In it, the sultry gold digger implores a Sugar Daddy Santa Baby to bring an impressive list of luxury gifts; a fur coat, a '54 convertible—light blue—a duplex, checks, decorations for her tree, bought at Tif-fa-ny—and especially, a ring, meaning bling.

Before I knew it, I was up and vamping around the shop, swishing an imaginary feather boa and humming along with Eartha.

But it wasn't until Elvis came on that I had my brainstorm.

Blue Christmas!

Screw the fruits and nuts. Screw vernacular. Screw tasteful. Screw the judges and the rules! I was gonna have a blue Christmas this year. And I'd by God have fun doing it.

CHAPTER 7

Blue, blue, blue, I chanted as I drove around town in a last-minute shopping spree. And maybe some silver. Yes, definitely silver. I hit Target and in the seasonal aisle loaded up on plain silver and metallic-blue glass tree ornaments. I bought boxes and boxes of silver garland, aluminum tinsel, and ten strands of old-fashioned-looking big bulb lights, all in blue, of course, to supplement the white twinkle lights I already had at home. Thank God the big box stores had discovered retro!

At Hancock Fabrics, my mind was reeling with songs with blue in the title. I heard Bobby Vinton singing "Blue Velvet," Diane Renay singing "Navy Blue," Willie Nelson crooning "Blue Eyes Crying in the Rain," even Elvis doing "Blue Hawaii."

My hands trailed across the racks of fabrics. I'd need a big effect for just a few bucks. Regretfully, I turned away from a

bolt of midnight blue velveteen—at $14.99 a yard, it was way too pricey. Blue satin was out of the question, and blue denim, still too high at $7.99 a yard, was too modern for the look I was going for.

But at the back of the store, in the bridal department, I hit pay dirt. Tulle! At eighty-eight cents a yard the price was right. But the colors—white, green, and red, were all wrong.

Still, I thought, eighty-eight cents a yard! I grabbed four bolts of the white tulle, all they had, and headed for the cash register, grabbing a bottle of blue Rit dye on the way.

At home I loaded the washing machine with what seemed like miles of netting, and spun the regulator dial to the gentle cycle. As the tub filled with water, I carefully added half a cap of blue dye, then a capful, then throwing caution to the wind, I went for two capfuls.

Blue foam filled the tub. I let the wash cycle run for only five minutes before manually switching to the machine's rinse and then spin cycle.

As soon as the machine slowed, I jerked open the lid of the washer. Blue! I had a gorgeous wet glop of bright blue tulle, which I unceremoniously dumped into the dryer, also set for the gentle cycle.

But I had no time to waste sitting by the dryer.

Back at Maisie's Daisy, I stripped the shop's window of everything but the aluminum Christmas trees, trimmed with my hoard of Shiny-Brite ornaments and the tiny white twinkle lights. I draped the big blue bulbs in swags across the front of the window.

Then I lugged the shop's one display bed, a vintage white

iron twin bed, and set it up in the window, draped with a white chenille bedspread with bright blue and green peacocks. I added a pile of pillows stuffed into old pillowcases trimmed in crocheted lace, and stepped back to study the effect. Not bad.

In the stockroom, I rummaged around until I found the big old "portable" record player I'd picked up at an estate sale, along with the funny round black record caddy I'd found at another sale, still full of some long-ago teenager's collection of 45s. I had my own stash of albums, 78s, that I'd collected just for the album covers. I set the record player up on the floor at the foot of the bed and fanned the 45s and the albums around the record player.

I studied my vignette. It was cute, yes. But it wasn't telling me anything. I needed story. I needed drama. I needed teen angst.

Back to the stockroom. I found a pile of old magazines that I had kept because I liked the graphics and the illustrations. There was a sixties issue of *Look* magazine with Jackie Kennedy on the cover. Too modern. Several old copies of *The Saturday Evening Post* with Norman Rockwell illustrations. Too corny. Half a dozen copies of Archie comics. Yes! I'd always identified with Betty, hated Veronica. I passed over some *TV Guide*s and some great *Field & Stream*s from the forties, till I came to the bottom of the stack, where my quest was rewarded with three like-new copies of *Silver Screen* magazine from 1958. The lurid headlines about Marilyn Monroe, Lana Turner, and Tab Hunter would be just the thing for my teen tableau.

As I was gathering up the magazines, I spied a pink

princess telephone. Pink was a prized color for a princess phone, but I frowned. Wrong color for a blue Christmas.

I could spray-paint it blue, but that would ruin the resale value, which was around sixty dollars. I turned the phone over and found the scrap of masking tape with the price I'd paid for it. Fifty cents.

My honor was at stake here. I took the phone out into the alley behind the shop, set it on an old copy of the *Savannah Morning News,* and quickly created an adorable, if now worthless, powder blue princess phone.

It was time to check on my dye job. The blue netting was absolutely heavenly. I gathered it up in my arms and was on my way out the back door when I spotted one of the many silver-framed photos of family and friends I had scattered all over the town house. This particular picture was of me and Daniel at the beach. I scowled at Daniel. He hadn't even called yet to find out if Jethro was all right.

Looking at the picture of my boyfriend took me right back to my own teenage angst. I turned the frame over and slipped the picture out of the frame, leaving it on the kitchen counter. I took the frame into the den, sat down at my computer, and did a Google image search. Five minutes later I was printing out a black-and-white photo of Elvis Presley in his army uniform. I inserted Elvis into the silver picture frame, gathered up the netting, and headed back to the shop.

For the next three hours I worked as fast and as hard as I'd ever worked before. I stapled and styled, draped and swagged and glue-gunned, until I was ready to drop. At four o'clock I forced myself to call it quits. The judges would be

making their rounds at six, and I still had to assemble all the refreshments for the open house, and bathe and dress.

When I got out of the shower, I moaned at how little time I had left. My original plan had been to get myself up in some glam outfit from my collection of vintage clothes. Maybe a red chiffon cocktail dress from the sixties, with a gold lamé cinch belt. But there was no time now for primping and, anyway, glam wouldn't go with my theme.

Instead, I slicked my wild mane of red hair into a perky ponytail and caught it up with a big blue tulle bow. I pegged the hems of my blue jeans, rolling them calf-high, and slipped on a kitten-soft pale blue beaded cashmere sweater from my vintage collection that had been my Meemaw's. But Meemaw had never worn a push-up bra and left the top three pearl buttons undone like I did that night. Briefly I mourned again for the missing blue Christmas tree pin that had started this whole thing.

But I still had the old jewelry box the brooch had come from. I looped three different strands of the faux pearls around my neck and tripled another strand of pearls for a bracelet.

Bobby socks and saddle oxfords would have finished off my outfit, but I'd long ago tossed out the hated black-and-white shoes that had been a required part of our uniform at St. Vincent's Academy, the all-girl Catholic high school I'd attended. Instead, I slipped on a pair of black ballet flats, and as a last-minute thought, grabbed my daddy's old maroon Benedictine Catholic High School letter sweater.

I was heading back downstairs to start gathering up the

trays of food to take over to the shop when I heard a noise coming from the kitchen. I stopped abruptly on the last stair.

Footsteps, light but audible, were coming from the kitchen. I heard the sound of the heavy door of my Sub-Zero refrigerator door open and then close.

For a second, a chill ran down my spine. Somebody was in my house! Then I relaxed. Daniel. My prodigal boyfriend had come over to apologize for his uncaring attitude the night before.

"Daniel?" I called. "Are you on a mercy mission? Did you bring over the dessert trays you promised for the party?"

No answer. Quick footsteps, and then I heard the sound of the back door closing.

"Daniel?" I peeked around the door into the kitchen. It was empty, except for Jethro, who was crouched under the kitchen table, his tail thumping softly on the wooden floor.

I darted over to the back door just in time to see the wrought-iron garden gate swinging shut. I stepped outside to look. The only truck parked in my two-car carport was my own. The lane was empty.

Another chill ran down my spine. I walked quickly back to the kitchen, stepped inside, and locked the door behind me, throwing the latch on the dead bolt for good measure.

My hands were shaking, I realized. Jethro scooched forward on his belly and licked my bare ankle.

"Jethro," I scolded. "Why didn't you bark at the bad man?"

Thump thump went the tail.

I checked the refrigerator. Damn! The silver tray on which I'd carefully arranged five pounds of concentric circles

of bacon-wrapped shrimp now held only a limp leaf of lettuce and a hollowed-out lemon half holding the cocktail sauce.

I ran into the dining room and pulled the drawer of my mahogany sideboard open. My grandmother's wedding silver, all eleven place settings of the Savannah pattern, were intact. My collection of sterling candlesticks on the dining room table was undisturbed.

In the living room, I picked up my purse from where I'd dropped it in the chair by the front door. My wallet was still stuffed with cash and credit cards. My checkbook was untouched.

I went back to the kitchen and picked up the phone and called Daniel's cell phone. I almost never disturb him when he's at the restaurant, especially this time of year, but this, I decided, was an emergency. I needed to be reassured by the sound of his voice.

"Weezie?" he said, answering after the second ring. "What's up?"

"Hi," I said, willing myself to stay calm. "Were you here just now?"

"No. Where? At your place? No. I'm asshole-deep in shrimp bisque here. Why?"

"Funny you should mention shrimp. Because mine are missing," I said, sinking down onto a kitchen chair. "Somebody was here," I said slowly. "In my kitchen. I'd just gotten dressed and I was coming downstairs when I heard somebody in the kitchen. I heard the refrigerator door being opened and closed. I just assumed it was you. But when I called your

name, whoever it was left. I think I spooked him. They slipped out the back gate. With all my bacon-wrapped shrimp."

"Are you all right?"

"Fine," I said. "They left. That's all I care about."

"Was anything else taken? Did you call the cops?"

"No, I called you first," I said. "All my silver is still here. My purse was out in plain view. Nothing in it was touched, and I had the day's cash from the shop in my billfold, around five hundred bucks."

"Jesus!" he said. "How did they get in?"

"I don't know," I admitted, walking to the front of the house as I talked. "The front door still has the security latch on. Nobody got in that way." I walked back to the kitchen. "When I came in from the shop, I came in the back door. I've been running back and forth from the house to the shop all afternoon ―"

"Well, did you lock the door the last time you came in?" he demanded.

"I can't remember," I wailed.

"Weezie!"

"I was in a big hurry," I said, near tears. "The judges are doing the historic district decorating contest at six, and I still needed to shower and dress, and get the food out for the open house―"

For the first time, I looked at the other silver trays of food I'd laid out on the kitchen counter, all neatly covered with plastic wrap. The platter of spinach-and-feta-stuffed mush-rooms had been decimated. Likewise, the sausage cheese

balls had been pillaged, and the mini crab quiches.

"Damn!" I cried. "They got the sausage balls. Not to mention the shrimp. Do you know how much I had to pay for jumbo shrimp?"

"Christ!" Daniel bellowed. "Forget the sausage balls and the judges. This is serious, Weezie. Somebody broke into your house while you were in the shower. You scared them off, otherwise. . . . Look, hang up and call the cops. Right now. I'm coming over there."

"No!" I shouted. "I'm fine. Nothing else was taken. Nobody was hurt. If you want to help me, send over something for me to feed this crowd of people I'm expecting. A cookie tray or something."

"I'm coming," Daniel insisted.

"No way," I said stubbornly. "You need to work. I need to work. Just . . . chill. Please? Okay? Maybe it was BeBe. In fact, I'm sure it was BeBe. She's supposed to come over and help me set up the food and bring her silver punch bowl for the Chatham Artillery Punch. It was BeBe, I'm positive. Which is probably why Jethro didn't bark."

"Jethro didn't bark? Somebody came in your house and he didn't bark?"

"Not a yip," I said, leaning down to scratch Jethro's ears.

"He still barks his head off when I come in the door," Daniel said darkly.

"That's different. You're a man. He thinks he's defending my honor."

"Well . . . lock the door."

"I did. I will."

"Promise me you won't forget again," he said. "There's bad guys running around downtown, Weezie. I had a customer robbed at gunpoint yesterday just after he left the restaurant at midnight."

"I'll be careful," I promised.

"Good," he said, his voice softening. "So, Jethro came home last night?"

"Yeah," I said. "That's another strange story. In fact, a lot of strange stuff has been happening around here the last couple days."

"You can tell me tonight," he said. "I'm staying over. And I'll send one of the busboys over with some appetizers and a cookie tray for your party. Okay?"

"That would be great," I said.

"Good luck with the decorating contest," Daniel said. "Knock 'em dead, kid."

CHAPTER 8

After I hung up the phone I got down on all fours and went eyeball to eyeball with my little furry buddy. "Did you eat up all my expensive appetizers, Jethro? Did you, Ro-Ro?"

Thump thump went the tail. He was the sweetest, most loyal dog God had ever created, but he was also, alas, one of the dumbest. Anyway, he was in the clear, since his breath smelled like Kibbles 'n Bits, not garlic and shrimp.

"Yoo-hoo!" BeBe was banging on the back door. I went over and unlocked it, and she struggled in under the weight of a heavy silver punch bowl, on top of which rested a huge white cardboard box.

"I've brought pecan tassies and chocolate chewies from Gottlieb's Bakery," she said, setting the boxes on the counter. "I figure if you can't win the decorating contest fair and square, we'll just bribe the judges with these little goodies."

"Thanks for the vote of confidence," I told her. "Were you just here a few minutes ago?"

"No," she said, looking puzzled. "I stopped at Gottlieb's first, and I just now drove up around back. Why?"

"Somebody was here," I said grimly. "Right here in this kitchen, while I was upstairs getting showered and dressed. I heard footsteps, and the refrigerator door opening and closing. I called down, thinking it was Daniel, and whoever it was took off out the back door."

"Good Lord," BeBe said, clutching her purse. "Burglars! Did you check your jewelry?"

"I'm wearing the only good jewelry I own," I said, gesturing at the diamond stud earrings that had been a birthday gift from Daniel. "Relax. All they got was the sausage balls." I gestured toward the half-empty party platters. "And the stuffed mushrooms and the bacon-wrapped shrimp."

"Not the shrimp," BeBe moaned. "They're my absolute favorites. I've been thinking of those shrimp all afternoon."

"You'll get over it," I said. I transferred the contents of one half-empty platter to another and rearranged the garnish and the plastic wrap. "Come on. We've got to start getting set up at the shop. The judges will be here in half an hour."

BeBe picked up the punch bowl and the cookie box and followed me out the door, giving a backward glance at Jethro. "You're sure your burglar wasn't the four-footed kind?"

"Positive," I said, locking the door behind us. "Jethro can't open the refrigerator. Or the back door. And I distinctly heard somebody do both."

"Oh," she said, following me over to the shop's back door. "Did you call the cops?"

"To report a case of purloined sausage balls? I somehow think the Savannah police have higher-priority cases than that these days."

"Spooky," BeBe said, stepping aside to let me unlock the door, which, I noted with satisfaction, was securely locked.

"You don't know the half of it," I said, stepping inside. "All kinds of creepy stuff has been happening around here."

But BeBe hadn't stopped to hear my story. She'd put her contribution to the party down on the big pine table at the back of Maisie's Daisy, and gone straight outside. I could see her, standing outside on the sidewalk, staring rapturously in at the window.

I smiled and switched on all the shop lights. The forest of aluminum trees lit up, and the thousands of tiny white lights I'd wrapped the shop's walls and ceilings with, hidden behind the mists of blue tulle, shone like little stars in a darkened sky. On the shelf above the cash register, I punched a button, and the shop's sound system started playing the special Christmas compilation CD I'd burned earlier in the day, after downloading my favorite oldies off the Internet. Brenda Lee's "Rocking Around the Christmas Tree" wafted through the store and out to the sidewalk, courtesy of the mini speakers Daniel had mounted on brackets over the shop's front door.

"It's perfect," BeBe said, when I joined her outside on the sidewalk. "Oh, Weezie, it's like a little movie set."

She glanced over at me and laughed. "Now I get why you're dressed like Rizzo from *Grease*."

"Not Rizzo," I corrected her, adjusting my pearls. "More like Sandra Dee."

"Whatever," she said, turning back to the window. "If those

judges don't give you first place, I'll have 'em impeached. I'll demand a recount."

All modesty aside, the window *was* divine.

I'd set two of the aluminum trees on either side of the front door of the shop, decked out in the cheap blue and silver glass balls and big blue lights. I'd spray-painted the previously rejected grapevines with flat white paint, draped them with more of the blue tulle, and wrapped them with white twinkle lights. And the color wheel I'd hidden at the base of each tree bathed the front of the shop in a deep blue light.

From inside the window, the halo effect of all that gauzy blue tulle artfully bunched in soft drifts gave the whole scene a dreamlike quality.

"It reminds me of one of those little dioramas we used to make in shoe boxes for school book reports," BeBe said. "But this one's called Blue Christmas, right?"

"So you get it?" I asked, delighted.

"How could I not?"

Inside the window, the blue lights on the aluminum trees had an almost eerie effect. On the other side of the window, I'd styled a fantasy fifties teenage girl's bedroom, complete with the silver-framed picture of Elvis on the nightstand. Beside Elvis, I'd placed an old-timey glass Coke bottle with a straw sticking out the top, and beside that was a paper plate with a slice of pizza, all of it illuminated by a kitschy formerly pink poodle lamp I'd mercilessly given the blue paint treatment to.

The blue princess phone was in the middle of the bed, waiting for that call from that special boy. Beside the phone

I'd propped up my own much-loved childhood teddy bear. His little black shoe-button eyes gleamed with some sort of secret amusement. And beside Teddy, I'd placed an open diary with a feather-tipped pen.

"Perfect," BeBe said, nudging me. "You should go in and lie on the bed and pretend to be a mannequin."

"That reminds me," I said, darting back inside the shop. I tiptoed into the vignette and took off the heavy gold Savannah High class ring that had been a gift from a long-forgotten boyfriend, and set the ring on the page of the open diary. Then I lovingly draped my daddy's letter sweater across the foot of the bed.

I heard a pair of hands clapping and, looking up, saw BeBe outside, where she'd been joined by a small knot of bystanders. One by one, they started clapping too, until I realized I was being given a standing ovation.

Modestly, I bowed low, and when I straightened up, I saw Judy McConnell, the president of the downtown business association, pinning a First Place ribbon to the wreath on the door. Appropriately enough, it was blue.

CHAPTER 9

The punch," I cried, suddenly jolted back into my role as shopkeeper and hostess. "We can't have a Christmas open house without the punch!"

I first tasted Chatham Artillery Punch as a fourteen-year-old kid, when I snuck a cup of it at a family wedding and spent the rest of the evening passed out under the piano at the Knights of Columbus hall. My mother, certain that I'd been abducted and sold into white slavery, was on the verge of calling the cops, when my cousin Butch found me curled up underneath the Steinway.

Chatham Artillery Punch isn't something you pour out of a couple of cans of fruit juice and call it a day. No, sir. The recipe I've always used, which is my adaptation of the one in the Savannah Junior League cookbook, the one with the great Ogden Nash limerick in the front, suggests that the hostess start the base of the punch at least two months ahead of time, preferably making it in a forty-gallon drum.

I hadn't started two months ahead of time, nor did I have any empty forty-gallon drums at my disposal.

Instead I'd mixed up my batch the previous week in a brand-new galvanized tin trash can, bought especially for this purpose.

My recipe calls for the following:

2 liters of rum
1 liter of gin
1 liter of bourbon
1 liter of brandy
3 bottles of rosé wine
¼ pound of green tea steeped in two quarts of boiling water
2 ½ cups of light brown sugar, dissolved in the hot tea
2 cups of maraschino cherries
2 large cans of chunked pineapple in their juice
Juice of 9 lemons

The original, classic recipe also calls for a pinch of gunpowder for that final, explosive charge, but I'd decided my version was explosive enough without the gunpowder.

I'd made the base, covered it with the lid, which I'd tightened with a bungee cord, and stashed it out on my patio all week, where the cool weather kept it nicely. After five days, I'd siphoned the punch off into washed and emptied plastic gallon milk jugs.

"Jeez," BeBe said, holding the punch bowl steady while I poured in my brew, "This stuff smells like a whole distillery. What's the alcohol content, do you think?"

"Lethal," I assured her. I went back into the stockroom, to the freezer compartment of the shop's refrigerator, and retrieved the cherry-and-lemon-encrusted ice ring I'd stashed there the day before.

Once the ice ring was floating in the bowl, I added the finishing touch, a bottle of champagne.

I filled two cups with the punch, handed one to BeBe, and kept the other for myself. BeBe clicked her cup against the side of mine. "To the victors go the spoils," she declared.

"Yowza!" she said after her initial sip. "I haven't really drunk any of this stuff since my debutante ball."

"What happened that night?" I asked.

"No idea." She grinned. "I shotgunned a couple snorts of the stuff, and when I woke up the next day, I'd taken a road trip to Jacksonville with the bass player from the rock band Mama'd hired for the party. She made me have the tattoo removed too."

"Take it slow," I advised, blinking at the depth charge from my own sip. "I'm counting on you staying sober back here at the refreshments, while I mind the store."

As soon as I unlocked the front door and announced the open house was officially open, people began to stream inside.

Judy McConnell was the first one in the door. "You know you broke all the contest rules, right?"

"Silly little rules," I said. "And yet you gave me first prize anyway."

"I want that aluminum tree in the window," she said, taking out her checkbook. "How much?"

I shook my head. "Sorry. It's not for sale. All the stuff in the window is from my personal collection."

She cocked her head and gave me a winning smile. "And yet we gave you first prize."

"Ninety bucks," I said quickly. "But you can't pick it up until Saturday. And if you tell anybody about this, I'll have to kill you."

"Deal," she said. "We would have given you first prize anyway. Your window rocks. Way more original than anything else we've seen in years."

I couldn't resist. "What about Babalu? The snow queens didn't grab you this year?"

"Having the children's choir from Turner A.M.E. Church dressed up in white robes singing 'Walkin' in a Winter Wonderland' was too over the top. Even for me," Judy said, wrinkling her nose. "And we lost a judge who slipped on that awful artificial snow they're blowing and wrenched her ankle."

Within a matter of minutes, Maisy's Daisy was full to capacity. The music played, and the punch got drunk, and people seemed to be in a very merry, non-blue mood. I saw lots of our regular customers, like Steve the banker, who stops by the shop every Wednesday afternoon. He's bought every old oscillating fan and Bakelite radio I've ever had. Tacky Jacky, my upholsterer client, came in too, and left with an armload of the vintage barkcloth drapes and cutter quilts she buys to make the designer throw pillows we sell in the shop.

But lots of the other customers were tourists, drawn in by

the irresistible music that spilled out onto the sidewalk, and of course, by our prizewinning decorations.

While BeBe doled out the punch and kept the appetizer platters refilled, I manned the cash register, which jingled merrily with all the purchases people were making. Our customers seemed to be grabbing up and buying everything that wasn't nailed down. And so many people kept trying to dismantle the display window to buy stuff, I finally had to scrawl a big sign on the back of a paper sack that said "Sorry! Window Display Is from Owner's Personal Collection—Not for Sale!"

By ten o'clock, an hour past our posted nine o'clock closing time, I finally had to physically escort Steve the banker out the front door. He had two huge shopping bags full of merchandise in each hand, but he wasn't done yet.

"But, I've really got to have the blue princess phone from the window," Steve was saying. "It's the perfect thing for the beach house at Tybee. It'll be a Christmas present for Polly."

"Not for sale, Steve," I said firmly.

He pressed his face to the glass. "Not even for Polly?"

His wife, Polly, was an old friend from high school days.

"All right." I sighed, giving in. "Thirty bucks. But you can't pick it up until Saturday. And if you tell anybody I sold you anything from that window, I'll have to kill you."

"Deal," he said, grinning ear to ear. "And what about the turntable?"

"Don't push your luck." I pulled down the window shade to end the discussion.

CHAPTER 10

Daniel arrived at the town house just in time to help wash up the last of the empty platters from the party and to play the role of chef and waiter to BeBe and me, serving up steaming bowls of sherry-laced she-crab soup to us in front of the fireplace in the living room while we conducted our usual party postmortem.

"I'm whipped," I announced, pushing my bowl away. "I want to go to bed and sleep for a year."

Daniel shoved me over on the sofa and plopped down beside me. "The bed part I can arrange. The year's worth of sleep I can't guarantee."

"Did you notice the shop's display window?" I asked, putting my feet in his lap.

He took the hint and started massaging my calves.

"It looked great," he said. "Congratulations on winning. It was kinda unusual though, huh?"

"Originality," I said. "It's all about originality. And I have you to thank for the idea."

"How's that?" he asked.

"You and your Christmas funk," I said lightly, deliberately avoiding the cause of his holiday moodiness. "Blue Christmas. It made me think of the Elvis song, and then, I just kinda spun it into this whole story line about a teenage girl missing her boyfriend at Christmas."

"I think I saw a photographer from the newspaper taking pictures tonight," BeBe volunteered. "You're gonna be famous."

"And I promise not to forget the little people I stepped on along the way," I said. Daniel gave my toes a playful squeeze.

"Anyway, it was a great party," BeBe said, mopping up the last of the soup with a chunk of French bread. She wriggled her sock-clad toes on the ottoman in front of her chair. "Daniel, you saved the day with that food you sent over."

"Just so you let everybody know it came from Guale," Daniel said. "I'm all about promotion, now that I own the joint."

"I was handing out the menus to everybody who came near the food table," BeBe promised. "And everybody just inhaled your crab dip and the deviled oysters. I've never seen so much food disappear so fast."

"And merchandise," I said gleefully. "I think I had my biggest day in the history of the shop tonight."

"How big?" BeBe asked.

"Big enough that I can afford to forget about that twenty-five-hundred-dollar table you sold for two fifty yesterday."

She stuck her tongue out at me, and I returned the favor.

"I didn't even get any of the desserts you brought, BeBe," I said. "They were all gone by the time I made my way through the crowd to the food table."

"They were a hit, no doubt about it," BeBe said. "I almost forgot to tell you. I saw one woman filling up her tote bag with the pecan tassies and chocolate chewies."

"One of my customers?" I asked, indignant. "Why didn't you say something about it to me?"

"You were busy. And I didn't want to make a federal case out of it. Anyway, I doubt she was one of your regulars."

"Are you sure she didn't slip anything else in her purse? Something more valuable than some cookies?" Daniel asked. "You know, Weezie scared off a burglar here earlier today."

"I kept my eye on the woman the rest of the night," BeBe said. "She knocked back a lot of that punch though. I don't know how she could even stand up, let alone walk, with as much as she drank. But she seemed fine. She mostly just walked around and around the shop, smiling and taking it all in."

"What did she look like?" I asked.

BeBe scrunched up her face in concentration. "Nothing special or out of the ordinary. Maybe mid-sixties. Short salt-and-pepper hair that was kind of wavy. Her clothes weren't what you'd call stylish. She was wearing like a brown sweater, and baggy, sort of blue wool slacks. And instead of a real pocketbook, she had one of those canvas tote bags, like they give you at bookstores sometimes. Oh yeah, I thought this was cute. She was wearing this little blue Christmas tree pin

on her sweater. I noticed it, because it fit in so well with the theme of your window, Weezie."

Daniel sat up straight on the sofa, and we exchanged startled glances.

" A blue Christmas tree pin?" I asked. "That's too much of a coincidence. It's got to be my pin. Damn! She must be the one who stole it out of my truck."

"What are you talking about?" Daniel demanded. "You never told me somebody broke into your truck. When did this happen?"

"Last night," I said. "After I got back from James and Jonathan 's party and went searching for Jethro."

"You should have called me," Daniel said. "I would have come right back. This is serious, Weezie. Your truck first, and then your house. I want you to call the cops right now and have them come over and fill out a police report."

"I'm not even sure the truck was broken into," I protested. "And I didn't tell you because I haven't had time. But I'm telling you now."

"What happened?" BeBe asked. "I still don't get when all this took place."

I took a deep breath. "It started last night, after Daniel dropped me off here. We'd had a fight—"

"It wasn't really a fight," Daniel interrupted. "You were pissed because I had to go back to work. You don't seem to understand how busy the holidays are at a restaurant."

"Maybe it wasn't a full-fledged fight, but I was definitely still pissed at you," I said evenly. "I do realize how busy you are at work, but I really wish you weren't such a cranky old

bastard around the holidays. You know how much I love Christmas."

"Hey!" BeBe called, holding up her hands in a defensive gesture. "This isn't supposed to be couples counseling here. Just tell me about these weird break-ins."

"I know you love Christmas," Daniel said. "But I can't help it if I don't. And I think you could be a little more understanding about the reasons why I'm not exactly all into the whole damned jolly holly-day deal."

"The break-ins," BeBe repeated. "Just stick to the facts, ma'am."

"Okay," I said, taking a deep breath. "When I got back here last night, Jethro took off out the front door. I drove around downtown, for hours, looking for him, but he'd just disappeared. I was heartsick. I slept on the sofa, so that if he came home, I'd hear him at the door and let him in. But he stayed out all night. He's never done anything like that before."

"Boys will be boys. Maybe he has a lady friend," BeBe suggested.

"Maybe," I said dubiously. "This morning, when I went out to get the paper, I looked up, and there was Jethro, inside my truck!"

"How'd he get in the truck?" BeBe asked.

"Somebody had to have put him there," I said. "There was a little piece of old string tied to his collar, and they'd loosely tied the other end to the steering wheel. And the windows were cranked down a little, so he'd have enough air." I gave Daniel a defiant look. "I know I didn't leave those windows

rolled down. It was cold last night. I even had the heater on."

"I believe you," Daniel said apologetically. "Go on."

"Jethro was fine. There wasn't a scratch on him," I said. "And I didn't realize until later on today that something was missing from my truck."

"The blue Christmas tree pin," BeBe suggested.

"I wore it to the Christmas party," I said. "Pinned to my black velvet shawl. But I left my shawl in the truck overnight," I said. "And it was right there, where I left it, when I found Jethro the next morning. He'd used it as a bed. But the pin was gone."

"What else?" Daniel asked. "Was anything else taken?"

"Not a thing," I said. "Nothing else was touched, as far as I know."

"You've got to be more careful about locking up," Daniel began. "The crime rate downtown—"

"Don't start," I warned. "I usually do lock the truck. And the house. It's like somebody was watching, waiting for the opportunity to break in, the one time my life is especially hectic, and I let down my guard."

"Was the pin especially valuable?" BeBe asked.

"No," I said. "Like I told Daniel, hundreds of thousands of those pins were made by dozens of manufacturers from the forties through the sixties. The pin I bought in the box lot at the auction was nicely made, but it was definitely costume jewelry. I could go on eBay right now and buy another one just like it, probably for under fifty bucks."

"Maybe you just think it's junk jewelry," BeBe said, starting to warm up to her theory. "Maybe the pin was made of

real sapphires. And gold. And the person who stole it knew what it was worth. Maybe they tried to buy it at the auction, and when you got it instead, they decided to follow you home and steal it from you."

"Back away from the Nancy Drew mysteries, BeBe," I suggested. "I bought three boxes of stuff at that auction in Hardeeville, for which I paid a grand total of seven dollars. The only other bidder was a redheaded lady named Estelle, who wasn't willing to pay more than five bucks, which is how I ended up with the winning bid."

"Oh," BeBe said.

"Although," I said slowly. "I think somebody else did follow me over to Hardeeville yesterday."

"Who?" BeBe demanded.

"Manny Alvarez."

"Who?" Daniel asked.

"One of the guys who own Babalu, the shop across the square. He just showed up at the auction, out of nowhere. None of the other Savannah dealers go over there, except me. It's like my secret source. But that day, Manny showed up. He outbid me for this great old Sunbeam bread display rack," I groused. "You should have seen the damn smug expression on his face. I could have throttled him when he hit two hundred dollars."

"Maybe Manny Alvarez broke into your truck," BeBe exclaimed. "Maybe he was just as pissed about you winning as you were at him."

"Impossible," I said, shaking my head. "He wasn't there when I bought the box lots. He left as soon as he paid for the

bread rack. And, anyway, he wouldn't have known the Christmas tree pin was there. It was in a jewelry case in the bottom of the last cardboard box. Trader Bob didn't even know what all was in those boxes. I bought everything pretty much sight unseen."

"Maybe he was skulking around outside, waiting for you to leave," BeBe said, persisting in her conspiracy theory.

"Why would this very successful, independently wealthy antiques dealer break into my truck and take only a silly, kitschy little pin?" I asked. "And for that matter, why would he walk into my kitchen—knowing I'm home, and steal my appetizers? Why?"

"Sabotage," BeBe said darkly. "He wanted to sabotage your open house. He's jealous of all your success. He can't stand it that you out-decorated him. I mean, he's a gay guy. Nobody out-decorates gay guys."

I yawned and stood up. "You're crazy. And I'm tired." I pulled Daniel to his feet.

"Bedtime," I said meaningfully.

CHAPTER 11

Daniel's breathing was as steady and reassuring as the ticking of the Baby Ben alarm clock on my nightstand. So why wasn't I asleep too? God knows, I was tired. And I had fallen fast asleep after a gentle, lazy session of lovemaking. Now I propped myself up on one elbow and examined Daniel's face in the moonlight streaming through the bedroom's lace curtains.

His dark, wavy hair needed cutting again, and although I knew he shaved every night before going on duty at Guale, his five o'clock shadow was already in evidence. His skin, still tanned from a summer and fall of fishing, crabbing, and working on his cottage at Tybee Island, shone dark against the bleached white cotton sheets. A study in black and white. Light and dark. Why, I kept wondering, was his soul so dark at this time of year? And what, if anything, could I do to change him?

I heard a light scratching at the bedroom door and sat up, as Jethro pushed the bedroom door open with his nose.

"You too?" I asked, getting out of bed and following him downstairs. We went through the kitchen, and I unlocked the back door and let him outside, shivering in the blast of cold air that met me.

Jethro barked a short, happy bark, and when I looked out, he was gone. The garden gate was swinging in the wind.

"Damn." I moaned. I'd checked and double-checked that all the doors were locked after BeBe had gone home and before we'd gone to bed. But I'd forgotten to remind BeBe to make sure the gate latched securely behind her when she went to get her car.

I shoved my feet into a pair of beat-up loafers I keep by the back door for gardening, and ran out through the garden to the lane. It was empty.

"Damn," I repeated. Upstairs, I threw on a pair of flannel pajama bottoms and the sweater Daniel had worn earlier in the evening. But he was sleeping so soundly, I didn't have the heart to wake him.

Just as I'd done the night before, I trolled the squares around Charlton Street in my truck, softly calling Jethro's name out the window, searching in the dark for my prodigal puppy.

An hour later, I'd spotted dozens of cats, one terrified-looking 'possum, and half a dozen homeless men and women stretched out on park benches and in the bushes in the squares, but no black-and-white mutt.

I drove home and parked the truck at the curb in front of

the town house, being careful to leave the truck's doors unlocked. Maybe Jethro's guardian angel would find him and bring him home again. Maybe he'd even leave behind my blue Chrismas tree pin. And maybe, I thought ruefully, if pigs had wings they wouldn't bump their butts when they tried to fly.

Sleep came quickly this time around, and when my doorbell started buzzing noisily a few hours later, I had no idea what time it was, or where I was.

Still in Daniel's sweater and the plaid pajama bottoms, I stumbled downstairs and opened the door.

"Jethro!" I exclaimed.

He was sitting on his haunches, looking up expectantly, almost like he was peddling hairbrushes door-to-door and had finally reached a cooperative housewife.

"Eloise!" Standing slightly to the right of Jethro, looking extremely peeved, was my neighbor and sworn enemy, Cookie Parker.

I glanced at my watch. It was barely eight o'clock, but Cookie was dressed in immaculate black wool slacks and an enormous Burberry plaid sweater. A matching plaid tam-o'-shanter was perched on his pumpkin-size pate.

"You found Jethro," I said, grabbing both his hands and shaking them. "Thank you so much for bringing him home."

"I found him, all right," Cookie said coolly. "He was assaulting my Ruthie!"

I rubbed the sleep out of my eyes and yawned.

"Assaulting?"

Cookie blushed. "You know what I mean."

"No," I assured him. "I don't. You mean they were fight-

ing?" I knelt down and took a closer look to assess Jethro's wounds. But I didn't see any.

"He was humping her, all right?" Cookie blurted. "Is that crude enough for you?"

"Jethro?"

Noncommittal, he licked his privates. Jethro, that is. Cookie just stood there, quivering with rage and indignation.

I stood up and yawned again. "Well, what do you want me to do about it? I mean, I'm sorry, okay? I got up around one this morning, to let him outside, and I guess my friend forgot to latch the garden gate. We had a pretty busy, late night last night."

Cookie pursed his lips. "We were well aware of your enchanted evening. I suppose congratulations are in order." He thrust out his hand and shook mine limply.

"Thank you," I said.

"It was an amusing display, I'll give you that," Cookie allowed. "Manny and I were just saying last night that the judges must have decided to go with camp this year, rather than beauty or artistic vision."

I supposed this was his version of a compliment. I decided to accept it, but then I had the impulse to giggle, which I managed to stifle.

"I thought Babalu looked beautiful, from what I saw of it," I said.

He shrugged. "It wasn't that big a deal to me. But Manny! The poor dear was devastated. He really puts his whole heart into these little competitions. He's been planning this winter wonderland tableau since July."

It was cold. Really cold. I looked down. My toes were turning blue. I edged them up under Jethro's butt, grateful for the borrowed warmth.

"Well," I said, anxious to go inside and back to bed. "Better luck next time. And I really am sorry about Jethro's, um, lapse in judgment. I don't know what's gotten into him lately. This is the second time in a week he's run away like this."

Cookie bit his lip. "I just hope Ruthie's not . . . well . . . you know."

"Not what?"

"Enceinte," he said, blushing violently. "This is only the second time she's come into . . ." He blushed again and stared at something above my head. "You know."

I blinked. "Oh. Wait. You mean your bitch is in heat? Oh, no."

"Yes," he said quietly. "Exactly."

I prodded Jethro with my bare foot. "Bad boy!"

He thumped his tail in perfect agreement.

"Wait," I said slowly. "If your dog was in heat, what was she doing out?"

"She never goes outside without one of us. Ruthie has two *very* protective papas. But last night, after the judges left and we found out *you'd* won the decorating contest, well, Manny was so distraught, I had to do something to take his mind off our rather crushing disappointment. We were supposed to have our open house last night too. But we just couldn't put on our happy party faces. I called the caterer and told her to come and take all the food to the children's home. Then I took Manny over to the Pink House for a quiet, intimate fire-

side dinner. Long story short, our garden gate got left unlatched too last night. Although I don't quite understand how or when. Manny got up sometime in the night to let Ruthie out, and then just stumbled back to bed without checking on her again."

His lips pursed. "Let me tell you, Mister Macho won't be making a mistake like that again anytime soon. Ruthie could have been dognapped."

Cookie sighed. "Latin men! You love them because of their fiery, passionate lust for life. But you forget, or at least I do, that the downside to all that passion is a darker, deeper despair than most Anglo men feel."

All this, I thought, over a decorating contest.

"As a result," Cookie continued, "Manny, I'm afraid, got absolutely *trashed* on mojitos."

My lips were twitching again. To cover, I yawned.

"And then he acted out," Cookie said, lowering his voice.

"How?"

"He stripped down to his Tommies and went skinny-dipping in that fountain in the middle of Lafayette Square!" Cookie said. "Can you imagine—if the bishop had looked out his window and seen something like that?"

Living as he did in the historic district, I felt fairly sure that the bishop at Cathedral of St. John the Baptist, which fronted Lafayette Square, had probably seen worse. But I kept that to myself.

"No," I said sympathetically.

"It was not an attractive display," Cookie said. "When I finally hauled him out of there, he insisted on coming over

here. To your place. I think he was somehow planning to vandalize your window. As revenge."

Alarmed, I stepped out of the house to see what, if anything had happened to my shop.

"Not to worry," Cookie said. "I managed to drag him away before he did any harm."

"I'm glad of that," I said.

"Although," he went on, "I'm afraid Manny did manage to wake up your employee. She looked pretty startled, and who can blame her? A dripping-wet, half-naked gorgeous Cuban man brandishing a can of spray paint at two in the morning."

"Employee?" I was drawing a blank.

"Or maybe one of your customers or party guests got overserved and decided it was safer to stay right where she was."

"Cookie," I said finally. "What are you talking about?"

"I'm talking about the woman who was sleeping in that bed in your shop window last night," he said. "Tucked in tight, teddy bear and all."

CHAPTER 12

I pulled the collar of Daniel's sweater tighter around my neck, to ward off the sudden chill.

"Is—" I gulped. "Is she still there?"

"I don't know," Cookie snapped. "I cut through the square to get to your place, so he"—he glared down at Jethro—"could stop and do his business there, instead of on my doorstep."

He thrust a plastic Kroger bag at me. "This is for you."

It was still warm. I held it at arm's length. "Thanks. And, again, I'm sorry about Jethro's bad behavior."

"Sorry just doesn't cut it," Cookie said, his nostrils flaring in anger. "You should have had that dog fixed. There are enough mutts running around loose downtown—"

"Look," I said angrily, shoving Jethro inside my door, "we'll have to continue this discussion some other time. If there's somebody sleeping in my window, I need to get over to the shop and see about it."

"I should hope so," Cookie said, and he turned and flounced off, his tam-o'-shanter bouncing with every step.

After depositing Jethro's poop in the kitchen trash can, I took the stairs two at a time, calling out as I went.

"Daniel! Wake up! One of the neighbors says he saw somebody sleeping in the bed at Maisie's Daisy."

No answer. Daniel is such a sound sleeper, he could—and has—slept through a hurricane.

"Daniel!" I yanked the blanket and sheet off the bed, and shook his bare shoulder repeatedly. "Wake up!"

"What?" He rolled onto his stomach and buried his head under the pillows.

"You've got to come over to the shop with me," I said, stepping out of the pajama bottoms and pulling on a pair of jeans. "That was Cookie Parker at the door just now. He says he saw a woman sleeping in the display window in the shop earlier this morning."

"Why?" Daniel swung his legs over the side of the bed. I tossed his jeans at him.

"Come on. Hurry up and get dressed. I'm not going over there by myself."

"Crazy," Daniel muttered, but a minute later he was right behind me on the stairs. When we got to the front door, he reached out and grabbed my hand.

"You better stay here," he said quietly. "If this is the same person who broke into your truck, and then the house, there's no telling how crazy she is. Just stay here. Call the cops."

"What? No cops. I'm coming with you," I insisted.

He put both hands on my shoulders. "Please? Just this once, listen to me?"

I shook my head. "It's probably just a harmless little old lady. The same one BeBe saw snitching cookies last night. We can't call the cops on her. They'll lock her up in jail. I don't want that on my conscience. Not at Christmas."

"Christmas again!" But he stood aside to let me out the door.

"Not all these homeless people downtown are the quaint little hoboes you seem to visualize," he said. "There're a couple of guys who were coming around the back door at the restaurant at closing time, mooching food. The busboys felt sorry for them, were giving them some of the leftovers we donate to the food bank. But a couple of nights ago, one of them started demanding money. He actually threatened Kevin with a knife."

"Lock the door," I said over my shoulder, already down the front steps of the town house. "I know you're worried about my safety, and I appreciate it. But this isn't some knife-wielding psycho. Cookie said it was a woman. And she was asleep—clutching my teddy bear."

"Probably had a revolver under the pillow," he said darkly when he caught up with me on the sidewalk outside the shop.

"She's gone." I was surprised at how let down I felt, staring in at the display window.

"Thank God," he said.

We both stood there, staring at my vision of a Blue Christmas.

"It's just like I left it," I said. And it was, mostly. The chenille spread was smooth, the pillows were arranged just as I'd placed them the night before. The feather pen was still poised atop the open diary. The class ring was still there. The blue princess phone, the poodle lamp, even the records were fanned out in the same order around the phonograph. Elvis's upper lip still curled up at me from the silver-framed picture.

"We'd better go inside and see what's missing," Daniel said. "And I don't care if they do have to lock somebody up, if anything's been stolen, we are calling the cops."

"Okay," I said meekly, knowing that a call wouldn't be necessary.

Daniel followed me inside, walking every inch of the shop, peering inside cupboards, checking the bathroom, he even got down on his hands and knees and looked under the bed, until he was satisfied that it was empty.

"This Cookie guy, was he sure he saw somebody in *your* shop?" he asked, yawning. "I mean, is there any chance he was mistaken?"

"Well, he admitted he and Manny had been drinking," I said. "Actually, he said Manny was so upset at losing the decorating contest that he got shit-faced last night over cocktails at the Pink House."

"The Pink House!" Daniel's eyes narrowed.

I knew immediately it had been a mistake to mention Guale's closest restaurant competition downtown.

"Anyway," I added hastily, "Manny got so trashed he stripped down to his skivvies and went for a dip in the Lafayette Square fountain. And then he came over here,

apparently to spray-paint graffiti on my windows. Fortunately, Cookie got him calmed down and put a stop to it. But that's when they both saw the woman asleep in my display bed."

Daniel yawned again.

"She's gone now, that's for sure. *If* she ever really was here. I know the bartender at the Pink House. She makes drinks strong enough to stop a bull moose in his tracks. I think she thinks it helps her tips."

I nodded thoughtfully, following Daniel out the front door and stopping to lock up. But he was already in front of the town house, standing on my front stoop.

"I'll make us breakfast," he offered. "French toast. You've got eggs and milk, right?"

"Yeah," I called back, looking in at the shop window again. My gaze lingered on the iron bed's footboard, where my father's high school letter sweater had hung the night before. The sweater was gone, and in its place was a threadbare brown sweater with a glittery blue Christmas tree brooch pinned to the collar.

CHAPTER 13

Three days before Christmas, and I still hadn't finished my shopping. Still, when BeBe offered to feed me dinner if I'd come over and help her wrap her gifts, along with my own, it was an offer I couldn't refuse.

BeBe is strictly a wrapping paper-and-ribbon girl, while I have always been one of those demented souls who insist on making every gift a perfect little work of art. Which meant that by ten o'clock that night, we'd drunk two bottles of wine, finished dinner and dessert, and wrapped all her gifts, while I was still slaving away over mine.

I was hot-gluing a string of fake pearls to a glossy black box to which I'd already affixed a vintage scrap of lace collar when BeBe came back into the study of her town house with another glass of wine.

"That looks amazing," she said. "Who's it for?"

As an answer, I opened the box and held up the contents.

BeBe winced. "The dreaded seasonal sweater. For your mother, right?"

"I know," I said. "But she just loves these things. And Valentine's Day is the only holiday she doesn't already have a sweater for. So . . ."

She scratched a fingernail against the appliquéd calico hearts on the pocket of the hot pink cardigan, then pointed at the white satin cupid shooting an embroidered arrow across the sweater's chest.

"Eloise," BeBe said sternly, "this is the most atrocious garment I have ever seen. Where in God's name did you buy the thing?"

"The Internet, natch."

"What's the site called, TackyTogs dot com?"

"Worse," I said, laughing. "The Kitten's Whiskers."

She put the top back on the box and pushed it away in distaste.

"I know you bought your dad another power tool, and I saw those beautiful leather books you wrapped up for James and Jonathan, but what did you buy for Daniel?"

I put the glue gun down and flopped onto my back on BeBe's Oriental carpet.

"Nothing," I wailed. "You know he's always hated Christmas. And it's worse than ever this year. He says he doesn't need anything, and he doesn't want me to buy him anything at all. It's so Grinch-y. But he's absolutely adamant about it."

"Ridiculous," BeBe said. "It's just a typical male ploy to get out of buying *you* a good present. Like an engagement ring," she said meaningfully.

"No," I said quickly. "I really believe he means what he says. You know he buys me wonderful birthday gifts, and even silly little no-special-occasion gifts. So I know it's not that. Besides, I don't want a ring. Not for Christmas, anyway."

"It's that whole weird family thing of his, isn't it?" BeBe asked.

She was intimately acquainted with Daniel's family saga, since it was she who'd uncovered the whole sad story back when Daniel was still working for her at Guale.

"Yeah," I said glumly. "His father left at Christmas. His brothers still live here in town, but Eric and Derek are busy with their own lives, and for Daniel, the restaurant just seems to eat up all his free time."

"Don't I know it," BeBe said. "That's one reason I finally decided to let Guale go. I wanted a chance at having a real life with Harry."

BeBe had inherited Harry Sorrentino, along with a broken-down mom-and-pop motel out on Tybee Island, less than a year ago, through an unfortunate encounter with a gorgeous con man who ultimately fleeced her. But, in typical BeBe fashion, she'd managed to track the guy down, get her money back, and keep and refurbish the inn into a money-making proposition.

Unquestionably, Harry, the only charter boat captain I know who reads Wodehouse and John D. MacDonald, was the best part of that particular acquisition.

"Speaking of which," I said. "What are you giving Harry? I know we wrapped a bunch of boxes."

She giggled and blushed. "Harry is the world's easiest lay.

He likes everything. So I went a little nuts, even though it is our first Christmas together. Let's see. Of course, there's that Hawaiian shirt you bought him at that yard sale down in Florida."

"For two bucks," I reminded her.

"Right. Harry loves a bargain as much as you, so I left the price tag on it. Oh yeah. I got him a fancy Shimano reel, and a new pair of Top-Siders to wear when he's out on the *Jitterbug*, and this one's my favorite: I commissioned a portrait of Jeeves."

"BeBe!" I exclaimed. "That's a great idea."

Jeeves, Harry's Yorkshire terrier, was like Harry's child, and although BeBe always professed to hate dogs, I knew she secretly adored the little guy.

"But where is it? I didn't wrap any paintings."

"The artist just finished it today. The paint's not even dry. I've got it hanging on a nail up in the attic."

"And what's Harry getting you? A ring?"

"No way!" she exclaimed. "He's been talking about it. And Lord knows, my grandparents are after me to let him make an honest woman of me, but after three trips to the altar, I still can't get used to the idea that marriage could be a good thing."

"It can be," I assured her. "And Harry's the one. The only. You can't judge marriage by what you had before. Those marriages don't even count."

"Bless you," BeBe said dryly. "Harry says the same thing. Only you have to consider the source."

I helped myself to a sip of BeBe's wine. "I'm just stumped when it comes to Daniel and Christmas," I said. "He doesn't

need any new clothes. And usually he buys anything he needs before I even know it's something he'd like."

"Hmmm." She took the wineglass from me and sipped.

"Books?"

"He never has time to read anything except cookbooks, and he buys those himself."

"Music?"

"I did get him the new Eric Clapton CD. But that's the only thing I've bought for him."

"Cooking stuff?"

I shook my head. "He has enough gadgets to open a store of his own."

"Okay. I give up. You're right. He's impossible."

"It'll come to me," I said, though not really convinced. "But in the meantime, I'm having the best time playing Secret Santa."

"For who?" BeBe asked, getting up to turn down the flame on the gas logs in the fireplace.

"Apple Annie," I said, reaching into the shopping bag I'd brought along and dumping out its contents.

"That's not her real name," I explained. "I don't know her real name, so that's what I've been calling her."

"And how did you meet Miss Apple Annie?"

"I haven't. Not officially. But you have."

"Me?"

"At the open house at Maisie's Daisy," I said. "Remember the bag lady who was snitching cookies? Did I tell you, I think she came back and slept in the shop's display bed that night?"

"You never said a word!" BeBe said. "Is this the same woman who stole your blue Christmas tree pin? Are you insane?"

"I'm not insane," I said calmly. I reached into my pocket-book and held out my hand for her to inspect the contents.

"The pin! Where'd you get it?"

"She gave it back," I said. "Actually, I guess it was a swap. She took my daddy's BC letter sweater that night and in its place left her own sweater. With the Christmas tree brooch pinned to it."

"What's this about your playing Secret Santa to her?" BeBe said suspiciously.

"It's just little things," I said. "Nothing expensive. After that first morning, when I found the pin, I wanted to thank her for giving it back."

"Thank her for giving back what she'd stolen from you!" BeBe said. "Weezie, this woman broke into your house and stole food. Then she broke into the shop. Wait, how did she break in?"

"I don't know. It's the weirdest thing. The doors hadn't been jimmied. The locks hadn't been tampered with. And whenever she's come and gone, Jethro hasn't made a sound. That's why I'm pretty sure she's the same one who brought him back that night and locked him up in the truck. He trusts Annie."

"Annie!" BeBe hooted. "Has it occurred to you that this woman slept in your shop? Don't you think it's just possible that she's a crazy, lunatic stalker? She could let herself into your house at any time and slash you to ribbons, and Jethro

would probably lick her foot and show her where the silver's hidden."

"Gee, BeBe," I said, my voice dripping sarcasm. "That thought hadn't occurred to me before, but I sure will sleep well now, thinking about that possibility."

"Weezie!" BeBe said, giving my shoulders a shake. "I'm serious. You shouldn't encourage this woman. You should call the cops and tell them what's going on."

"You sound just like Daniel," I said, calmly spreading out the contents of my shopping bag. "He's convinced she's some knife-wielding loony tune. He's such a cynic. Promise me you won't tell him about the Secret Santa thing."

"You are such an idiot," BeBe said.

"Promise," I begged.

"All right," she said grudgingly. "But don't come crying to me if you get murdered in your sleep."

She pointed at my heap of goodies. "What's all that?"

"Just some little treats for Annie," I said. "Hotel soaps and shampoos I've picked up on buying trips. A toothbrush and toothpaste. A pair of warm woolen socks. A candy bar. We know she has a sweet tooth! After I wrap them up, I put them in ziplock bags. So they won't get ruined in the rain."

"Of course," BeBe said in a mocking voice. "And where does Annie's Secret Santa leave her goodie bags?"

"You're making fun of me," I said.

"Absolutely," she agreed. "Best friend's prerogative. Where do you leave the stuff?"

"In the truck," I said. "Late at night. And it's always gone the next morning."

"Oh, there's a surprise," BeBe said. "You live in the historic district, which is headquarters for every homeless man in Savannah, and amazingly enough, when you leave stuff in your unlocked truck, it's gone the next day."

"I always put the presents in the glove box," I said. "Nobody but Annie would know to look there."

"Except for the army of homeless people who camp out in Colonial Cemetery, which is what? A block from your place? Anybody could be watching while you do your little Secret Santa thing."

"But they're not," I said stubbornly. "Annie is the only one who knows. Anyway, who else would leave presents for *me*?"

For once, BeBe was speechless. But only for a moment.

"A homeless woman leaves you gifts?"

"Wonderful gifts," I said. "Yesterday she left me a huge hotel key. From the old DeSoto Hotel."

"They tore that place down more than thirty-five years ago," BeBe said.

"I know. And she must know how I love anything from old Savannah," I said smugly.

"She probably stole it years ago," BeBe said flatly. "She was probably a hotel thief before she became a homeless thief. What else has she given you?"

"One morning, there was a huge pinecone. From a ponderosa pine, I think. It was the biggest pinecone I'd ever seen. Another time, it was the tiniest, most perfect little baby conch shell. No bigger than my thumbnail. But today's present was the best of all."

"I can't wait to hear," BeBe said in a perfect deadpan.

Ignoring her sarcasm, I reached back into my purse and brought out Apple Annie's gift.

"A bottle," BeBe said. "That's appropriate. For an old alkie."

"Not just any bottle," I said, turning the deep blue container over to show her the marking on the bottom. "This is a John Ryan soda bottle." With my fingertip I stroked the bottle, its finish worn to velvet.

"And?"

"Look at the date here," I instructed.

She scrunched up her eyes and examined the bottle's bottom.

"Eighteen sixty-seven. Is this thing really that old?"

"Yeah," I said softly. "You know I don't deal in old bottles. That's really more of a guy thing. But there are lots of bottle diggers and dealers around town. I know just enough about old bottles to know that I don't know enough. So I mostly leave them to the boys. Still . . ."

"This bottle is worth more than a million bucks," BeBe said. "And a homeless woman gave it to you. Just like that."

I gave her an annoyed look.

"I knew that John Ryan bottles were highly collectible," I said finally. "This one was filled with soda right here in Savannah. And yes, in 1867. So I did some research. It's *not* worth a million bucks. But the cobalt color is really desirable. This one, unfortunately, is missing the wire bail that would originally have been around the neck, to cap it. And there are some chips around the lip, and a hairline crack. I found a similar bottle on the Internet, that one was perfect. And it sold for ten thousand dollars."

"For an old soda bottle."

"I don't make the prices," I said. "I'm just telling you what the market is. Anyway, this bottle is nowhere near perfect. Not for a collector. But for me, I wouldn't take any money for it."

She sighed, picked up her wineglass, and drained it.

"You don't get it, I know," I said. "But Annie knows me. She knows I love anything that was made here in Savannah. Where *I* was made. And she knows blue is my favorite color. I think she must have found this somewhere. Maybe dug it up herself, somewhere around town, although that is totally illegal. But I don't care. It's the perfect Christmas gift."

"And it came from a wino," BeBe said.

"That's it!" I said, jumping up. I reached down, grabbed her hand, yanked her to a standing position, and gave her a huge hug.

"What?"

"Wine!" I said. "That's what I'll give Daniel. I got a flyer in the mail today. From Trader Bob. He never sends out flyers. But when he was up in the North Carolina mountains, he bought out this old guy's wine cellar. And he's selling all the wine bottles. Tomorrow morning! You know what a wine snob Daniel is. I'll run over there first thing tomorrow and buy him the best bottle of wine I can find."

"You don't know diddly about wine," BeBe said.

"No," I said, hugging her again. "But you do."

CHAPTER 14

I picked BeBe up at her place at eight the next morning. It had rained a little the night before, but this morning was sunny and colder than it had been earlier in the week. It really was beginning to feel like Christmas.

She walked unsteadily to the truck, and wobbled a little as she slid into the front seat, clutching a huge mug of coffee in one hand and a rolled-up magazine in the other.

"Not feeling well?" I asked, pulling away from the curb.

She shot me the look. "Do you know how much wine we put away last night?"

"A lot?"

"Three bottles. And I think I took care of more than my share."

"Sorry," I said.

"Not as sorry as me." She shuddered. "I don't think I can stand to look at another bottle of wine again. Ever."

"Well, you're going to," I said brightly. "Leuveda, she's Trader Bob's sister? There was a message from her on my answering machine when I got home last night. She says there are, like, two thousand bottles being auctioned off this morning."

BeBe closed her eyes and leaned her head back. "You are the only person in the world who could get me to go to a wine auction the way I'm feeling today."

I glanced over at the rolled-up magazine in her lap.

"Uh, BeBe? I don't think you're gonna have time to catch up on your reading at the auction. Trader Bob really moves these things along. And since I don't know a thing about wine—"

"Relax," she said, unrolling the magazine without opening her eyes. "This is *Wine Spectator*. Their annual price guide. It's research, sweetie."

"Oh. Good." I took a sip of my own coffee. "So I've given it some thought, and here's what I've come up with. If the prices are decent, I'd like to buy two really good bottles of wine. A bottle of red—you know how much Daniel likes red wine—and a bottle of really good champagne."

"Champagne!" She moaned. "Oh, God. The only thing worse than a wine hangover is a champagne hangover."

"Forget hangover. Concentrate on helping me find Daniel a great Christmas present."

She opened one eye. "Red. Is that the best you can do? I mean, can you be a little more specific? Does he like bordeaux, burgundy, what?"

"Just red," I said. "You know me. I'll drink any old thing.

Daniel, on the other hand, likes the good stuff. So we're looking for something spectacular. Also the one thing I do know is the vintage."

"Yes?"

"Nineteen seventy," I said. "It's got to be a bottle from 1970."

"Impossible," she said flatly.

"Why?"

"There is no spectacular red wine from 1970," she said. "Pick another year, please."

"But I can't. That's the year he was born. It's the year I was born. It's got to be a 1970 vintage. Surely not everything from that year is awful?"

She yawned. "Well, it's certainly not 1961—the birth year of the most fabulously drinkable Château Latour—and the amazing Harry Sorrentino."

"What? Everything made that year sucks?"

She opened her eyes. "I didn't say they all suck. What I mean is, it wasn't a truly spectacular year, for the most part. Don't get your panties in a wad. I'm sure we'll find something drinkable at your little auction."

"Don't forget the champagne. I want a really nice bottle of champagne."

"Cristal's nice."

I made a face. "Isn't that what all the rappers and rock stars drink? I want something Daniel couldn't just pick up at Johnny Ganem's liquor store. Something for when we have something to celebrate."

"Hmm." Her eyes were closed again. "We'll see."

"I'm running out of time here," I reminded her. "Christmas is the day after tomorrow. And the whole family's coming over tomorrow night, and then I'm going to midnight mass."

Her eyes popped open again.

"Mass? Family?"

"I know," I said. "The mass thing is a Christmas gift for Mama. She's been saying novenas that I'll find my way back to the fold. So everybody, Jonathan and James and Miss Sudie, Mama and Daddy, is coming over to my house for supper on Christmas Eve. That's my gift to Daddy."

"Because?"

"That way he doesn't have to eat Mama's cooking for twenty-four hours. I've promised him a ham, and turkey, and oyster dressing and all the fixings. He'll have leftovers for days. And no heartburn, hopefully."

"Very Christian," BeBe said approvingly.

"And I want you and Harry to come over too," I said.

"Hmm."

"Please?" I tugged on the sleeve of her sweater. "At least for supper. That way, it won't be Daniel all alone with my bizarre family."

"Not everybody in your family is bizarre," she pointed out. "James is quite normal. And your daddy is a lovely man."

"But not a brilliant conversationalist. All Daddy ever talks to Daniel about is his old mailman war stories. And cars. You know Daniel doesn't give a rat's ass about cars. If you come, Daniel will have somebody else to talk to besides Daddy. And Mama—who keeps pumping him about when we're going to get married."

"Maybe," BeBe said. "I'll mention it to Harry. See what he thinks. I know we're definitely spending Christmas morning at my place. My grandparents are coming over, and I think one or more of my brothers may show up. And we're going out to the Breeze in the afternoon for an oyster roast, if the weather stays nice."

"Great," I said, beaming at her. "You'll even get a chance to meet Daniel's family."

"Daniel's family?" She raised an eyebrow.

"Derek and Eric and their wives and kids," I said. "It'll be the first time anybody in my family has met anybody from Daniel's."

"Does Daniel know about this?"

"It's a surprise," I said. "I've been planning it for weeks."

"All right," she said finally. "We'll come. I can't wait to see Daniel's family up close and personal after all these years."

"I'm getting a little nervous about it," I admitted. "It'll be a big help if you come."

"Great," she said, paging through her *Wine Spectator*. "I'll spend Christmas Eve refereeing the Foley Family Feud."

She spent the rest of the ride over to Hardeeville reading and dog-earing her magazine, and I spent the rest of the ride listening to Christmas carols on the oldies station I keep the truck radio tuned to.

"Ho-Lee Ca-rap," I said slowly as we pulled up to the parking lot at Trader Bob's.

A huge tractor-trailer rig was parked in the middle of the old cornfield, and at least fifty people were milling around the field. A makeshift wooden gangplank led from the field

into the interior of the truck, and people were walking in and out of the trailer.

We parked, and I made my way through the crowd to a card table set up outside the door of the auction house. Leuveda Garner sat behind the table, wearing a fur Santa Claus hat and a moth-eaten mink stole. A stainless-steel coffee urn sat on the table beside her, along with a mountain of foam coffee cups. Folding chairs were stacked on the ground beside the table.

"Hey, Weezie!" she called out. "You got my message."

"I did," I agreed, looking around at the crowd. "Looks like a lot of other people did too. What's with the big rig?"

"That's the wine we're auctioning off," Leuveda said. "That whole truck is loaded to the rafters. There was so much of it, we didn't have time to unload everything. So Bob's just gonna set up and do his thing right there in front of the truck."

She handed both of us a thick sheaf of typed paper.

"This is the catalog," she said. "Don't pay any attention to my spelling. All those French words really had me flummoxed. You can walk up that ramp to the truck. We've got lights rigged in there, and you can take a look at the wine. Bob's got a helper in there, he can move the crates, if there's something in particular you want to see. "

BeBe was leafing through the catalog, running a finger down the listings. "Wow," she said admiringly. "There's some decent stuff here." She looked up at Leuveda. "Is any of it drinkable?"

Leuveda shrugged. "Don't know. Don't care. What you

see is what you get. We've never done a wine auction before. Bob only agreed to do this one as a favor to the family."

"Two thousand bottles of wine," I said, glancing down at my list. "And it all belonged to one guy?"

"Oh, this isn't even half of what he had in his basement and stashed around the house," Leuveda said. "We brought this much because it's all that would fit in the biggest truck we could rent. If this goes well, Bob may bring the other stuff down and auction it off after the holidays."

"Who has this much wine lying around his house?" BeBe asked, suspicious as always.

"A nut," Leuveda said promptly. "Wine nut, his family calls him. Of course, they had no idea he'd been collecting this much wine. He was kind of a shut-in. It wasn't until he got sick and had to be moved to a nursing home against his will that they discovered his whole house had been turned into a walk-in wine cellar. You should have seen the place, Weezie. He had the windows all covered with black cloth, and the thermostat set real low. Most of the furniture was gone. He had a bed and a recliner, and everything else was just cases and cases of wine."

"Sad," I said. But I had been to hundreds of estate sales over the years, and I had seen how a collecting mania could take over a person's life. Especially a person who was estranged from any kind of outside life or interests.

"Yeah," Leuveda agreed. "Funny thing is, the poor guy didn't even drink. He came from a family of real foot-washing fundamentalists. The wine was his idea of an investment plan. Of course, now he's dead, and the foot-washing funda-

mentalists are mortified about having to get rid of all that sinful wine."

BeBe laughed. "I'll bet they'll be willing to spend the money y'all make selling the wine though."

"Of course," Leuveda agreed. "Money talks, bullshit walks."

From the other side of the field, we heard a buzz of static electricity, then the voice of Trader Bob Gross booming through the mists still rising from the field.

"All right, folks," he called. "What was it those Gallo brothers said? We will sell no wine before its time? Well, it's high time, folks. So let's sell some wine."

"I'll get our chairs and set them up front as close as I can get," I told BeBe. "Why don't you run over to the trailer and take a look to see if any of it looks any good?"

"Okay," she said, seeming dubious. "I can look, but if they won't let us take a taste, all I'll be going on is the appearance of the bottles and the corks."

While BeBe sprinted toward the tractor trailer, I took two chairs and set them up in what was becoming the second row for the auction. I exchanged greetings and nods with other auction regulars I knew—Janet, the Hummel lady, who always showed up to bid on Hummel porcelain figurines with a stack of price guides in tow; Waldo, a long-haired hippie type who usually bid on comic books, old records, or any kind of toy or board game related to sixties or seventies television shows; and, inevitably, Kitty, the knitting lady. I didn't know any of these people's full names of course, and I'd made up Kitty's name, but this was as far as our auction relationship went.

I tried reading the wine listings, but none of it meant anything to me, with the exception of a Château Margaux listing, which I recognized because I'd read somewhere that Margaux Hemingway had been named for the wine her parents drank the night she was conceived.

Just as Bob was tapping his microphone for the second time to signal that he was about to start the auction, BeBe came strolling up.

"We're good," she said tersely, looking around to see if anybody was eavesdropping.

"You found a wine for me to bid on?"

"Mmm-hmm. Absolutely," she said. "Now, pay attention. If they auction the wine in the order it's listed—"

"He will. Bob always does things in order."

"Okay. Well, this bottle is listed number twelve. So pay attention. Get that bid paddle of yours ready to rock and roll."

"That good, huh?"

"It's a 1970 Château Pétrus pomerol," BeBe whispered. "*Wine Spectator* rates it a must buy."

"Right year, right color," I said, nodding approval.

"There's just one thing I should tell you," she added. "It's not cheap."

"This is Daniel's Christmas present," I said. "Money is no object."

"Good," she said. "Because the last bottle anybody bought of this particular vintage, they paid a thousand bucks for it."

CHAPTER 15

"Folks," Trader Bob intoned, "here's the ground rules for today's auction. All bottles of wine are sold 'as is' with no guarantees on my part that any of it will taste any damn good."

Chuckles and guffaws rippled through the field. The sun was out, but it was chilly, and I was glad of my heavy denim barn jacket with the big patch pockets, where I'd stashed a couple of granola bars and my checkbook and billfold.

"Due to the nature of this auction, and by request of the estate's family," he continued, "we're operating on a strictly cash-and-carry basis. What that means is, what you buy today, you take away today. And we will not be accepting checks or credit cards."

"No!" I gasped. BeBe glanced over in alarm.

"They always take checks," I said. "And the flyer didn't say anything about cash only. Well . . . shit."

"Also," Bob said, "nothing except coffee and sodas are to be consumed on our premises today because I don't want the sheriff on my tail."

He reached out to one of the helpers who were busily surrounding him with a growing hill of cardboard wine cartons and took a slender green bottle that he held up to the light.

"Let's start with this little beauty right here. It's a . . ." He frowned, pushed his glasses to the end of his nose, and squinted at the label.

"Ah, hell," he said finally. "It's bottle number one, lot one, listed right there on your catalog."

BeBe rolled her eyes and grimaced. "Liebfraumilch. And a strictly mediocre one, at that. It's a good thing the guy who bought this stuff died before he had to start living off his wine investments."

"We got three cases of this stuff here," Bob said smoothly. "And I'll take one money for all three. Let's see. That's twelve bottles a case, thirty-six bottles, let's say thirty bucks a bottle."

"Let's don't," BeBe said.

"Round it to a thousand bucks for the lot," Bob said. "Come on. One money, thirty-six bottles of pure drinking pleasure. Who'll give me a K?"

The field was quiet.

"Twenty a bottle?" Bob asked. "Seven eighty. Gimme seven eighty."

Trader Bob cupped his hand to his ear. "Mighy quiet out there. Are y'all awake, or sleepin' one off?"

He exchanged a questioning look with Leuveda.

"Don't ask me," she drawled. "You know I drink Cold Duck, my ownself."

"Gimme ten," Bob urged. "Ya can't hardly buy nothin' for that these days. And think of all the Christmas joy you could be spreading."

The crowd's reaction was a deafening indifference. In fact, the only thing I heard, aside from BeBe's snort of derision, was the steady, hypnotic clicking of Kitty the knitter's needles.

"Five?" Bob clutched his hand to his chest, as though a knife were being thrust through it, but still no bid paddles were extended.

"All right," he said finally, a beaten man. "We got a lot of wine to move this morning. Let's get this thing rolling. Somebody gimme an offer."

"Five bucks a case, Bob," called a gnomish man standing off to the right. He wore a set of green camouflage coveralls and a bright orange Elmer Fudd cap with fur earflaps.

"Fifteen bucks for all that delicious fruit of the vine?"

Elmer Fudd nodded and held up his paddle to officially register the bid.

"All right. We got fifteen. Gimme sixteen," Bob chanted. Paddles went up. Bob's chant accelerated until he'd gaveled the first lot down for an underwhelming thirty-six dollars, or as Bob put it, "a pitiful buck a bottle."

BeBe nodded her approval.

The next few lots of wine didn't fare much better. The top individual bottle sold for sixty bucks, and to get that, Trader

Bob, wheedled, cajoled, and once threatened to walk off his podium, "And call the whole damned thing off."

Through it all, BeBe alternated glances between her well-thumbed copy of *Wine Spectator* and the catalog, noting each winning bid in the catalog with her slender silver Mont Blanc pen.

"This is looking good," she said after the tenth lot had sold. "That last case of chenin blanc should have brought at least thirty bucks a bottle."

"But the whole case only went for two hundred dollars," I pointed out. "So I should get my bottle cheap, right?"

"Hopefully. Of course, that chenin blanc is sort of a sleeper. Not a lot of people have heard of the winery it came from. Unfortunately, the wine we want is quite well known and sought after. It's one of the classiest ones they're selling off today. So it could be that everybody's just holding out, waiting for the good stuff to come up."

I turned around in my chair to appraise the competition, and was surprised to see that the crowd had grown appreciably since the auction started. All seventy or so chairs were full, and more people were milling around the trailer and standing at the back of the rows of chairs.

My heart sank when I saw a familiar Burberry plaid tam-o'-shanter.

"Shit," I exclaimed, slapping my thigh with the rolled-up catalog.

"What?" BeBe turned and craned her neck.

"Cookie Parker is here," I said. "And Manny. I should have guessed they'd somehow find out about this."

"Which ones are they?" she asked, half standing to get a better scan of the crowd.

"Standing right by the trailer," I said. "Cookie's wearing a goofy plaid hat and a tan coat with a fur collar. And Manny's the one in the—"

"—tightest blue jeans I have ever seen on a grown man," BeBe exclaimed, openly staring. "Also the gaudiest cowboy shirt ever made. Sequins before noon! Who *are* these guys?"

"My worst nightmare," I said gloomily. "Gay guys with money."

"And questionable taste," she added, standing up. "We'll just see about this."

"Wait," I said. "What are you going to do? My wine is coming up pretty soon."

"You just concentrate on buying that pomerol," BeBe instructed. "According to the catalog, there are three bottles of it and they'll each be sold separately."

"How high should I bid?" I asked, suddenly unnerved by the prospect of bidding in such unfamiliar territory.

"How much cash did you bring?"

I dug in my jacket pocket and brought out a wad of bills, which I quickly counted.

"Looks like one hundred seventeen dollars," I wailed. "Not enough. Not nearly enough."

"I've got two hundred right here," she said, patting her pocketbook. "Think of me as your own personal ATM."

"But you said the last bottle sold for a thousand bucks."

"At a black-tie charity auction in Sonoma Valley, California," she said. "Whereas, *we* are standing in a cornfield in

Hardeeville, South Carolina. Don't spend more than three hundred dollars. There's still a bottle of champagne, a Krug blanc de blanc Clos de Mesnil, 1985, that I've got my eye on. It's on the third page, and it won't be cheap."

"It doesn't matter," I said, slumping down in my metal chair. "Manny and Cookie will be bidding up everything. We might as well leave right now."

"Is there any coffee left in your thermos?" she asked.

"Yeah, it's still half full," I said, wondering what this had to do with my current predicament. I unscrewed the cap and sniffed the steam rising from the vacuum jug.

"Gimme," she said.

I handed over the thermos. "Leave it up to me," BeBe said, giving me a wink. "I always get my man."

She shrugged out of her own flannel-lined jean jacket and I shivered on her behalf. The wind had picked up a little, and the sun was suddenly playing hide-and-go-seek behind a bank of clouds. The sky was cold, and promising, if not snow, some nasty icy rain.

I watched while she sashayed across the field in the direction of the trailer and the Babalu boys. She saw me watching and jerked her head in the direction of Trader Bob, reminding me that I needed to pay attention to the ongoing auction.

Bob finished hammering down a half case of a wine I'd never heard of and was pausing to read off the description of the lot I'd been waiting for.

"Folks," he drawled, "this next wine is the real deal."

Heads jerked to attention. My own hand clenched the bid paddle so tightly I felt my fingertips go numb.

"This here," he said, holding up a bottle to the light, "is the kind of wine they tell me is one of a kind. It's a bordeaux. That much I can pronounce. And it's got a pedigree out the ying-yang. They say a bottle of this stuff here will sell for a thousand bucks."

"Yeah. In your dreams, Gross," yelled one of the hecklers standing by the trailer, his fists jammed into the front pockets of his jeans.

Bob shrugged. "All right. I figger somebody out there is an educated wine connoisseur. And that somebody will be willing to pay the price for a one-of-a-kind bottle of bordeaux. We got three bottles, and I'm selling 'em for one money. Y'all can keep one, sell the others off, whatever you want. But I'm looking for twenty-five hundred dollars. That's way less than the going price."

His head swiveled to and fro, surveying the bidders. I turned and tried not to stare at Cookie and Manny, who had their heads together, in rapt discussion about something. BeBe stood off to the side, watching them intently.

"Two thousand?" Bob asked.

The crowd was quiet, but I heard a distinct, low-level buzz. People were interested, trying to decide when the time was right to jump in.

"I'll give you fifty, Bob," Kitty hollered, holding up her paddle in one hand, but not bothering to drop her knitting.

"Fifty?" Bob sounded wounded. "For that, I'll take it home and drink it myself."

"Ya gotta start somewhere," Leuveda advised. "Or we'll be here all day."

"Sixty," somebody in the back yelled.

"Seventy-five," called Waldo the hippie.

The bids were coming fast and furious now, and Bob was straining to keep up.

It stalled out a little when the bidding hit $150, and for the first time I raised my paddle.

"Weezie, got you at one fifty," Bob called, nodding his approval.

"One sixty." I recognized Cookie's voice instantly.

Gritting my teeth, I nodded at Bob. "One seventy."

"One eighty." This time it was Manny doing the bidding.

Bob cocked an eyebrow at me.

I nodded. "One ninety."

A woman's voice called out from the front. "Two hundred."

Damn, now it wasn't just the Babalu boys bidding me up.

"Two ten," Cookie called.

"Two twenty," the woman said coolly.

I bit my lip. "Two thirty."

I glanced over at Manny and Cookie just in time to see BeBe sashay past in the most casual of manners. Suddenly though, she tripped on something, and I saw, as though in slow motion, the coffee thermos go flying up in the air. Now a stream of hot coffee was raining down on Cookie.

A shrill, high-pitched scream pierced the air. Heads turned.

"Two forty?" Bob asked, impervious to pain or injury or anything else that distracted from a sale. "Anybody for two forty?"

I was too stunned to do anything but watch. BeBe had picked herself up off the ground and was now busily trying to blot coffee off Cookie's chest.

"Leave me *alone*!" Cookie cried. "Ohmygod. This coat is cashmere."

"It's ruined!" Manny chimed in.

"Two forty," the woman in the front row called.

I glanced over at BeBe, who jerked her head in the direction of Bob.

"Two fifty," I prompted.

"I'm so sorry," I heard BeBe wail. She stuck a pencil and a pad in Cookie's face. "Here. Write down your phone number. I'll pay for the cleaning. I'll replace the coat."

"He's burned!" Manny wailed, pulling Cookie's damp shirt away from his chest. "I think we need a doctor."

"Two sixty," my new female nemesis called, sounding bored with the whole drama.

Bob cocked his head. "Weezie?"

"Two seventy," I said, reminding myself that this was Daniel's Christmas present. Out of the corner of my eye, I saw Manny hustle Cookie off in the direction of the parking lot.

"Three hundred!" the woman in front called triumphantly.

I closed my eyes for a moment and gave it some deep thought. If I went any higher, there was no guarantee I'd win the bordeaux. And there was still the champagne to consider. Maybe by the time it came up, the crowd would have thinned out, and I'd get it at a bargain. Maybe.

"Weezie?" Bob asked.

I kept my eyes closed and shook my head no.

"Three hundred fifty!"

It was BeBe's voice. I opened my eyes and saw her striding up the aisle in my direction. Her shirt was soaked with coffee, and she had that look in her eye.

"Three sixty?" Bob asked.

Silence.

"All right then," Bob said quickly. "Three fifty once, twice, sold! To—"

BeBe grabbed my bid paddle and held it triumphantly over her head.

CHAPTER 16

The first drops of rain started falling as I counted out our hard-won cash to Leuveda, including two crumpled twenty-dollar bills that BeBe pulled from a secret compartment in her right boot.

"Don't ask," she said darkly, when I was about to. "Ever since my episode with poverty, I go nowhere without a couple twenties tucked in my shoe for a rainy day."

I glanced up at the charcoal-tinged sky and flipped up the hood on my jacket. "And this definitely looks like it's going to be one of those days."

"Here," I said, shoving one of the bottles at BeBe, along with the keys to the truck. "Get the heater going. I'll be back in a few minutes."

A few turned into twenty, and it had started to drizzle, but when I climbed into the driver's seat, it was with a smug grin on my face and the bottle of champagne tucked inside my jacket.

"What took so long?" she grumped.

I handed her the Krug and two twenties and started to thread my way out of the lot.

"How?"

"I sold off the other two bottles of bordeaux to the woman who was bidding against me," I said. "For two hundred bucks. I had to go eighty to get the Krug."

She shook her head in admiration. "And you still broke even. Weezie Foley, you are a mess!"

By the time we were on the road, the rain was coming down hard and the temperature had dropped at least twenty degrees.

BeBe shivered and buttoned her jean jacket up over her bra. "What I wouldn't give for some of that hot coffee right now," she said through chattering teeth.

"Was Cookie really burned?" I asked, wincing at the memory of his screams.

"No way," she assured me. "I left the top off the thermos for five minutes. It was barely lukewarm. He's just a big ol' baby. Gay or not, did you ever meet a man who wasn't a big ol' baby?"

"You're the authority," I agreed.

BeBe turned up the heat a notch and sat back and rubbed her hands in glee. "Anyway, we both did what we had to do. I can't believe you got the wine *and* the champagne. It's a fabulous gift. Daniel will love it."

"He'd better," I said. "Anyway, that's a huge load off my mind. Now I'm done. My last Christmas gift!."

"Speaking of gifts," she said. "What did you get from Annie?"

"Annie?" My mind was a blank.

"Apple Annie. Your charity case."

"Jeez," I said. "With the excitement of the auction, I completely forgot to look. Open the glove box and see what's in there."

I glanced over once, but mostly kept my eyes on the road. Driving over the humpbacked Talmadge Memorial Bridge that crosses the Savannah River gives me a bad case of the heebie-jeebies on a good day, but now with the rain and the gusting winds, I was more nervous than usual.

BeBe punched the lock on the glove box and brought out a festive red plaid gift bag tied with a jaunty black velvet bow.

"Hey," she said, holding it in front of me. "Look. Apple Annie's got your gift-wrapping gene."

I frowned. "That's not *for* me. It's *from* me. Look again. Is there anything else in there?"

BeBe rummaged around in the glove box and held up her findings. "Screwdriver."

"Check."

"Flashlight."

"Check."

"Hoo-hoo!" she chortled, bringing out a small cardboard box. "Condoms! Annie must know you better than I thought."

"Give me those," I said, snatching the box away from her and stashing it under my seat.

"I take it those are also not from Annie?" BeBe asked in a teasing singsong.

"Not another word."

"Well, there's nothing else in the glove box," she concluded, shutting it.

"I don't understand," I said. "The truck was unlocked. Why didn't she take her gift?"

"Maybe she was busy getting her hair and nails done for the Symphony fund-raiser," BeBe quipped.

I shot her a dirty look, but BeBe just tossed her hair and fidgeted with the top button on her jean jacket.

"This isn't like Annie," I went on. "I've been leaving her those little presents every night for a week. And she hasn't missed picking them up. Not once. Till now."

"You're worried," BeBe said, rolling her eyes, "about a bag lady."

I nodded agreement, my mind already filling with a variety of possibilities to explain the gift's presence in my truck. None of them were pleasant.

"You think something bad could have happened to her," BeBe went on.

"She lives on the streets!" I exclaimed. "Of course I'm worried. She could be hurt. Or sick . . ."

"Or drunk. Look, Weezie, you said it yourself. This is Apple Annie we're talking about here. She's a street person. Maybe she just hit the road. Anyway, you don't know anything about her. Not really. So don't go making yourself sick worrying and inventing all kinds of tragic scenarios about why she didn't pick up her little care package."

I chewed at the inside of my mouth and stared out the windshield as the wipers sliced through ribbons of rain. I drummed my fingertips on the steering wheel.

BeBe sighed and shifted in her seat.

"You're not going to just forget about her, are you? You're going to make some desperate, well-intentioned, but totally futile attempt to track her down and patch her up. Aren't you?"

I stared straight ahead.

"She's not a stray kitten," BeBe warned. "Weezie, these street people live that way because they want to, most of 'em. They're fiercely independent and they totally resent any efforts to change their lifestyle."

I rolled my eyes.

"She's a human being," BeBe went on. "A complex and probably deeply screwed-up human being. You can't fix her."

"But it's Christmas," I blurted out. "Look, I know she's not some house cat I can just feed a bowl of milk to and tie a ribbon around her collar. I *know* that. But I can't help it. Yes, I'm worried about Annie. It's not like her to completely miss picking up her present. Or to miss leaving one for me. I swear, I don't want to fix her or adopt her. I just want to give her a lousy bag of soap and shampoo and some candy. Is that so awful?"

"Not if you're able to just leave it at that," BeBe said. "Anyway, if you want to give her something she can really use, you should have bought some of that rotgut buck-a-bottle wine back there in Hardeeville."

"Screw you, Ebenezer." I said it softly, mostly under my breath, but definitely loud enough to be heard.

We were just turning onto Charlton Street when BeBe finally spoke again.

"All right," she said with a martyred sigh. "I give up. Where do we start looking for Apple Annie?"

"The women's shelter," I said promptly. "You check there. I'll drive over to Reynolds Square, and then over to Franklin Square, where those homeless guys always hang out. If you find her, don't talk to her. Just call me on my cell phone."

She gave me a mock salute. "Aye-aye, captain."

CHAPTER 17

I drove slowly around Reynolds Square, looking for Apple Annie. But the square was deserted. Not even a pigeon would have braved this cold and rain.

The thought occurred to me, as I headed north to Franklin Square—where *do* homeless people go in this kind of weather? It was too early for the shelters to open yet. And for that matter, where do pigeons go when the weather's gruesome?

Franklin Square, which stood at the edge of Savannah's revitalized City Market district, wasn't any livelier than Reynolds Square. The homeless men who usually congregated on the park benches, playing checkers on upended buckets, had disappeared.

I sighed and headed slowly around the square. I spent the next hour cruising every downtown street and lane, looking for Annie.

Finally, when I was passing the soup kitchen at Emmaus House, on Abercorn Street, I noticed two shabbily dressed men crouching under the building's overhang, trying to stay dry.

I parked the truck illegally in front of a fire hydrant, and splashed through the puddles toward them.

The men were both white, but their faces were so caked with grime and their shabby knitted caps pulled so low over their foreheads, it was impossible to guess their ages.

"Excuse me," I said breathlessly. "I'm looking for a friend of mine. She's an older lady who, uh, lives on the streets around here."

"Yeah?" The shorter of the two men, whose cap was faded red, took his sock-covered hands out of his pockets and rubbed them together. "What's she done?"

"Nothing!" I said. "I've, uh, got something I need to give her. But she's not around. I wonder if either of you have seen her? Maybe here at the soup kitchen?"

The taller man, whose hat was olive drab, coughed roughly, and I jumped backward, instinctively.

He wiped his nose with his bare hand. "What's this lady look like?"

That gave me pause. I'd actually only glimpsed Annie once, that night of the open house at Maisie's Daisy.

"She's a white lady," I said hesitantly. "Probably in her sixties. Gray hair . . ."

"And?" Green Hat said impatiently, pulling a mangled half-smoked cigarette out of his pocket and lighting it with an orange plastic lighter.

Suddenly I remembered another, telling detail.

"She might be wearing a maroon BC letter sweater."

Green Hat exhaled smoke in my face, then coughed again. Cringing, I took another step backward.

"I'd remember better—" he said thoughtfully.

"—if we had some money," his red-hatted friend said, finishing the idea.

"Oh." I fished in my jacket pocket, then remembered, belatedly, Daniel's advice about giving handouts to homeless men.

I brought out the granola bars I'd stashed in my pocket for breakfast.

"I'm kinda broke," I said, flashing an apologetic grin. "But you can have these. They're chocolate chip and peanut butter. Protein, you know?"

"No, thanks," Red Hat snarled. "We're trying to cut back on sweets."

"Yeah," the smoker said. "We gotta watch our girlish figures."

I shrugged and started to turn away. "Sorry."

"Too bad," Red Hat said. He knocked on his forehead. "Aw, look. I forgot where I saw your lady friend. Earlier. Like maybe half an hour ago."

"You saw her?" I turned back. "Where?"

"We forget," the smoker said. He took a last drag on his cigarette and tossed the butt at my feet. It hit a puddle and sizzled a moment before dying out.

"That's not very nice," I said, giving them a reproachful look. "It's Christmas, you know."

"Yeah," Red Hat said. "We know."

"Well—" I sputtered, trying to think of a clever comeback. "Merry Christmas!"

The smoker stepped forward menacingly, and I turned and ran for the safety of the truck, locking the doors as soon as I slid onto the seat.

I was almost home before I noticed the white rectangle of paper stuck in the corner of my windshield.

"Damn," I cried. "Another stinking parking ticket."

It was past one by the time I pushed open the front door at Maisie's Daisy.

Mary, the blond-haired UGA student who sometimes helped out around the shop when she was home from school, looked up from the magazine she was reading. "Hey, Weezie," she called. "Wow. You're soaked."

"Pretty much," I agreed. I shrugged out of my jacket and pulled off my equally sodden boots and headed for the back room to try to dry off.

"Anything going on around here?" I called to her.

"Not much. It's been raining so hard, not a single person came in all morning."

I emerged from the back room with a towel wrapped around my wet hair.

"Figures," I said. "You can go on home if you want, Mary. I think I'll close up early. Nobody with any sense is coming out in this mess."

"Okay." She hopped down from the wooden stool behind the counter, grabbed her purse, and headed for the door.

"Wait." I opened the cash register drawer and took out a twenty, which I tried to hand her.

"Oh no," she protested. "You don't need to pay me. I

didn't do anything except read your magazines. The phone didn't even ring."

"I insist," I said, pressing the bill into her hands. "So nobody came by at all? You didn't happen to see a little homeless lady hanging around outside? Maybe wearing an old BC letter sweater?"

Her big blue eyes widened. "An old lady in a letter sweater? No, I didn't see anybody like that."

After Mary left, I wandered around the shop, doing some light dusting, straightening shelves, and making a list of merchandise I'd put on my After Christmas Clearance table.

The blue lights twinkled on the aluminum tree, and my retro Christmas tunes played away on the shop's CD player, but I somehow couldn't shake the melancholy that settled over me like a mist.

I kept a close watch on the sidewalk in front of the shop, and a couple times even went to the back door to look out to the lane, which was just as quiet. It was futile, I knew, but I still hoped maybe Annie would reappear.

It was nearly four when my cell phone rang. I ran to answer it.

"No go on the women's shelter," BeBe reported. "And they've never even seen a woman who fits the description I gave them of Annie. They said most of their 'guests' are younger."

"Okay," I said with a sigh. "I didn't find her either. I did find two guys in front of the soup kitchen at Emmaus House who tried to extort money from me in exchange for information. But they probably didn't really know her."

"Probably not," BeBe agreed. She hesitated. "You're not

going to let this Apple Annie thing turn into a full-blown obsession, are you?"

"No. You're probably right. I'm just going to forget about her."

"I'm definitely right," BeBe said. "Now go home and wrap some Christmas presents."

"I've only got two left to wrap," I reminded her. "But I am going to close up early and start cooking for tomorrow night."

"Thatta girl," she said. "What time do you want us?"

"Dinner's at eight. But you could come early and help keep Mama out of the kitchen."

"Just as long as you don't make me eat any of that fruit-cake," she promised.

I was standing at the front door, with my keys in hand, ready to lock up, when a tall woman in a rusty black ankle-length raincoat came dashing up out of nowhere.

"Don't tell me you're closed!" she wailed, spying the keys.

"Sorry." I flashed her a regretful smile.

"Please?" She pushed a damp strand of graying red hair out of her eyes. "I left work early just to come over here. I walk by every night on my way home, but you're always closed by then."

She pointed toward the display window. "The record player. How much is it?"

"Sorry," I repeated. "It's actually just a display piece. It's not for sale."

"Oh no." Her shoulders drooped.

"You can get very nice repro turntables at Restoration

Hardware now," I said helpfully. "Or you could probably buy one on eBay."

"No time," she said sorrowfully. "My bus leaves for Buffalo in a couple hours. I wanted it for my older sister," she explained. "She's got all these records, from when she was a teenager. They're the old forty-fives, but she's got nothing to play them on. Dad gave away her record player years ago, after my mom died and he sold the house."

"Oh." I didn't know what else to say.

"It's okay," she said. "I've got some perfume for her, and a book. She likes mysteries. Nothing gory. She likes romance novels better, but her husband left this summer. Took off with his twenty-eight-year-old secretary. So I don't want anything too sappy. Of course, everything makes her cry these days."

"What kind of music does your sister like?" I asked, unlocking the door and holding it open.

"Huh?"

"Come on," I said, shooing her inside. "If you're going to take the turntable, you might as well take the records too. How about Elvis? Does she like Elvis?"

The woman stood in the doorway of the shop, rain streaming onto the floor.

"Are you kidding? She loves Elvis. Chuck Berry. The Platters. Tams, Temptations."

I scooped the record player off the display bed in the window and took it and the records over to the cash register. I found a gift box under the counter, popped the record player inside it, and placed the records on top.

"Pick out your gift paper," I instructed, pointing to the rack of papers behind me. "Pink poodles? Penguins? Christmas trees?"

"Linda would love the red plaid," the woman said promptly. "She's still got her old red plaid lunchbox from when we were kids."

"To Linda," I wrote the name on the card with a flourish. "From?"

"Nancy," she said, reaching for her purse. "My name's Nancy. This is so sweet of you. Really. I can't thank you enough. How much?"

"It's on me," I said, feeling the melancholy melt away as quickly as it had come. I tied on a huge green velvet bow. "Merry Christmas."

CHAPTER 18

Daniel let himself in the back door of my town house around midnight, right as I was taking the last two pies—a pecan and an apple—out of the oven.

"Hey," I said, pleased and surprised to see him this early. Christmas business at the restaurant had been so hectic, he sometimes didn't get in until two or three in the morning.

"Hey, yourself," he said, touching a practiced fingertip to the crust of the already cooling lemon pound cake on a cake stand. He nodded approval.

Daniel kissed me briefly, then sat down at the counter, surveying my kitchen. All evening, I'd checked numerous times to see if Annie had shown up to collect her gift, my anxiety feeding a burst of nervous energy that I'd poured into chopping, stirring, and sautéing.

The counters were covered with cakes, pies, and cas-seroles, not to mention a big pan of oyster dressing and a

giant bowl of navel oranges which I'd spent the last hour peeling and cutting up for ambrosia.

"What's all this?" he asked, pouring himself a glass of red wine.

"Christmas dinner," I said, holding out my own glass for a refill.

"Did you invite the whole street? I mean, there's enough food here for Pharaoh's army."

"You know how I always overcook," I said lightly. "Mama says it's a sin to let a guest leave your table hungry."

"Eloise?" Daniel put down his wineglass. There were two bright spots of red on his cheeks. "Just how many people did you invite over for dinner?"

"Not that many," I said, busily grating coconut into the cut-glass bowl for the ambrosia. "Just family and a couple friends."

"Whose family? The Osmonds? This is a serious shitload of food here. And I seem to remember that you're an only child."

"Yes, but besides you and me and Mama and Daddy, there'll be Uncle James and Jonathan, of course, and Miss Sudie. And BeBe and Harry are coming, and Derek and Eric—"

"Whoa," he said sternly. "You invited my brothers for Christmas dinner without consulting me?"

"And their wives and kids," I said quickly, getting it out of the way.

"That's not a family dinner," he said. "It's a traveling freak show."

"It's Christmas. I just thought it would be nice to have both our families for dinner. Is that a crime? Our families have never met."

"Why do they have to meet? Ever?"

Quietly I set the coconut down on a clean plate. I wiped my hands on a dish towel. I took a deep breath.

"Our families need to meet each other because you and I are in a serious, committed relationship. Aren't we?"

"So far."

I ignored that.

"This will be my first Christmas cooking dinner in my own house. Every other year my mother has cooked. And before that, in the bad old days, when I was married to Tal, his mother cooked Christmas dinner." I shuddered involuntarily at the memory of those silent, chilly dinners in the Evans family dining room.

"Finger bowls," I said suddenly.

"Huh?"

"Tal's mother used to set the table as though the duke and duchess of Windsor were expected. Right down to finger bowls. Crystal knife rests, place cards. Four different forks, two knives, and three wineglasses. It was grotesque. I could never eat a bite without worrying she'd catch me using the wrong fork, or dropping peas on her Aubusson carpet."

I took another deep breath. "This year, I wanted to do something special. I know how you feel about Christmas. I know it has all kinds of bitter associations for you. And I want to change that. I want to make a beautiful holiday din-

ner for the person I love most in the world. For you. You're my family. And your family is my family."

I felt a little weak-kneed after finally giving my big speech, the one I'd been practicing in my head for days now.

"All right," he said finally. "If this means so much to you, I guess I can go along with it."

I leaned over and kissed his cheek.

"It won't be so bad. I promise. It'll be fun!"

"Like a root canal."

"Daniel!"

"Look. Eric's kids won't eat anything except dinner rolls, white rice, and vanilla ice cream," he said. "Their mother, Ellen, caters to this absurd behavior. And Derek's wife, Sondra, is diabetic. Not to mention a practicing vegan."

I smiled serenely. "I know all about your family's dietary peculiarities. Sondra faxed over a list of foods that are acceptable to her. I just left the butter and cream out of a couple dishes, and I fixed some pumpkin bars that are made with applesauce, instead of eggs. Also Eric volunteered to bring his kids' favorite rice dish, as well as the ice cream. See? I have everything under control."

"You wish," he said. "Did Sondra happen to mention that she and Ellen haven't spoken to each other since *last* Christmas, when Ellen had too much eggnog and told Sondra she needed to gain some weight because she was starting to look like an anorexic crack whore?"

I swallowed hard. "Uh, no. That didn't come up."

He gave me an evil grin. "It will. You might want to think

about writing up some place cards of your own, to keep those two from having a catfight."

He poured himself another glass of wine, topped off my glass, then stood up and took me by the hand.

"Come on, Eloise Foley. It's getting late. Let's go sit by the fire in front of that Christmas tree of yours and see if you can't put me in the holiday mood."

"Be right there," I promised. "Save me a seat. I just need to run out to the truck and check on something."

"In the truck?" He frowned. "At this time of night?"

"I had my arms full of groceries when I came in," I fibbed. "And I left the last bag in the front seat."

"I'll get it," he said, turning toward the kitchen door.

"No!" I said quickly. "It's, uh, a Christmas gift for you. A surprise."

"All right, but don't forget to lock the truck before you come in. I'm still not comfortable with all the weird things that have been going on around here lately."

I grabbed a sweater from a hook by the back door and hurried out to the truck. Opening the passenger-side door, I popped the lock on the glove box, still hoping.

But the red plaid bag, with its jaunty bow, was untouched.

I left the bag where it was and closed the door. I stood by the truck, wrapping my arms around myself for warmth. "Annie," I called softly. "Come out, come out, wherever you are."

CHAPTER 19

I smoothed my grandmother's starched white damask cloth over the battered pine harvest table in the dining room, and with my fingertips, traced the tiny patches where she'd so painstakingly mended it. If I looked closely, and I did, I could see the faintest ghost outlines of stains from family dinners long ago.

The pale pink splotch on one corner, I was sure, was the remnant of a red wine spill, probably from one of the bad uncles at Thanksgiving dinner. There were numerous small grease stains—my Meemaw served gravy on everything— even eggs. There was a single scorch mark near the middle of the rectangular cloth, and this, Mama had told me, was the result of my sixth birthday party, when I'd blown out the candles on my cake with such gusto that I'd sent one candle flying onto the tablecloth, where Daddy had extinguished the resulting flame with the remnants from a coffee cup.

I had plenty of beautiful linens I could have set the table with that night. Years of dealing and collecting old textiles had yielded a closet full of them. I'd considered using the gorgeous Irish linen cloth with the hand-tatted convent lace that had been a wedding gift to Mama, who, saving it for "nice," had never once used it before handing it down to me at my own ill-fated wedding to Talmadge Evans III.

But Meemaw's tablecloth, with all those tangible reminders of happy family occasions, was the only one that would do for such a special night.

Circling the table, I dealt out the dishes, not fine bone china, which I had plenty of as well, but instead, my favorite flow blue china in a pattern called Claremont, by Johnson Brothers.

I'd found three of the flow blue dinner plates years and years ago at the Junior League Thrift Shop in Atlanta, when Tal was still in school at Georgia Tech. At two dollars apiece, they were a big splurge at the time. Over the years, I'd managed to fill out those original plates to a service for twelve. I rarely buy Claremont anymore, though, as the plates now sell for close to $150 apiece.

We'd actually have thirteen at the grown-up table tonight, but I had another flow blue plate, from a different but similar pattern, that I would put at my own place at the table.

After the china was placed, I added etched wineglasses from several different patterns, and topped each plate with a heavy damask banquet-size napkin with a gorgeous rococo monogrammed *W,* and added my wedding silver, which I'd stubbornly kept buying long after my wedding was history.

I placed two cut-glass bowls of white roses down the center of the table and scattered about my collection of sterling candlesticks, no two of which matched.

"Wow," BeBe said, popping her head in from the kitchen. "It's beautiful, Weezie. Like a painting or something."

"It's not too fancy?" I asked anxiously, remembering those dreaded stiff dinners in the Evans family dining room.

"Elegant, but not off-putting," she declared, dragging in two of the wooden folding chairs she was loaning me for the children's table.

"But not too casual, right? I mean, I want it to be really special tonight. Daniel's brothers have never stepped foot in my house. I don't want them or their wives to think I'm poor white trash."

"They won't. You aren't," BeBe said, gazing down at the card table I'd set up for Daniel's four nieces and nephews with green Depression glass plates and a centerpiece of green-and-red gumdrop trees.

"This is cute," she said, flicking the edge of the tablecloth, a vintage forties luncheon cloth with a bright poinsettia motif border.

"This was in that box lot of stuff I bought at Trader Bob's," I told her. "The one that had the blue Christmas tree pin." I patted the collar of my cream satin blouse, where the brooch was now securely pinned. "And this," I said, pointing to the frilly white taffeta apron I'd tied over my black silk slacks.

"Something's dinging in the oven," Harry Sorrentino announced as he entered the dining room with a large silver bowl heaped high with boiled shrimp.

"Harry, you're an angel," I said, giving him a quick kiss on the cheek. "Are these your shrimp?"

"Yep," Harry said, blushing a little.

"Our shrimp," BeBe corrected. "You may have caught the little buggers, but I'm the one who headed 'em, deveined 'em, and marinated them in the lemon juice and capers."

"But it was my recipe," Harry countered.

Before the good-natured bickering could continue, I heard the key turn in the front door and Daniel stepped inside carrying a foil-wrapped platter.

"Thank God," I breathed, hurrying to take the ham out of his arms. "It's past seven. I was halfway afraid you were going to be a no-show."

He followed me into the kitchen, closing the door behind us.

I made room for the platter on the kitchen table and popped the foil off the ham, which smelled heavenly, with its dark brown maple-sugar-and-orange glaze. He'd even sliced the ham at the restaurant and garnished the platter with gorgeous clusters of sugared grapes.

"It's amazing," I said, kissing him gratefully. "You're forgiven for being late. Now get out of that jacket and give me a hand with the rest of this stuff."

He stepped out of my embrace and looked away.

"What?" I said, knowing in my gut what he was about to say.

"I can't stay," he said. "Eddie's car got T-boned on Eisenhower this afternoon. He's in the hospital."

"Oh no," I said, alarmed. Eddie Gonzalez was Daniel's

best line cook. He'd worked at Guale since the beginning. "Is he going to be all right?"

"Couple broken ribs and some cuts on his face," Daniel said. "But in the meantime, we're swamped. I gotta get back. Forgive me?"

I shrugged. This was the restaurant life, I knew, although I couldn't help but wonder if a part of Daniel wasn't glad to be missing out on this family dinner which he'd only reluctantly agreed to.

"Go," I said, shooing him out of the kitchen.

He gave me a grateful kiss. "I'll call you," he promised. "Maybe things will slacken up a little after nine."

We both knew that was wishful thinking.

I was lifting a bubbling earthenware dish of hot crab dip from the still-dinging oven when Mama and Daddy came in through the back door.

"Merry, merry," Mama chirped, holding out a gaudy green plastic tray.

"I made your favorite," she said.

Gingerly I lifted the edge of the linen napkin covering the tray to view something brown and vaguely cinnamon scented.

"Yum," I said, trying to sound enthusiastic.

"Zucchini bread," Daddy said glumly. "Here I thought she'd given it all away last summer, but there was still one last loaf on the bottom shelf of the freezer."

"Luckily," Mama said.

"Where's Danny?" Daddy asked, making me cringe involuntarily.

"You just missed him," I said lightly. "He brought the ham, then he had to dash back to the restaurant. They're booked solid tonight, and his best cook got in a car accident today."

Mama took her coat off and handed it to Daddy. "Never mind," she said. "Just put me to work instead," she ordered, rolling up the cuffs of her Christmas sweater.

"Oh no," I said quickly. "Out to the living room with the both of you." I gave them a little shove. "I've got my staff helping tonight. You and Daddy are strictly company. I forbid you to lift a finger."

From behind Mama's back, Daddy shot me a grateful wink.

"Come on, Marian," he said, taking her arm. "The front doorbell is ringing. You and I will be official greeters. Is that okay, Weezie?"

"Perfect," I said. I handed Daddy a tray with the crab dip and a basket of Triscuits. "And you can also pass this around and get everybody's drink orders when they come in."

"Just ginger ale for me," Mama said quickly.

"And cranberry juice," I agreed. "To make it look festive."

From the direction of the living room, I heard BeBe greeting our guests, and recognized James's and Jonathan's voices. Then the doorbell rang, and I heard more voices. Daniel's family. I untied my apron, put on some fresh lipstick, and went out to the living room to witness the meeting of the families.

"Well, hello strangers," I said, swooping down on Derek and Sondra, who were standing in the middle of the living room, still wearing their coats, with Sondra clutching a plastic-

wrapped casserole dish. I introduced them around, and Harry, bless him, took their coats and fixed them drinks.

"Daniel sends his regrets," I announced before anybody else could ask. "He's hoping to make it back here before dessert, if things slow down at the restaurant."

"Where are the children?" I asked, giving Derek a quick hug.

Sondra blinked. "Children? You mean Sarah Jo and Hollis? They're at my mother's house. They always spend Christmas Eve with their cousins there."

"But look who we did bring!" Derek said, reaching into the huge tote bag on Sondra's shoulder and bringing out the tiniest, most rodentlike animal I'd ever seen.

"Say hello, Barkley," he instructed, rubbing his nose against the animal's snout.

The dog's ears lay flat against his skull and he bared his little fangs and lunged in my direction.

"Rowrowrowrowrow."

"Jesus!" I cried, jumping about a foot in the air.

"Barkley!" Sondra said. She shook a finger at the animal. "That was naughty, naughty."

She laughed apologetically. "Barkley didn't mean it. Our vet says he's overcompensating for being the smallest of his litter with inappropriate aggression."

"Derek?" She narrowed her eyes at her husband. "Sweetie, did you give Barkley his meds tonight? You know he doesn't transition well without his Paxil."

"Wait," Derek said. "You mean Barkley gets the Paxil? Uh-oh. I thought he got the Flintstones chewables. I gave the Paxil to Sarah Jo."

"What?" Sondra shrieked.

"Just kidding," Derek said with a chuckle.

The look Sondra gave him would have melted cast iron.

Then the doorbell rang again, and Harry ushered in Eric and Ellen and their two children, Stoney, a seven-year-old who was too busy playing with his Game Boy to say hello, and five-year-old Stormy, who clung to her mother's side like stink on a dog.

Once Ellen saw Sondra, she and Stormy beat a hasty retreat to the den, where Daddy, Jonathan, and Uncle James had already retreated to watch football on television.

"I'll just put the ice cream in your freezer, Weezie," Eric said. "What about this rice? Where do you want Ellen's rice casserole?"

"Just put it on the dining room sideboard, please," I said.

When I turned around, Sondra had moved to the corner of the living room, standing ramrod straight, eyes focused on nothing in particular, still clutching her casserole dish. In her middle thirties, Sondra was thin to the point of emaciation, and had raven black hair and skin so milky pale you could see a fine network of blue veins in her face. Daniel referred to her as Morticia when his brother wasn't around.

"Here," Mama said, taking Sondra's dinner contribution. "I'll take this into the dining room. Mmm," she enthused. "It smells wonderful. What is it?"

"Tofurkey," Sondra said shyly.

"Oh." Mama's smile dimmed somewhat. "I don't believe I've ever eaten tofurkey before."

"You'll love it," Derek said, putting an affectionate arm

around his wife's shoulder. "Sondra is an amazing cook. You should taste her lentil cakes."

Eric returned to the living room, with two beer bottles in hand, one of which he handed to Derek.

"Yessir," Eric drawled. "Ol' Sondra here whomps up a mean tofu stew. I was just saying to Ellen on the way over here tonight, 'I hope ol' Sondra brings some of that make-believe meat of hers.'"

"Can it, Eric," Derek snapped. "You're not half as funny as you think you are."

"Hey," I said brightly. "Daddy and the other guys are watching the ball game in the den. Want to join them?"

Mama had somehow enticed Sondra to sit on the sofa beside Miss Sudie and BeBe, and I noticed with relief that they seemed to be having a pleasant conversation.

Just then Harry sauntered into the kitchen to get a beer.

"How's it going in the den?" I asked. "Is everybody behaving themselves?"

He popped the cap on a Heineken, took a long swig, and considered the question.

"So far so good, mostly," he said. "They're all hunkered down around Derek's videotape of the 1980 Georgia-Florida game. You know, their championship season. But at halftime I did overhear Eric telling a fag joke to your uncle James."

"Oh no." I moaned, covering my eyes with my hands.

"James was pretty cool about it," Harry said.

There was a scratching at the back door, and Harry went over and looked out. "Hey, Jethro, buddy," he called, opening the door.

"Wait!" I started. "He can't—"

But it was too late. Jethro bounded into the kitchen, delighted to be invited to the party, and hearing voices coming from the living room, he dashed off in that direction.

"Oh no. You'll have to help me catch him now. He can't stay in the house. There are too many people. And Sondra and Derek brought this little dog Jethro could swallow whole in one bite."

"Rowrowrowrow," I heard. We ran into the living room in time to see Jethro, on his haunches, backing away in terror from the attack midget hanging out of Sondra's tote bag, which she'd set on the floor beside her chair.

"Jethro! Here!" I called.

He turned, gave me a reproachful look, and retreated to his favorite hiding place, under the coffee table.

"Rowrowrowrow." Barkley was out of the tote bag, his ears twitching in indignation at this new interloper.

"Here, Jethro," Harry called, getting down on his hands and knees. "Come here, buddy. Come see Uncle Harry."

But instead of going to Harry, Jethro scooted out the other side of the coffee table, where he spied the hot crab dip on top of the table.

He was on it in a flash, wolfing down the entire contents of the bowl before anybody could stop him.

"Jethro! Bad!" I hollered.

He gave me that reproachful look again, and trotted off in the direction of the den.

"I'll get him," Harry volunteered.

"Sorry about the dip," I told the womenfolk. "But dinner's

almost ready anyway, and now you won't spoil your appetites."

"Well, I believe I'll just go out to the kitchen and help you get dinner on the table," Mama said, getting to her feet.

"Owowowow!" Barkley yelped.

"You stood on his tail!" Sondra cried, snatching the dog into her arms.

"Owwooooo," Barkley howled.

"Poor baby," Sondra cooed, cradling the dog in her arms. "Poor angel."

"So sorry," Mama said. "I didn't even see him there."

"You could have killed him!" Sondra said.

BeBe and I followed Mama into the kitchen.

"I should have killed him," Mama muttered. "Who brings a dog to a dinner party?"

"For that matter, who brings tofurkey?" BeBe chimed in.

I was transferring the real turkey to a serving platter when I heard a screech coming from the den.

"Good Lord!" Mama said. "What now?"

"I'll take care of it," I said, hurrying away. "Everything's ready to go out to the sideboard. Except the gravy. Let's leave it on the stove until everybody's seated."

In the den I found the men huddled tensely around the television, watching a twenty-six-year-old football game whose outcome was already etched in their brains. A glance at the screen told the tale—Georgia was trailing Florida 21–20. They were all on their knees, all except Eric. He and Ellen were trying in vain to quiet Stormy's sobs.

"What happened?" I asked.

"Your dog!" Eric shouted at me. "Your goddamned dog—"

Jethro cowered in the corner.

"He bit her?" I asked in disbelief. "Jethro's never bitten anybody in his life."

Wait. Suddenly I smelled it. A hideous, disgusting smell.

"No!" Eric said. "He puked all over my kid's shoes."

"Her brand-new patent leather Stride Rites," Ellen said, her lips tight.

"My shoeeeeees!" Stormy howled.

My crab dip, I wanted to cry.

For the first time, Derek turned away from the television to address his tear-stricken niece.

"Stormy, honey," he said kindly. "It's fourth down and there's less than two minutes left in the game. Buck Belue's fixin' to throw that tater to ol' Lindsay Scott, and your uncle Derek wants to hear Larry Munson scream 'Run, Lindsay, run,' but we can't do that until you shut the fuck up."

"Derek!" Ellen screeched, clamping her hands over her daughter's ears.

"My shoeeees," Stormy wailed.

I sighed and held out my hand to the child. "Come on, Stormy," I said. "Let's go upstairs and get you washed off. I'm sorry about your shoes. I'll buy you a new pair."

"I'll buy her a fuckin' pony if you get her out of here right this minute," Derek called over his shoulder.

CHAPTER 20

At nine o'clock, finally, we all gathered in the dining room, holding hands, seated around the tables.

"Uncle James," I said, nodding in his direction. "Would you ask the blessing?"

Big mistake. Never, ever ask a former clergyman to say the blessing over a holiday dinner. Not if you like your dinner warm, anyway.

Beaming, James started out strong. "Lord," he said earnestly, "we thank you for bringing these two families together tonight. We thank you for the opportunity to remember the reason for this season."

And he went on like that for the next ten minutes. It was a most un-Catholic-like prayer, especially coming from a former priest. James thanked God for the turkey, the ham, the oysters, and the final score of the 1980 Georgia-Florida game. All this time, Daddy was gripping my right hand so

tightly that it had gotten totally numb. BeBe, on my right, was giggling silently, her shoulders heaving from the strain of near hilarity. Stoney, at the far end of the children's table, was staring intently at the Game Boy on his lap.

When he slowed down a little, Jonathan jumped in. "And thank you for everything else. Amen!"

"Amen!" the others said in unison, sitting down and looking at me expectantly.

I went to the sideboard and started passing around the bread and cranberry relish.

"Hey," Eric said as I was leaning over to serve him. He reached out and touched the pin on my blouse. "Hey, Derek, did you see Weezie's pin?"

"I noticed that," Derek said. "It's just like the one we bought Mama for Christmas that year."

"I know," I said quietly. "Daniel told me the whole story about how you boys used all your lawn-mowing money to buy it for her."

"*We* didn't all buy it," Eric corrected me. "Daniel and I pooled our money. But hotshot over there," he said, pointing to Derek, "spent all his money buying an ankle bracelet for his girlfriend."

"Oh yeah." Derek grinned. "I remember the bracelet, but I can't for the life of me remember that little ol' gal's name."

"Hmmph," Sondra said, glaring at him.

"I can't remember her real name either," Eric said mischievously. "Only her nickname. Huffy."

"Huffy?" Ellen wrinkled her nose in distaste. "What kind of nickname is that?"

"Never mind," Derek said quickly. "Forget it. Ancient history."

"No, really," Ellen persisted.

"We called her Huffy," Eric said, guffawing now, "cuz every guy on our block took a ride on her."

"Eric!" Ellen said, blushing beet red. "There are children in the room. Our children."

"That's revolting," Sondra said.

"Thanks, bro," Derek said under his breath. "I owe you one."

"Who's ready for turkey?" I called, escaping into the kitchen.

That turkey was a thing of beauty. I'd soaked it overnight in a salt and herb brine, stuffed it with roast chestnuts and wild rice, tucked more herbs and butter and garlic under the skin, and basted it all morning with an apple cider glaze.

It was golden and regal, resting on my best Staffordshire platter on top of a bed of roasted potatoes, parsnips, carrots, and onions.

I set the platter down on the table with a flourish. "Daddy? Daniel usually carves the meat, but he's still stuck at the restaurant. Do you feel like carving tonight?"

"Oh no," Mama interjected. "Your father is terrible at carving. Ask somebody else."

Daddy glowered at her, but kept silent.

"I'll give it a shot," Eric volunteered. "I was the oldest in our family, so Mama always let me carve all the meat. I'm pretty good at it too."

"He really is," Ellen agreed. "He watches all those cooking

shows on FoodTV." She beamed at her husband, then reached into her lap and brought out a small plastic bottle of clear liquid. I watched, fascinated, as she squirted the liquid into her hands and rubbed them together briskly.

"What's that?" Mama asked. "Hand lotion?"

"Oh no," Ellen said. "Just Purell. It's a disinfectant." She called Stormy over, and the little girl held out her hands to be squirted. Stoney, unprompted, came over and held out his hands for his dose.

I watched, stunned, as she proceeded to polish my wedding silver with the contents of another plastic bottle that appeared from nowhere.

Ellen caught me staring.

"No offense," she said. "But you never know what kind of food-borne pathogens are lurking in the average American household. Poultry, especially, is vulnerable to a whole host of opportunistic bacteria. You've got your salmonella, your botulism, and of course, if the food's been prepared in anything less than totally hygienic conditions, you run the risk of cryptosporidium."

Everybody at the table suddenly put down their forks and looked at me expectantly.

"My kitchen is clean," I cried. "I always wash my hands."

Ellen shook her head sadly. "Unless you scrub under hot water for at least three minutes with an antibacterial soap, you're just inviting trouble."

Eric rolled his eyes. "Shut up, Ellen," he said. "I'm sure crypto-whatever is not on Weezie's menu tonight."

He picked up my stag-handled carving set and plunged the knife into the turkey breast.

"There's a real science to carving a bird like this," he began. "I like to start with the breast, putting the knife on the diagonal, like this."

As we watched, paper-thin slices of white meat fell obligingly onto the platter. The irresistible smell of roasted meat filled the room. People picked up their forks again. They sipped wine and passed vegetables. It was going well. I congratulated myself.

And then it happened.

Eric was demonstrating how he liked to separate the whole leg from the turkey carcass. He made an extravagant cut into the bird, then cried out.

"Oh shit!"

He held up his left hand. The tip of his pinkie dangled by a strand of flesh. Blood spurted onto his white shirtfront.

"Oh shit," he repeated, sinking down into his chair. Blood poured from his hand as he stared dumbly down at the spreading crimson pool on the turkey platter and the table.

"Here," James said, jumping up and running over to him. He grabbed Eric's hand and wrapped it in a damask napkin. "Keep the pressure on it," he said calmly.

"Eric!" Ellen cried. Her face went white and she slumped forward in her chair, striking her head on her dinner plate, and cracking it neatly in two pieces.

"Mama!" Stormy screamed. "My mama is dead!"

"Call an ambulance," Sondra cried. "My God, now she's bleeding too."

Eric tilted his head against his chair back. "No ambulance," he said weakly. "My insurance won't pay for an ambulance."

"Mama," Stormy wailed.

BeBe knelt beside Ellen, holding another napkin to a nasty gash in her forehead.

She looked up at me. "I'm no expert, but I think she's gonna need stitches."

"For God's sake." Derek jumped up out of his chair. "Come on then," he said. "Harry, can you help me carry Ellen out to my car? James, you and Jonathan get Eric. We'll take 'em both over to the ER at Memorial."

Sondra stood up too. "Why can't you take Eric's truck?" she said plaintively. "We just had your car detailed."

"Give me the keys," Derek ordered, holding out his hand.

"I want my mama," Stormy howled, latching onto Derek's knees. "Don't take my mama away."

"Stormy, honey," Derek said, leaning down and tenderly brushing away the tears streaming down the little girl's face. "Shut the fuck up."

CHAPTER 21

"Weezie, wake up!"

I opened my eyes slowly. Daniel was kneeling down beside the sofa, still in his grease-stained chef's smock. His thick hair was more rumpled than ever, and there were dark circles of fatigue under his eyes.

I yawned, sat up, and looked around. Had I dreamed this calamitous evening? One look at the living room told me that my nightmare was reality. The place was a wreck. Beer cans and wineglasses littered the tabletops, and a blood-soaked napkin had been discarded on the floor by the sofa where I'd fallen into a catatonic sleep after the untimely departure of my dinner guests.

"What happened here? Where is everybody?" Daniel asked.

"Where were you? I tried and tried to call you, but I never got any answer."

"Sorry," he said sheepishly. "The restaurant was a mad-house. I forgot and left my cell phone on the front seat of the truck. I only saw how many calls I'd missed after I locked up for the night."

He reached over and ruffled my hair. "I'm really, really sorry about tonight. Swear to God, I tried to get away earlier. Besides Eddie being out, half my waitstaff didn't show up for work either. I'm gonna kick some major ass come Tuesday. Just when it started to slow down, there were two parties of twelve apiece who decided to linger over coffee and dessert so long that I eventually had to come out of the kitchen and politely start stacking chairs on tables myself."

I sighed. I could have bitched him out, or given him the silent treatment, but that wouldn't solve anything. Owning a restaurant, in particular a successful one like Guale, meant hard work and long hours— especially on the holidays.

"It's okay," I said finally. "After all, you did give me fair warning about your family."

He put an arm around my shoulders and drew me closer. "What in God's name went on here tonight? Was there some kind of knife fight? There's a trail of blood leading from the street into the dining room. When I pulled up out front and saw the blood, I halfway expected to find you all dead or maimed in here."

I took a deep breath. "Where should I start? It's been a long, hairy night."

"Whose blood?" he asked, examining my arms for wounds.

"Oh, yeah," I said. "That would be the blood of your

brother Eric. He was demonstrating his prowess in turkey carving and managed to slice off the tip of his pinkie."

"Jesus!" Daniel said.

"That's what I said too. There was quite a bit of blood, as you could imagine. Then, when Ellen saw Eric's finger, she passed out cold—hitting her head on her dinner plate and splitting her forehead wide open. Not to mention breaking one of my hundred-fifty-dollar flow blue plates."

"I'll buy you a new plate," Daniel said. "What else?"

"Well, when little Stormy saw both her mama and her daddy bleeding like stuck pigs and being hauled off to the emergency room by her uncle Derek, she went into uncontrollable hysterics. We finally had to dose her up with some of Sondra's dog's Paxil."

"You gave doggy downers to my niece?" Daniel asked. "Was that wise?"

"It shut her up, and that's all we cared about at the time," I said.

Daniel buried his head in his hands. Suddenly I saw his shoulders quaking with emotion. I patted his back soothingly.

"Don't worry. Everybody's all right. James went to the hospital with them. They managed to reattach Eric's fingertip, and they got Ellen's forehead stitched up by the town's best plastic surgeon, whose mom happens to play bridge with Miss Sudie. Stormy's fine too, although they expect her to sleep till noon tomorrow."

Daniel lifted his head. Tears streamed down his face, and I realized he was actually choking on his own peals of laughter.

"I'm sorry," he said, gasping. "It's not really funny—but then again, in a really sick way, it is funny."

He kissed me. "Someday we'll look back on this night and laugh about it. But I do regret that you had to endure it all by yourself."

"At least BeBe and Harry were here," I said. "After the family cleared out, they helped me clean up the kitchen. And anyway, it's not like my family was entirely blameless."

"Don't tell me your mother took a drink," Daniel said.

"No, thank God. But she did step on Sondra's dog and almost killed it. And then Jethro ate the crab dip and puked all over Stormy's shoes. Also Mama caught Daddy feeding her famous zucchini bread to Barkley, Sondra's dog, and she got furious and demanded to be taken home."

Daniel was wheezing he was laughing so hard.

"What happened to your beautiful dinner? Did anybody get to eat?"

"No," I said succinctly. "Oddly enough, everybody's appetite was somewhat dimmed by the appearance of a turkey drenched in human blood. They cleared out of here so fast it made my head spin."

Daniel's face fell. "No turkey sandwiches? No turkey hash?"

"I pitched it in the garbage. There's plenty of ham, of course, and some oyster dressing in the fridge, and some veggies too. I'd offer you some of your sister-in-law's tofurkey, but she took it with her when she left."

"Tofurkey, phooey," Daniel said. He stood up and pulled me to my feet.

"There's still all that dessert—right? I didn't have time to eat tonight. I'm starved. Come on, let's go raid the fridge."

"There's still a lot of dessert left," I said. "But you can forget about the pumpkin pie."

"What happened to the pumpkin pie? You know it's my favorite."

"Stoney Stipanek happened to it. In the rush to get Eric and Ellen to the hospital, everybody forgot about little Stoney. I forgot about him myself until I went into the den to turn off the Christmas tree lights. He was sound asleep on the sofa, his damned Game Boy clutched in one hand and the empty pumpkin pie pan in the other."

"Pie-eating pig," Daniel muttered. "Just like his old man. When we were kids, Eric used to sneak back into the kitchen after everybody had gone to bed, and he'd eat every sweet in sight. One time he ate a whole can of Hershey's chocolate syrup. Kid weighed two hundred pounds in the fifth grade."

"You'd never guess that now," I commented. "Eric's thinner than you or Derek."

"You'd be thin too if you had to eat a steady diet of Ellen's cooking," Daniel told me, slicing himself a thick slab of pecan pie. "So where's Stoney now?"

"Home. Derek came back and fetched him."

His mouth full, Daniel nodded approval. "Good. You got any milk?"

"Soy milk," I said with a grin. "Sondra's contribution, natch. The kids drank all my real milk while the grown-ups were sniping at each other and watching the football game."

"Beer?"

"If your brothers and Harry didn't drink it all."

He was rooting around in my fridge for more food when the doorbell rang.

Daniel looked at the clock on the kitchen wall. "It's past eleven. You got any other family members expected for dinner tonight?"

"None," I promised. "Stay here and I'll get rid of whoever it is."

A Savannah police officer stood on my doorstep, his hand clamped firmly around the arm of a petite old lady dressed in a maroon BC letter sweater.

"Annie!" I exclaimed.

"Ma'am?" the cop said, looking from me to Annie. "I just apprehended this here suspect trying to break into a green pickup truck parked out here at the curb. She claims she knows you."

"She does," I said quickly. "And she wasn't really breaking in. She was picking up a gift I left for her."

"See?" Annie snapped at the cop. "What'd I tell you?"

The cop looked dubious. "You're leaving gifts in your truck for a bag lady? Ma'am, there's a lot of crime downtown. You don't want to be leaving your truck unlocked. These street people will steal you blind."

"Hey!" Annie said, squirming furiously. "I'm no bag lady. You see any shopping bags hanging off of me? You see me pushing a Kroger grocery cart?"

"She's a friend," I assured the cop. "Leave her with me. I'll personally vouch for her."

"All right," he said, obviously reluctant to relinquish his prisoner. "I'm releasing her to your custody."

The temperature was dropping, and an icy wind whipped down the street. "Come on in," I said, gently tugging at Annie's arm. "It's freezing outside."

"Hey!" Annie said, backpedaling as fast as she could. "Don't leave me here, officer. Go ahead, arrest me. I'll go quietly."

"One more thing," the cop added. He reached in his jacket pocket and brought out a small, bedraggled-looking teddy bear. "She had this too. I figure it's yours."

I looked from Annie to the cop. "Thank you," I said. "Merry Christmas." And then I closed and locked the door.

Annie looked wildly around the room, like a caged animal. "I've got to go," she said in a low voice. "Just let me leave, all right? No harm done. We both know you left that bag for me. That stupid cop wouldn't believe me. I tried to tell him—"

"Hey, Weezie," Daniel called, strolling into the living room, "who was at the door?"

Annie's face turned ghost white. She reached for the doorknob, but I reached it first.

"Don't go," I said softly. "I've been worried sick about you for the past two days. Come on. Stay. It's Christmas Eve. We were just going to have some dessert. I know you like sweets."

"No! I can't. Gotta go," she stammered. "I won't bother you again. Please?"

Daniel put his plate of cake on the console table by the door. "Who's this?"

I looked from Daniel to Annie and back again. Her hair was salt-and-pepper, with more salt than anything else, but it was still dense and wavy, and her eyebrows, thick for a woman, were set above very blue, very frightened eyes.

"BeBe and I have been calling her Apple Annie," I said apologetically. "I didn't know her real name. Not till just now."

"And?" Daniel said impatiently. "What is her real name? And what's she doing at your house on Christmas Eve? I swear, Weezie, you are a magnet for weirdness—"

And then he saw the teddy bear in my hand. Wordlessly, he took it from me.

"Where did this come from?"

I nodded in Annie's direction. "She brought it here," I said.

A single tear floated down the old woman's haunted face.

"You're Paula, right?" I asked. "Paula Stipanek."

She tried furiously to blink the tears away. "Not Stipanek. Not anymore. It's Paula Gambrell."

"Welcome home, Paula," I said. "I'd introduce you to the rest of your family too, but they had to leave early. I'm afraid it's just me and you. And your son."

"Danny." She whispered the name. "Oh, God. I should never have come back."

CHAPTER 22

Is this some kind of joke?" Daniel asked, his face ashen under the shock of hair that had fallen in his eye. "Are you for real?"

The old lady reached out and touched his hand, but he jerked away from her. "Danny?"

"I'll leave you two alone," I said, heading for the kitchen. "Coffee. I'll make some coffee. And, Annie, I mean, Paula, would you like some dessert? I've got cake and pie—"

Daniel grabbed my hand. "Stay." Then his face softened, and he gave my hand a gentle squeeze. "Please?"

"Only if it's okay with your mom," I said, glancing over at Paula.

She peeled off the BC letter sweater and thrust it at me. "Here. I'm sorry. I shouldn't have taken it. I shouldn't have come here and bothered you at all. I'll just go. All right?"

She was edging back toward the front door.

"Do what you want," Daniel said, looking down at the teddy bear. "But tell me something, what's this supposed to mean? Why did you come back after all this time? Why now?"

The old lady's eyes filled with tears again. "I've been back in Savannah for a couple months now. I came . . . I guess I came back because I had nowhere else to go."

She stared down at the floor. "Hoyt. My husband? He died in September. He'd been sick for a long time, ever since he went to prison. Heart disease."

"I'm so sorry," I said as I perched on the arm of the sofa. "Please, won't you sit down? And let me fix you something to eat and drink?"

"I'm really not hungry," Paula said with a sad smile. "We had a feast at the Salvation Army tonight. Ham and collard greens and mashed potatoes and pumpkin pie, and eggnog, without the whiskey, of course."

"I still don't understand what you're doing here," Daniel said, his jaw set in a hard, unforgiving line.

Paula shrugged. "I'm not sure I understand myself. I guess I needed to make sure you were all right."

"I'm fine," he snapped. "Anyway, you're a day late and a dollar short."

"Daniel!" I punched his arm angrily. "If you can't be polite, you can leave. This is my home and your mother is a guest of mine. "

Paula sat uneasily on the edge of the armchair nearest the door. "I don't blame you for feeling the way you do about me. I feel that way about myself. Worse, maybe, if that's possible."

"You don't know anything about how I feel about you

walking away and leaving us," Daniel said. "Leaving us for him. I felt something years ago. But I don't now. I don't feel one way or another about you."

"I wouldn't expect you to feel any differently," Paula said. Her hands were folded neatly in her lap. "But that doesn't stop me from caring about you. From worrying about you and your life. And your brothers."

"That's just a pile of crap," Daniel said angrily. "I don't want to hear any more."

Now he was the one who was standing up and walking toward the door.

"Dammit!" I said fiercely, grabbing his arm. "Just stay. Hear what she has to say."

He sank back down onto the sofa, crossing his arms across his chest. "I'm listening."

Paula's face softened and she almost smiled. "You used to do that when you were a little boy. You were the most mule-headed child I'd ever seen. If you didn't get what you wanted, you'd stick out that chin and cross your arms and just dig in your heels. People said you got that from me."

Daniel stared at the ceiling.

"I never meant to leave you for good," Paula said. "After Hoyt went to prison, I thought, well, I thought I'd send for you boys after things settled down. But there was no money. I was living in a tiny little apartment not far from the prison down in Jacksonville, waitressing in a coffee shop, working nights. Eventually, after a year or so, I did come back to Savannah. I meant to take you all back to Jacksonville with me. I'd been saving up to get a larger place, and I figured

Derek was old enough then, he could look after you younger boys while I worked."

"You came back?" Daniel seemed surprised. "Nobody ever told us."

"Nobody knew," Paula said. "Your aunt was furious with me for leaving. I didn't dare call her or come around the house while you were staying with her. I just kind of snuck into town. I rode past the house, and I actually saw you and Eric outside, shooting basketball at that hoop she'd tacked up on the garage. And you looked happy, you know? I drove past your school, and I watched Derek's football practice. I just . . . didn't have the heart to uproot you. You boys were settled in school, you had your friends, and your aunt. I couldn't ask you to make that move."

"You could have given us the option of deciding for ourselves," Daniel said, his voice icy. "Instead of playing the martyr."

"I was a coward," Paula said, sitting up very straight. "There'd been that big scandal, when Hoyt was arrested, and then the trial. It was so ugly. Everybody thought I was trash. I thought so too. And I thought, if I weren't around, eventually people would forget that I was your mother. Then . . . the longer I stayed away, the harder it seemed I could ever get my boys back."

"We did all right for ourselves," Daniel said. "All three of us. Despite what you did to us."

"You did more than all right," Paula said eagerly. Her face was glowing now. "I've seen the restaurant, how successful it is. And the children, Eric's and Derek's, so beauti-

ful. A friend here loans me a car sometimes, and I drive past their houses. I snuck into Stormy's dance recital last month." She sighed. "What I wouldn't give to hold those precious babies."

"You still can," I said, ignoring Daniel's icy glare. "The past is past. I bet if Eric and Derek talked to you, if they heard your side of things, they'd want to see you. Want you to get to know your grandchildren."

"No," Paula said hastily. "I don't have that right. Seeing them is enough for now."

"Paula? Can I ask you something?"

"Sure."

"Were you the one who broke into this house—and ate the appetizers?"

She blushed and nodded. "I didn't really break in. You left a set of keys on the seat of your truck one night. I took them so nobody else would. There's a lot of crime downtown, you know."

"I do now," I said, laughing.

"I ran off those street bums after they picked all the fruit off your beautiful decorations that night," she said proudly.

"If they were really hungry, they were welcome to the fruit."

"And I want to apologize about taking your goodies," Paula said. "I didn't realize you were having a party that night. I shared it with the girls over at the Salvation. They'd never seen such grand food in their lives."

"It's all right," I said. "As it turns out, there was plenty of food for everybody."

"And Jethro?" I asked. "You found him and brought him home?"

She nodded. "He was way down on River Street, rummaging through some garbage cans in back of one of the bars down there. He's a sweet old thing, isn't he? He came along just as nice as you please, once I tied that rope to his collar."

"So—" Daniel cut in. "You've been watching us? Me and Weezie? Why?"

"I was worried about you," she said simply. "Your brothers, they're settled down. Got nice wives and children and homes. And this young lady"—she gestured toward me—"you've been keeping her steady company."

Now it was my turn to blush.

"We'll settle down," Daniel said. "When the time is right."

"What makes you think the time is ever right?" Paula said. "You think God cares about your plans? I thought I'd have all the time in the world with your daddy. But I was wrong. About that and a lot of other things."

Daniel gave a derisive snort.

"Do you love her, son?"

His face darkened. "That's between us."

"Just answer, please. As a favor to an old lady."

He reached over and took my hand. "I've loved her since I was eighteen years old."

Paula nodded at me. "And you?"

I smiled and nodded. "He kind of grows on you, doesn't he?"

"He was an ornery baby," she said. "Beautiful, but ornery."

"Still is," I agreed. "Paula, where have you been the past

few days? When you didn't pick up your present, I was really worried."

"Present?" Daniel asked.

"Your mother and I have been exchanging Christmas gifts for the past few days," I said. "She gave me some wonderful gifts. A room key to the old DeSoto Hotel. A tiny seashell. A gorgeous blue John Ryan bottle. And this," I said, touching the Christmas tree brooch pinned to my collar.

"But you bought that pin. At the auction," Daniel said. "And she stole it."

"Borrowed it," Paula and I said at the exact same time.

"And I gave it back," Paula added. "Weezie's given me gifts too." She held up the red plaid gift bag. "First gifts anybody's given me in years."

"But where have you been?" I asked.

"Jacksonville," Paula said. "I took the bus back down to Jacksonville. I was going to stay down there too. I'd seen about my boys. They were doing just fine. Even Daniel."

"Then why come back?" Daniel challenged.

"I had all my things in storage, in the prison chaplain's basement," Paula said. "Not that there was very much. I've learned to live lean since Hoyt died. I was going through my things, and I found that," she said, pointing at the bear. "And I wanted you to have it, son."

"Old bear," Daniel said, holding the tattered stuffed animal in both hands. "I'd forgotten about him."

"You slept with him until you were six, and your brothers teased you so for being a baby, you threw it in the trash,"

Paula said. "I rescued him, and I've been saving him all this time. Do you remember the song he plays?"

Daniel turned the bear over and wound a key protruding from his back.

"Teddy bear," he said as the tinkling mechanical tune began. "Just wanna be your teddy bear."

"Elvis again?" I asked.

"Yes, ma'am," Paula said proudly. "I was always a huge Elvis fan. I was at his last concert here in Savannah, February 1977, right here at the Civic Center, last one he gave here before he died."

"I like Elvis too," I said. "Always have."

"Danny here was named for a character Elvis played in a movie. Did you know that, son?"

"You're kidding."

"No sir. You were named for the boy in *King Creole*. Best movie he ever made."

"I love that!" I said gleefully.

"Nobody calls me Danny anymore," he said accusingly.

"I do. Sometimes," I said.

"You're a gal who appreciates the good things," Paula said approvingly. "Like that pin."

I touched the Christmas tree brooch. "It's not . . . the same one, is it? The one your boys gave you?"

"See for yourself," she said, reaching into the pocket of her worn brown slacks. She held her hand out, palm open for us to see. In it was another blue Christmas tree pin. Not exactly the same as mine, but close.

"That was the real reason I went back to Jacksonville,"

Paula said. "To see if I could find that pin. When I did, I started to think. What could happen if I came back to Savannah? Could I make a difference to my boys?"

We both looked expectantly at Daniel.

"He hates Christmas," I told Paula. "That's how I got the idea for the Blue Christmas theme for the antiques shop."

Daniel shook his head. "She probably hates it too. Seems like everything bad always happens around the holidays."

"Not everything," Paula said. "Sometimes good things happen. Sometimes, if you work at it, you can find what you lost at Christmas."

I heard a faint scratching from the front door.

"The cops again?" Daniel said.

When I opened the front door to investigate, I was assaulted by a blast of freezing air and a small, wet bundle of black fur that shot inside the door.

At the same time, Jethro, who'd been asleep under the coffee table, raised his snout, took one look, and leaped to his feet.

"What the hell?" Daniel said as the black dog raced past him into the kitchen, followed by Jethro.

"That's Ruthie," I said, peeking into the kitchen, where the two dogs were crouched side by side over Jethro's food bowl. "She belongs to Manny and Cookie. You know, the guys across the square who own Babalu. She must have gotten loose. I guess I better take her home. She's their little princess. They'll probably assume she's been dognapped."

"Stray dogs and bag ladies," Daniel said, shaking his head. "The joys of living downtown."

"I am *not* a bag lady," Paula said indignantly. She picked up her gift and buttoned the cardigan she'd been wearing under the letter sweater. "I'll be glad to take Ruthie home," she volunteered. "I know right where she lives."

"What about later, Paula?" I asked. "Where will you stay tonight?"

She shrugged. "Not at the Salvation, thanks to that cop who hauled me in here. They lock the doors at eleven sharp. Nobody gets in after that. But don't worry about me. I'll find a place. I always do."

I shot Daniel a helpless look.

"You can't sleep on the streets," he said gruffly. "It's freezing out there. And from the looks of that dog, it's starting to rain too. Come on. I'll drop you at a motel."

"I can't."

"It's on me," Daniel said. "Christmas present."

Just then the doorbell rang. The three of us turned to stare at it.

"Now what?" Daniel muttered.

CHAPTER 23

This time my guests were human.

Manny and Cookie, dressed in soaking-wet formal wear, stood huddled together on my doorstep, rain streaking down their faces.

"Ruthie's gone," Manny blurted. "We just got back from candlelight services at the Cathedral. I don't know how she got out—"

"She'll freeze to death," Cookie cut in. "She's not used to being out without a jacket—"

"We had a workman in, dealing with the hot water heater, and he must have left the back gate open," Manny said. "We don't know how long she's been out—"

"She's here," I said quickly. "In the kitchen, sharing Jethro's dinner."

"Thank God," Cookie exclaimed.

I led them into the kitchen, where Jethro and Ruthie were curled up asleep on Jethro's bed, snout to snout.

"My precious!" Manny whispered, tugging at Cookie's sleeve. "Would you look at this? Did you ever?"

"Does this remind you of—"

"Lady and the Tramp!" Manny said. "Forbidden love. And yet—"

"They're very sweet together," Cookie concluded. "I don't even have the heart to wake her up and take her home, she's so warm and cozy."

"She can stay tonight," I offered. "I'll bring her home in the morning."

"What do you think?" Manny asked his partner.

Cookie shrugged. "What's one night? All right. She's already knocked up. So she can stay. Thank you."

"You're welcome," I said, hesitating a moment. "Look. I was just making some coffee. And we've got all this pie left from dinner. Would you like to join us?"

Cookie nudged Manny. "Tell her," he whispered.

"Tell me what?"

"We're sorry," Manny said, twisting the tasseled ends of the white silk scarf tossed casually around his neck. "We haven't been very good neighbors to you. And now that we're practically in-laws, well, we'd like to start over. We got all off on the wrong foot, and acted like pissy little queens. And that is so *not* who we are."

I blushed. "I haven't been very friendly either. The two of you are so creative and talented, I guess I felt threatened by your success with Babalu."

"Us, creative?" Cookie hooted. "Sweetie, lamb, when we saw that Blue Christmas display of yours, we were just knocked for a loop. We have *never*—"

"—seen anything as fabulous!" Manny said with a giggle. "Are you sure you're straight?"

"Positive," Daniel said, walking into the kitchen. "She's definitely straight. I can vouch for that." He leaned down and scratched Ruthie's ear, and she wagged her tail in bliss.

"Daniel," I said, "these are my neighbors. Cookie and Manny."

"Friends," Cookie corrected. "We're your friends."

"And in-laws," Manny added.

"The boys were just going to join us for some coffee and dessert," I said.

"Great," Daniel said.

"So I'll just go drop Paula off at a motel and be right back."

"No motel," I said. "It's Christmas Eve. She stays here tonight."

"May I speak with you in the other room?" Daniel said, his voice tense.

"Your mother is in the other room," I reminded him. "Do you want her to hear us fussing about where she's staying?"

"That's your *mom*?" Cookie asked.

"What about it?" Daniel snapped. "Not that it's any of your business, but she left my brothers and me when we were kids. We were raised by an aunt. Now she waltzes back into town and expects me to feel all warm and fuzzy."

"Oh puh-leeze," Cookie drawled. "My mama beat me with a hairbrush when she caught me waxing my eyebrows in tenth grade. And Daddy still tells people that Manny's my 'business associate.' "

"Hard-shell Baptists, through and through," Manny said

with a sigh. "Neither one of them would set foot at our commitment ceremony," he added. "Although they did send a place setting of our good silver, which was very generous, considering. But so what? They're our family. My folks are dead. So we're stuck with Ma and Pa Parker."

"You don't understand," Daniel said. "There's a lot more to it than that."

"Puh-leeze," Cookie repeated. "Grow up and get over yourself."

I wrapped my arms around Daniel's waist and leaned in close. "One night," I said. "Just let her stay one night. For me."

He kissed the top of my head, which I took as a good sign.

"One night," he repeated. "Just for you. But I have to tell you, this solves nothing."

"Thank you," I whispered. Flushed with good cheer, I went to the living room, to ask Paula what she wanted in her coffee.

She was gone, but my daddy's letter sweater was still draped over the back of the chair where she'd been sitting.

Back in the kitchen, Cookie and Manny were admiring my heart-pine cabinets and Sub-Zero refrigerator, while Daniel poured coffee into the mugs I'd set out.

"Daniel!" I said sharply. "She's gone."

He sighed and set down the coffeepot. "All right. Let me just get my coat and gloves."

"Can I ask you guys a favor?" I asked, turning to my new-found friends.

"Sure," Cookie said. "If you tell me where you found these nickel-plated faucets."

"Deal," I said quickly. "Paula's gone. Daniel and I are going out to look for her. Can you stay here, in case she comes back?"

Manny was lifting the foil from a tray of dessert. "Oh no! Pecan pie," he moaned. "A moment on the lips, a lifetime on the hips."

"Knock yourself out," I said, grabbing the keys to my truck.

CHAPTER 24

The cold and rain seemed to have swept the historic district's streets clean by the time the bells at St. John's and the Lutheran Church of the Ascension tolled midnight.

Daniel drove my truck and I kept my face pressed to the passenger-side window, looking for some glimpse of Paula. Neither of us said much until we'd worked our way all the way north to Bay Street.

"How old do you think she is?" I asked.

"Who?"

"Your mother," I said, exasperated.

"No idea."

"Well, how old is Eric?"

He had to think about it. "Thirty-nine?"

"How old was she when she married your father?"

His face flushed.

"What?" I asked.

"They had to get married, okay? She was a junior and my old man was, like, nineteen. She never even finished high school."

"So she was probably no more than seventeen when she had Eric. My God, Daniel, do you realize your mother isn't even sixty yet?"

"So?" He drummed his fingers impatiently on the steering wheel. "This is useless, Weezie. For all we know, she could have hopped a dog by now to head back to Jacksonville."

"Good idea," I said. "Let's check the Greyhound station."

He turned the car west, toward Martin Luther King Boulevard and the bus depot.

"Paula's not even sixty, but she looks as old or older than my mama, and she's seventy-two," I pointed out.

"Back in the day, my mother was a real knockout," Daniel said. "There was a picture of her in a bathing suit at the beach, standing by the edge of the water, in an old family album. I always assumed the girl in the picture was a movie star until Aunt Lucy told me it was . . . Paula."

We pulled into the bus station parking lot and peered through the brightly lit picture window. We could see a few people standing around, and a maintenance man, pushing a floor-waxing machine. Before Daniel could object, I hopped out of the truck and dashed inside.

Less than five minutes later, I was back, shivering from the rain and cold.

"No luck," I said, trying to catch my breath. "There aren't any buses to Jacksonville tonight. The last one left at eight."

Daniel turned the heater up and pulled away from the curb. "This is hopeless. I'm taking you home before you catch pneumonia."

I didn't dare point out that his mother was out in this weather alone, wearing nothing warmer than a moth-eaten sweater.

"She was just a kid when she had you," I said. "Barely into her twenties. And all of a sudden, after your dad left, she was a single mom with three little boys to take care of."

"Lots of people become single parents at a young age," Daniel said. "They don't abandon their kids when they find a new partner."

"What were you doing when you were in your early twenties?" I asked.

He snorted. "That's different. I was in the Marines. I was partying, raising hell, like every other guy I knew."

"Think about what Paula's life was like," I urged. "Just out of her teens, saddled with three little boys. She's working at the sugar plant, and she meets some smooth-talking boss who sweeps her off her feet—"

He glared at me. "Why are we having this discussion? You don't know anything about her. Anyway, she said it herself. She was a selfish coward."

"It's Christmas," I said, wanting to change the subject. As we rounded the square by the Cathedral of St. John the Baptist, we saw people emerging from the church, umbrellas unfurled like a forest of mushrooms. "And I promised Mama I'd go to mass with her this year."

"Was she mad at you for not going?" he asked.

"No. I think she understood that when dinner went hay-wire I wasn't going anywhere. She might be disappointed, but not mad."

"No guilt trip?"

I smiled. "Well, maybe a little one."

We were on Charlton Street now, and it pleased me to see the blue glow of my shop windows reflected in the rain-slicked street in front of the shop.

"Hey," I said suddenly. "I've got an idea."

We parked at the curb and walked over to the shop, and stood in the rain to look at Paula Stipanek Gambrell, sound asleep in the display bed.

Daniel slipped an arm out of his jacket and pulled it over my head to shield me from the worst of the weather.

"She doesn't look all that evil," I observed.

"Not even sixty," he said. "But she's been all beat up by life."

Paula's skin looked dark and leathery in the pale wash of lights from the windows, her short-cropped hair dark silver against the white bed linens.

"She's much smaller than I remembered," he said. "And her hair! Look how gray. It used to be jet black. She wore it long, almost to her waist."

He shook his head, and raindrops splattered on my cheek. "She's nothing like I thought she'd be now. Hoyt Gambrell was a rich man before he went away to prison. I always pictured her living on some golf course, playing bridge with a bunch of rich country-club women."

I slid an arm around his waist. "Maybe she did you a favor—leaving you with your aunt. You guys had a home in a

decent neighborhood. A middle-class upbringing. She couldn't have given you that."

He clutched me tightly to his chest, and I could hear the even in and out of his breathing. I looked up, and he looked away.

"That last Christmas, before she left? It was the best one we'd ever had. Hoyt must have slipped her some extra money. Derek got an NBA regulation basketball and Eric got a slick skateboard. We all got new clothes and sneakers."

"What about you? What'd you get?"

He laughed. "What I'd been begging for. An Easy-Bake Oven. And a Popeil Pocket Fisherman like I'd seen on television. I was a weird little dude, huh?"

"You were a prodigy," I protested.

"What should we do?" he asked haltingly. "Chase her off? Wake her up and take her back to your place?"

I had a ready answer for that one, but I managed to choke it back. "It's your call."

"Let her sleep," he said finally, steering me toward my own front door. "If she's not gone by morning, we'll figure something out."

"We?"

"Yeah. All of us. My mom. You and me. And my brothers."

The living room was dark when we stepped inside. We found Manny and Cookie in the kitchen, sipping eggnog and giggling like a couple of teenagers.

"Hope you don't mind," Manny said, jumping up to greet us.

"Did you find her?" Cookie asked. "Is she coming back here?"

"She was asleep. At my shop," I said.

"It's late," Daniel said pointedly.

When they'd finally gone, we locked the front and back doors, and checked a final time on the dogs curled up together on Jethro's bed.

"You sleepy?" Daniel asked as I headed toward the stairs.

"Not really," I admitted. "I was tired earlier, but I think I'm too keyed up now to sleep."

"It's officially Christmas," he said, pointing to the clock on the mantel. "Maybe Santa came while we were out."

"The way things have gone around here tonight it's more likely that the Grinch came and shoved all our presents and the roast beast up the chimney while little Cindy Lou Who was asleep," I said. "But we could check."

I reached for the light switch in the darkened den, but Daniel caught my hand. "Let's leave 'em off," he suggested. He went over to the fireplace and switched on the gas logs, then slowly lit the dozen or so candles I'd arranged on the mantel. While he was lighting the candles, I found the remote control switch for the Christmas tree and clicked it on.

When I saw the lit tree, I burst into laughter.

"What's so funny?" Daniel asked, turning abruptly.

"The tree," I said, pointing at the eight-foot Fraser fir.

"It's beautiful," he said, coming to stand beside me. "Prettiest tree you've ever decorated."

"Except I didn't decorate it this way," I told him. "Look at the way those strands of twinkle lights are draped in precise six-inch loops."

"So?"

"So I just threw 'em on there any old way. And where are my big ol' gaudy colored lights? And my tinsel? I had about a ton of tinsel on this tree earlier. And now there's not even a smidge. Not to mention the way the gifts are so artfully arranged under the tree. Look at it! It looks like something out of a magazine."

"I don't get it," Daniel said. "If you didn't do this, who did?"

"A couple of elves named Manny and Cookie."

"Damn," Daniel said.

"I know. We've been the victims of a drive-by redecorate."

"It's still a beautiful tree," he said, his dark blue eyes suddenly serious. "Perfect for a beautiful woman."

"Sweet," I said, kissing him. "Is this you, apologizing?"

"Yes." He nodded. "I've been a prick. About Christmas. And family. And everything."

"You have been pretty awful," I agreed.

He wrapped his arms around my waist. "I'm going to do better. I swear it, Weezie."

"I know," I said, kissing him.

"No, really," he said. "You make everybody around you happy. You make me happy. I don't tell you that enough, but you do."

"That's quite a speech," I said, nuzzling his neck. "Is that my Christmas present? Because if it is, it's a really good one. I've got a good present for you too. Wanna see?"

"I'm not done yet," he said carefully. "I've been thinking about this all night. Even before Paula—I mean, my mother—

showed up. I'm tired of blaming other people for the way my life turned out. Because it didn't turn out so bad, you know?"

"I know."

"I've got a home, and a great business. A family—even though they drive me nuts, I've got a family. And I've got you. I can't imagine what my life would be like without you."

"Even though I drive you nuts?"

"Especially because you drive me nuts. I get to choose—whether to be happy or miserable. I choose happy. I choose you, Weezie Foley."

He kissed me, long and slowly and thoroughly.

"I choose you back," I said when I came up for air.

Without warning, he sank down into the big leather armchair by the fireplace and pulled me onto his lap.

"Is this the part where you ask me if I've been a good little girl this year?" I asked, giggling and fumbling with his belt buckle.

"We'll get to that part," he said, kissing me hungrily and running his hands up under my sweater. "Although, to be honest, I have to say I prefer you naughty. Actually, I was thinking we'd do the present part now."

"I do *love* presents," I said, working on his shirt buttons.

"We'd better do the presents first," he said, pushing me upright. "Or we might not get around to it tonight."

"Me first," I said.

Fortunately, Manny and Cookie's redecorating scheme had left Daniel's little pile of presents at the front edge of the tree. I gathered them into my arms.

"All that for me?" he said, his face falling. "I only got you one."

"Only one of these is really special," I assured him. "The others are nothing. They can wait till tomorrow."

I climbed back onto his lap, carrying only the tall, cylindrical gift that I'd wrapped in heavy gold paper with a thick blue velvet ribbon. "Open it," I commanded.

He untied the ribbon with a single tug and slipped the bottle out of the paper.

"Wow," he said, reading the label aloud. "A 1970 pomerol. My God, Weezie, this is an amazing bottle of wine. Where'd you find it?"

"An auction," I said anxiously. "You like it?"

"I will," he said, running his fingertips over the cork.

"It's a 1970," I said. "Because of the year you were born. I wanted to buy you a special bottle, and BeBe said this would be good."

"Better than good," he said. "Life-altering." He shifted, sliding out from under me and standing up. "Stay there. I'll be right back."

When he came back, he was carrying a corkscrew and two wineglasses. Before I could stop him, he'd plunged the opener into the cork.

"Wait!" I protested. "Daniel, this is a once-in-a-lifetime bottle. You don't know what I had to go through to buy it. I mean, I love that you're excited about it, but don't you want to save it for a special occasion?"

He poured a few drops into one of the glasses, rolled it around, then held it to his nostrils, inhaling deeply and smil-

ing widely. He tasted, nodded, then poured a glass and handed it to me.

I sniffed dutifully. And sipped. It was very good wine, as far as I could tell. But then, I thought the screw-top stuff I bought at Kroger was good too.

Daniel sipped his, then carefully set his glass down on the coffee table.

My heart sank. "Not so hot, huh? I've got some champagne too, but maybe we'd better wait on that."

"Later," he said. "Now it's my turn." He scooted me over to one side and raised a hip to reach into his pocket.

He brought out a small black velvet box and held it out to me. "Sorry about the wrapping," he said. "I was going to wait until tomorrow. But you said I should save the wine for a special occasion. This is as special as it gets."

My hands were damp and shaky, and my fingers couldn't quite work the tiny silver clasp on the box.

"Here," he said impatiently. He took the box and flipped the top open.

A circlet of blue sapphires winked and sparkled in the reflected light of the Christmas tree, and in the center of the sapphires sat one perfect square-cut diamond.

"I know they're not your birthstones, but you love blue, and they're sapphires, and just a diamond didn't seem like enough—"

"Shut up," I said, kissing him quiet.

"Yes?" he asked, a little while later, taking the ring from the box and fitting it on my trembling left hand.

"Yes," I whispered. "Oh, *hell* yes."

Foley Family Irish Corned Beef Dip

The way you class up a recipe calling for canned corned beef is to serve it in a hollowed-out bread round that you buy at the best bakery in your neighborhood—preferably the bread should be rye, pumpernickel, or sourdough.

2 loaves unsliced bread
1 ⅓ cups sour cream
1 ½ cups Duke's mayonnaise
2 teaspoons dried minced onion
1 can corned beef
½ teaspoon horseradish

Combine all ingredients except the bread, mashing with a fork to create even consistency. Spoon into a hollowed-out bread round. Serve with cut-up chunks of the second loaf of bread.

Red Roosters

A Christmas-y cocktail that will make your guests crow with delight. Just remember to make it the night before your party so that the juice mixture has time to freeze. And remind guests that this potable is mighty potent. Supposedly makes ten servings. As if!

¼ cup granulated sugar
½ cup water
1 cup frozen lemonade concentrate
1 cup frozen orange juice concentrate
2 cups cranberry juice
2 cups vodka
4 cups ginger ale

Bring sugar and water to a boil in a saucepan over low heat, stirring until sugar dissolves. Add all juices and vodka and stir to blend. Freeze mixture in pitcher or freezer-safe container. One hour before serving time, add ginger ale to pitcher. As mixture thaws, break into slush with a long spoon.

MORE CHRISTMAS CHEER
from Mary Kay Andrews

MY BLUE CHRISTMAS

For years our neighborhood sponsored a "holiday decorating" contest. And for years, tasteful, tiny white lights and Williamsburg-style natural decorations, with pine boughs and cranberry and orange wreaths, dominated our neighbors' seasonal greeting displays.

But one year, I'd had enough of tasteful. I wanted tacky, I wanted tasteless. I wanted fun. I wanted . . . Elvis.

My Blue Christmas was born from that one crazy idea. I started with yards of lights—big-bulb light strands. All blue. And they were racing. Like the kind you see in a roadside used-car lot. I strung them across our front porch and along the roofline. I added blue lights to the small potted evergreens on either side of the front porch steps. At the point of the porch gable, I fixed a gigantic silver-foil wreath wound with blue satin ribbon and a big poofy bow. Shining out from the middle of the wreath was a blown-up photo of the King. Elvis.

My kids loved our Blue Christmas. My husband wanted to change his name and address. Needless to say, we didn't win the contest that year. But some of our neighbors admired my subversiveness, and for years referred to us as "The Elvis House."

When my editor asked me to write a novella set in Savannah at Christmas, I knew I'd write about antiques picker Weezie Foley, and that Weezie would have her own version of a Blue Christmas. Way back in 1977, when I was a newbie reporter at the newspaper in Savannah, I'd covered Elvis's last concert there. So I knew Elvis would return—at least in spirit—for Weezie's Christmas story. As a child of the fifties, I collect vintage midcentury Christmas decorations, so I knew Weezie would share my passion for these dime-store treasures from the past. I also knew there would be a vintage Christmas-tree pin involved in this stor—one similar to the brooch we found in my mother-in-law's home after her death a few years ago. And the one thing I knew for certain was that this would be a very special Christmas for Weezie and her boyfriend Daniel, and the rest of her nutty but loving family.

I hope you'll love reading *Blue Christmas* as much as I enjoyed writing it. However you celebrate your own holidays this year, I hope yours will be full of love, light, and warmth — and maybe, just a touch of tackiness.

Mary Kay Andrews

MARY KAY'S TIPS
for Keeping the Happy in Holidays

• At family gatherings, do try to find something nice to say about your brother-in-law's new girlfriend—even if it's only that all her tattoos are spelled correctly.

• The holidays call for cheerful, uplifting conversation. So remember—Christmas dinner is probably not the optimum time to announce a divorce, pending indictment, or gender change.

• When hosting a large family get-together, tactfully suggest that your guests leave firearms at home.

• Gift-giving should never be an occasion for helpful hints about the recipient's lack of hygiene, questionable morals, unfortunate taste in clothing, or recent huge weight gains.

• Remember to update Christmas-card addresses on a regular basis. Nobody likes getting a card addressed to Mister and Missus after the Mister has taken another Missus.

• If you must re-gift, make sure the new recipient lives in a different zip code from the previous giver. And always check to make sure you've removed all those pesky little gift cards that might have slipped down inside that root beer–scented candle given you by Aunt Gladys.

• Fruitcake: Just say NO!

Mary Kay's Cool Yule Playlist

Merry Christmas, y'all. I hope you'll enjoy my Christmas playlist. If you've already got a copy of the all-time best Christmas compilation ever—*A Christmas Gift for You from Phil Spector*, which Weezie listens to in her shop in *Blue Christmas*, you might not even need my playlist. Still, there are some goodies here. And some great trivia nuggets connected with them.

Enjoy!

Number one on my list, of course, is **Blue Christmas**, by the King, Elvis Presley. Did you know that when this song was released, Irving Berlin, the composer of "White Christmas," was so infuriated he mounted a letter-writing campaign to radio stations across the country, suggesting that they ban it? Didn't work, of course.

I love Darlene Love's version of **White Christmas** on the Spector album. Did you know that Darlene, of the Blossoms, and then later of the Crystals, was a backup singer for the

televised Elvis 1968 comeback special? And that she had an uncredited role in *Change of Habit*, Elvis's 1969 movie costarring Mary Tyler Moore as a nun? Watch for Darlene to appear on *The Late Show with David Letterman* in late December, as he usually has her on to sing his favorite, **Christmas (Baby Please Come Home)**. She also appeared in all four Lethal Weapon movies as Trish Murtaugh, Danny Glover's wife.

Did you know that Ronnie Spector, of the Ronettes, had a disastrous (and violent) marriage to Phil Spector? Just adore that trademark wall of sound on their version of **I Saw Mommy Kissing Santa Claus**.

Lots of artists, including Madonna, have covered **Santa Baby**, but my favorite version is by Eartha Kitt, who was one of several actresses who played Catwoman on the old *Batman* television series.

Novelty songs are great, but occasionally I like a maudlin holiday tune, and for me, nothing fills the bill as well as Judy Garland's achingly sad **Have Yourself a Merry Little Christmas,** which she first sang in the 1944 movie musical *Meet Me in St. Louis*. Garland, who later married the movie's director, Vincente Minnelli (Liza's dad), refused to sing the original lyric of the song, which had her singing to child actress Margaret O'Brien, *"Have yourself a merry little Christmas. / It may be your last."*

I've always loved Booker T. & The MG's, so I've included their version of **Jingle Bells.** You do know, don't you, that "Jingle Bells" was written by James Pierpoint, who copyrighted the song in 1857, when he was a church organist living in Savannah? Pierpont's grave, with a "Jingle Bells"

marker, is located in Savannah's historic Laurel Grove Cemetery.

Baby, It's Cold Outside has been covered by tons of duos, including Louis Armstrong and Ella Fitzgerald, but I've included Dean Martin's version because it's so laugh-out-loud lascivious, and as a shout-out to my late dad, who sorta resembled Dino.

THE LIST

"**Blue Christmas**" — Elvis Presley, 1968

"**Jingle Bell Rock**" — Bobby Helms, 1957

"**Santa Baby**" — Eartha Kitt, 1953

"**Christmas (Baby Please Come Home)**" —
Charles Brown, 1965

"**I Saw Mommy Kissing Santa Claus**" — The Ronettes, 1963

"**White Christmas**" — Darlene Love, 1963

"**Jingle Bells**" — Booker T. & The MG's, 1966

"**Little Saint Nick**" — The Beach Boys, 1963

"**The Bells of St. Mary**"
Bob B. Soxx and The Blue Jeans, 1963

"**Have Yourself a Merry Little Christmas**" —
Judy Garland, 1944

"**Sleigh Ride**" — The Ventures, 1965

"**Run, Rudolph, Run**" — Chuck Berry, 1958

"**Baby, It's Cold Outside**" — Dean Martin, 1959

Junior League Cheese Pennies

The beauty of these lil' darlin's is that you don't have to mess with those tricky cookie-press doohickeys. I don't know about you, but when I try to make cheese straws, they come out "all whompy-jawed," as my grandmother would say.

½ cup softened butter
2 cups grated sharp cheddar cheese
2 cups all-purpose flour
¼ tsp. salt
½ tsp. cayenne pepper
½ cup very finely chopped pecans
Paprika

Cream butter and cheese together, using an electric mixer. Sift flour, salt, and cayenne, and then add the cheese-butter mixture and the pecans. Roll into 1-inch-diameter logs, wrap in wax paper, and refrigerate until firm. Slice crosswise into "pennies." Bake on an ungreased cookie sheet at 350 degrees for 10 to 15 minutes, keeping close watch so they don't burn.

Dust with paprika before cooling.

Chatham Artillery Punch

ALERT! Chatham Artillery Punch (CAP) has been known to cause bad behavior in unsuspecting victims. This behavior can include French-kissing your best friend's husband (in front of her), goosing the minister at your cousin's wedding, and dancing the dirty gator at your child's junior high mixer when you were supposed to be the chaperone. The Chatham Artillery is the oldest military unit in Georgia. Legend has it that this drink started as a harmless fruit punch prepared by wives and sweethearts of the unit's members, which was then spiked with a different variety of alcohol by each man who passed the punch bowl.

2 cups red Catawba wine
2 cups strong green tea
⅔ cup rum
½ cup dark brown sugar
½ cup rye whiskey
½ cup orange juice
⅓ cup gin
⅓ cup Hennessy brandy

⅓ cup lemon juice
1 bottle dry champagne
1 can pineapple chunks
1 small bottle maraschino cherries

A week in advance of your soiree, mix all the liquids and the brown sugar—except for the Champagne—in a large container. Refrigerate. The night before the event, add in the pineapple and cherries and refrigerate again. Just before serving, stir in the Champagne. And stand back!

· A NOTE ON THE TYPE ·

The typeface used in this book is a version of Sabon, originally designed in the 1960s by Jan Tschichold (1902–1974) at the behest of a consortium of manufacturers of metal type. As one who began as an outspoken design revolutionary—calling for the elimination of serifs, scorning revivals of historic typefaces—Tschichold seemed an odd choice, but he met the challenge brilliantly: The typeface was to be based on the fonts of the sixteenth-century French typefounder Claude Garamond but five percent narrower; it had to be identical for three different processes, working around the quirks of each, such as linotype's inability to "kern" (allow one character into the space of another, the way the top of a lowercase f overhangs other letters). Aside from Sabon, named for a sixteenth-century French punch cutter to avoid problems of attribution to Garamond, Tschichold is best remembered as the designer of the Penguin paperbacks of the late 1940s.